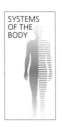

SYSTEMS
OF THE
BODY

THE
RESPIRATORY
SYSTEM

SYSTEMS OF THE BODY

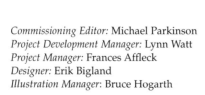

Commissioning Editor: Michael Parkinson
Project Development Manager: Lynn Watt
Project Manager: Frances Affleck
Designer: Erik Bigland
Illustration Manager: Bruce Hogarth

THE RESPIRATORY SYSTEM

Andrew Davies PhD DSc
Professor of Physiology, University of Glamorgan, Pontyprydd, UK

Carl Moores BA BSc MB ChB FRCA
Consultant Anaesthetist, Royal Infirmary of Edinburgh, Edinburgh, UK

Illustrated by Robert Britton

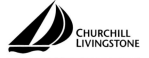

CHURCHILL
LIVINGSTONE

EDINBURGH LONDON NEW YORK OXFORD PHILADELPHIA ST LOUIS SYDNEY TORONTO 2003

CHURCHILL LIVINGSTONE
An imprint of Elsevier Science Limited

First published 2003

ISBN 0 443 062315

British Library Cataloguing in Publication Data
A catalogue record for this book is available from the British
Library

Library of Congress Cataloging in Publication Data
A catalog record for this book is available from the Library of
Congress

Notice
Medical knowledge is constantly changing. Standard safety
precautions must be followed, but as new research and clinical
experience broaden our knowledge, changes in treatment and
drug therapy may become necessary or appropriate. Readers are
advised to check the most current product information provided
by the manufacturer of each drug to be administered to verify the
recommended dose, the method and duration of administration,
and contraindications. It is the responsibility of the practitioner,
relying on experience and knowledge of the patient, to determine
dosages and the best treatment for each individual patient.
Neither the Publisher nor the author assumes any liability for any
injury and/or damage to persons or property arising from this
publication.
The Publisher

ELSEVIER
SCIENCE
your source for books,
journals and multimedia
in the health sciences
www.elsevierhealth.com

The
publisher's
policy is to use
**paper manufactured
from sustainable forests**

Printed in Spain

Students of medicine and related vocations frequently have difficulty in seeing the relevance of preclinical subjects to their final goal of becoming a practitioner. They also have difficulty in integrating these subjects to form a coherent picture of normal function, which is essential if the effects of disease are to be understood.

In order to address these problems, this book, like others in the Systems of the Body series, adopts an integrating approach based upon function. Into the description of normal function and its relation to structure, a description of the effects of the disruption caused by disease is integrated.

To enable students to learn effectively they must have a good idea of what is expected of them, and what is to be learned should be broken up into manageable and coherent amounts. These aims are fulfilled by including Objectives at the beginning of each chapter and by providing chapters which are of content that the experience of many years teaching this subject convinces us are a coherent and essential description of that particular aspect of the respiratory system.

There is no single disease which illustrates all the aspects of the subject covered in any chapter and so, rather than choosing a general condition which loosely relates to the subject, we have selected clinical cases which clearly illustrate an important aspect of the subject of that chapter.

So as to acknowledge that many students using this book may have had little clinical experience at this early stage of their course we have highlighted important terms. These are shown in bold in the text on their first occurrence and we have provided a Glossary to define those that can be succinctly explained.

To help with that bane of student life – examinations – some typical questions are included at the end of each chapter.

The authors wish to thank Drs Doris Redhead, Suzanne Guy and J.T. Murchison, all of whom are from the Radiology Department, Royal Infirmary, Edinburgh. They would also like to thank Dr Pat Warren, University of Edinburgh, for her helpful comments on the manuscript.

CONTENTS

CONTENTS

INTRODUCTION

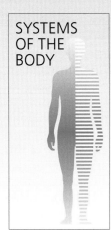

SYSTEMS
OF THE
BODY

Chapter objectives

After studying this chapter you should be able to:

① Define respiration.

② Explain the role of respiration in human homeostasis and its disorder in specific pathology.

③ Explain the interaction between respiration and the circulation.

④ Describe the pivotal role of diffusion in respiration.

⑤ Give examples of the importance of named physical phenomena in specific clinical conditions.

⑥ State the gas laws necessary to measure lung function in specific tests for disease.

⑦ Explain the rationale of respiratory symbols.

Introduction

The aim of this book is to provide an understanding of the respiratory system: its structure, function, and the diseases and conditions that may affect it. In attempting to do this we are adopting the philosophy of the new curriculum in medicine, which involves bringing to bear on a particular topic all the sciences relevant to that topic. To include in one book all that a student should know about the anatomy, histology, physiology, pharmacology and medicine of the respiratory system would result in a gigantic and intimidating tome. Equally unsatisfactorily, all these subjects could be treated superficially. We have adopted the policy of basing an understanding of the respiratory system on a full description of its physiology and anatomy, with specific topics of particular clinical importance being expanded upon in terms of clinical sciences.

For students to learn effectively, the material they must master should be broken down into manageable portions with a coherent theme: these are the chapters of this book, with each theme being based on a particular function of the respiratory system.

Students must also know what is expected of them, and each chapter is preceded by a list of aims and objective – things you should be able to do when you have mastered the material of that chapter. To provide experience of that bane of student life, **examinations**, each chapter contains questions of the type you might be asked at an undergraduate level.

What is respiration?

That depends on the context in which you use the word. Biochemists use it to describe the energy-producing chemical processes that take place in tissues, cells or even parts of cells. In this book we will use the physiologist's definition, which is 'An interchange of gases between an organism and its environment'. To all intents and purposes, for human beings this means 'breathing' (Latin, *spiro*, 'I breathe'). The movement of air into and out of the lungs, which most people call breathing, is called by physiologists **ventilation**. Breathing is brought about by specific structures of the body, including (but not exclusively) the lungs. A description of these structures at a macroscopic (anatomical) and microscopic (histological) level helps us to understand the processes of the respiratory system and the disruption of these processes and structures (pathology) that brings about disease.

The part of our environment involved in this 'interchange of gases' mentioned above is of course the air around us, and our need for air must have been obvious to even our most distant ancestors. This need is recorded in some very ancient writings. For example, Anaximenes of Miletus (*c.* 570BC) observed that air or *pneuma* (Greek, 'breath') was essential to life.

What was not clear to the ancients was what the air was used for. Aristotle, drawing on theories dating from the 5th century BC which noted the rapid and repeated movements of the heart, relegated the function of the lungs to a sort of radiator, and stated with his usual authority:

> …as the heart might easily be raised to too high a temperature by hurtful irritation (by its rapid movements) the genii placed the lungs in its neighbourhood, which adhere to it and fill the cavity of the thorax, in order that air vessels might moderate the great heat.

Galen (130–199AD), probably more by an accident of metaphor rather than on any scientific evidence, came close to describing the true nature of respiration when he compared it to a lamp burning in a gourd:

> When an animal inspires it is, I think, similar to a perforated gourd, but when respiration is prevented at the appropriate place on the trachea, you may compare it to a gourd unperforated and everywhere closed.

If Galen had had the benefit of modern gas analyzing facilities he would have found even closer parallels between breathing and burning, with oxygen (O_2) being consumed and carbon dioxide (CO_2) being produced in both cases.

The 'bottom line' of an account of the complicated process of respiration begins with a flow of

OXYGEN IN and ends with a flow of CARBON DIOXIDE OUT.

These two flows are the first and final results of the complex metabolism of the body, and this book describes the respiratory system that facilitates these flows.

The need for respiration

One definition of the success of a species of organism, in evolutionary terms, is how well it can maintain constant the composition of the fluid surrounding its individual cells (its internal environment) despite changes in its external environment (surroundings getting dryer, colder, warmer etc.). This process is called **homeostasis** and requires energy. Most of the energy generated by our tissues is the result of oxidation of food substrates, and this is the reason we need a flow of OXYGEN IN. Neophytes in physiology often emphasize the role of the respiratory system in providing this oxygen, and certainly an uninterrupted supply is important, particularly for the nervous system, but of more immediate importance is the removal of CO_2. The word oxygen means 'acid producer' (Greek, *oxy*; acid; *gen*, to produce), and the major product of our oxidative metabolism is the acid gas CO_2. The accumulation of CO_2 would result in acidification of the body fluids. The importance of removing this CO_2 can be demonstrated by rebreathing from a plastic bag for a few minutes. The unpleasant sensation that forces you to stop this rather dangerous experiment is due to overstimulation of the reflex that controls breathing to get rid of this gas. You will see later (Chapter 8) that CO_2 produces its acidic effect by reacting with water to form carbonic acid.

Ventilation of the lungs would not fulfil the needs of the cells of our bodies if the results of this ventilation did not diffuse into the blood, which is then carried close to the cells of the body by the circulation.

Diffusion in respiration and the circulation

The flows of O_2 and CO_2 into and out of the body take place as a result of one very basic physical phenomenon: **diffusion**, which results in the movement of molecules in liquids and gases from regions of high concentration to regions of lower concentration. Because they are small, microscopic organisms such as the humble amoeba in its pond can rely on this phenomenon alone to carry O_2 to and remove CO_2 from its single cell. Multicellular creatures are too large to rely on diffusion alone: the distances gases would have to

diffuse are too great, and the movement of gas therefore too slow to maintain life.

Although in human beings the same passive mechanism of diffusion alone supplies and removes these gases from our bodies (there is no active chemical transport), the phenomenon of diffusion is maximized by complicated respiratory and circulatory systems which accomplish what the pond water does for the amoebae in providing a supply of and a sink for these gases. The lungs promote diffusion by having an enormous surface area, which is very thin, through which diffusion can take place easily. A surface of over $90\,m^2$ is enclosed in a lung volume of less than 10 L. This functional $90\,m^2$ is often reduced in disease, by thickening of the membrane, excess fluid in the lungs, or by a reduction in the supply of air or blood. The circulation of the blood forms the transport link between the diffusion site of the lungs and the diffusion site of the capillaries within the tissues. The distances involved in this link are enormous in molecular terms, and diffusion would be totally useless to transport gas over the metre or so between the lungs and distal tissues of our bodies. This transport is accomplished in seconds by the circulation.

Timing in the circulation and respiration

The processes of breathing and the beating of the heart are both cyclic events. One involves the inhalation of air and then its exhalation; the other involves filling of the heart with blood and then its ejection into the circulation. The time courses of these two cycles are very different: at rest you may take 12 breaths in the minute the heart beats 60 times, ejecting 5 L of blood through the lungs.

The composition of air in the lungs changes as a result of two effects: during inspiration it is altered by the addition of fresh air to that already in the lungs and the effects of exchange with the blood passing through the lungs. Expiration in this context is the equivalent of breath-holding, because no new air is added: the only effect is due to exchange of gas in the lungs with that in the blood. These changes in the composition of the air in the lungs are picked up by the blood flowing in the pulmonary circulation, which therefore shows cyclic changes in its composition that coincide with the breathing cycle.

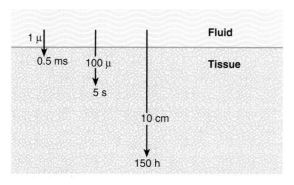

Fig. 1.1
Time course of diffusion over increasing distances.
This Figure illustrates how the time needed for diffusion to take place increases as the distance involved increases. The absolute times shown in this example would be for a fairly large molecule such as a neurotransmitter.

Basic science of respiration

All these changes, just like all the events in respiration, are properly described in terms of the basic sciences physics and chemistry. These are generally not the favourite subjects of students of the basic medical sciences. We have therefore included at the end of the book a short section (Appendix) on the most relevant parts of physics and chemistry that a student should understand in order to understand respiration. That section is not obligatory to students confident with these subjects. The Appendix, which is intended to aid

not torment, will repay scrutiny by students who have any doubts about their grasp of basic science. That this basic science is integral to understanding normal respiration and diseased states is illustrated when we take an overview of human respiration and point out where the phenomena we describe apply (Fig. 1.2).

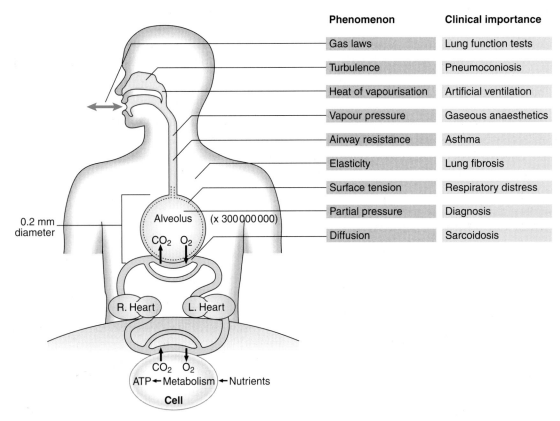

Phenomenon	Clinical importance
Gas laws	Lung function tests
Turbulence	Pneumoconiosis
Heat of vapourisation	Artificial ventilation
Vapour pressure	Gaseous anaesthetics
Airway resistance	Asthma
Elasticity	Lung fibrosis
Surface tension	Respiratory distress
Partial pressure	Diagnosis
Diffusion	Sarcoidosis

0.2 mm diameter

Alveolus (x 300 000 000)

CO_2 O_2

R. Heart   L. Heart

CO_2 O_2

ATP ← Metabolism ← Nutrients

Cell

Fig. 1.2

An overview of respiration, showing the physical phenomena that make it up and the clinical situations where understanding these phenomena is important.

Introduction Box 1

Clinical boxes

Each of the chapters of this book is illustrated with a clinical example of respiratory disease. The respiratory conditions relate to the anatomy and physiology that are discussed in that chapter and are designed to deepen your appreciation of 'normal' physiology as well as illustrating why a sound knowledge of basic science is so important in understanding disease processes.

In this chapter, rather than discussing a particular respiratory condition, we will consider the symptoms of respiratory disease that patients complain of, we will

discuss how the respiratory system is examined, and we will look at the features of a normal chest X-ray.

This review is not comprehensive: it is not the place of this book to teach you how to take a history and examine patients; rather, the clinical boxes in this chapter are designed to provide you with enough background information to understand the clinical cases in later chapters.

Symptoms of respiratory disease

Patients with respiratory disease complain of symptoms which fall into a few broad groups.

① *Cough* Cough is probably the commonest symptom of respiratory disease and is usually a response to irritation of the respiratory tract. Cough is one of the most important features of chronic bronchitis, and also occurs in patients with chest infections as well as in asthmatics, where it may be particularly common at night.

② *Sputum* Sputum is the substance coughed up from the respiratory tract. The colour of sputum may give a clue as to its cause: for example, respiratory infection usually results in yellow or green sputum, whereas pink, frothy sputum may indicate pulmonary oedema.

③ *Haemoptysis* Haemoptysis means coughing up blood. Haemoptysis may indicate a chest infection, but may be a symptom of more serious respiratory disease such as tuberculosis or bronchial carcinoma.

④ *Breathlessness* Breathlessness is a symptom of a range of respiratory diseases as well as being a symptom of cardiac failure.

⑤ *Wheezing* Wheeze is a characteristic musical sound caused by gas flow through narrowed airways. Patients may complain of wheeze and it may be audible on auscultation of the chest. It is characteristic of pulmonary diseases such as asthma, chronic bronchitis and chest infection, all of which can result in airways narrowing.

⑥ *Chest pain* In certain respiratory conditions patients may complain of chest pain. Such conditions include infection, pleuritis, pulmonary infarction and pneumothorax.

Introduction Box 2

Examination of the respiratory system

A clinical examination of the respiratory system includes examination of the hands, tongue, neck and chest wall, as well as percussion (tapping) and auscultation (listening with a stethoscope) of the chest.

These are the important findings in a clinical examination of the respiratory system:

① *Finger clubbing.* Inspecting the hands is an important part of examining the respiratory system. As well as looking for peripheral cyanosis (see below) it is important to look for finger **clubbing**. Clubbing is present when the normal angle at the nailbed is lost, the curvature of the nail is increased and there is increased mobility of the nail on the nailbed (the nail is **fluctuant**). (Fig. 1.3). It is not known for certain why finger clubbing occurs, but it is present in a number of respiratory diseases, including bronchial carcinoma, bronchiectasis and pulmonary fibrosis. Clubbing is also present in some non-respiratory diseases.

② *Cyanosis.* Cyanosis means a blue tinge to skin or mucous membranes and indicates the presence of deoxygenated haemoglobin (p. 111). Cyanosis may be either **central** or **peripheral**. Central cyanosis means blueness of the lips and tongue. Because these organs are covered in mucosa rather than skin, cyanosis is more evident there than in the face, for example. Blood does not travel far from the heart to reach the tongue and lips, and so if they are cyanosed it suggests that blood leaving the left ventricle is deoxygenated, either because of lung

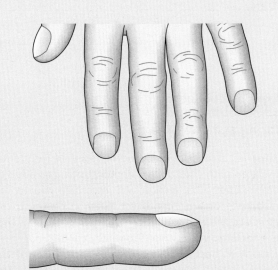

Fig. 1.3
Finger clubbing. In clubbed fingers the angle of the nailbed is lost and there is increased mobility of the nail on the nailbed.

disease or as a result of certain forms of heart abnormality. Peripheral cyanosis means blueness of the extremities and is usually most evident in the fingernails and toenails. In the absence of central cyanosis it usually suggests inadequate circulation to the periphery.

③ *Trachea.* The trachea can be felt in the neck above the sternum and it is examined to assess whether it is lying in the midline or deviated to one side. Tracheal deviation can occur in a number of lung diseases, including pneumonia and pneumothorax.

④ *Inspection of the chest.* Examination of the chest itself starts with inspection. The shape of the chest may be abnormal: for example, in asthmatics the chest is often unusually expanded and rounded – so-called barrel chest. Surgical scars or other abnormalities of the skin on the chest wall may be present. The patient is asked to take a deep breath and the movements of the chest wall are noted. Movements of the chest wall may be limited by abnormalities of the spine or chest wall itself, or by abnormalities of the underlying lung.

⑤ *Percussion.* Percussion essentially means tapping the patient's chest and listening to the sound that is produced. Normally, the chest sounds hollow or **resonant** if the underlying lung is filled with air, but a **dull** sound is heard if there is fluid in the intrapleural space (**pleural effusion**) or if the alveoli of the underlying lung are filled with fluid. If there is a pneumothorax and there is air between the chest wall and the lung, then percussion may **hyper-**

resonant, in other words the chest sounds more hollow than normal.

⑥ *Auscultation.* Auscultation means listening to the lungs with a stethoscope. Normally, it is possible to hear air quietly entering and leaving the lungs without there being any added sounds. Breath sounds like this are called **vesicular**. Breath sounds may be absent or very quiet if there is a pleural effusion or a pneumothorax. There may also be sounds present in addition to breath sounds. Where gas passes through narrowed airways a sound like a musical note may be produced. These sound are called **wheeze** or **rhonchi**, and are usually heard during expiration and are most likely to be heard in asthma or chronic bronchitis, although if airway narrowing is very severe, no gas flow takes place and there is no wheeze. **Crackles** or **crepitations** may also be heard on auscultation. Crackles probably represent the opening of closed airways and are most commonly heard in chronic bronchitis, pulmonary fibrosis and pulmonary oedema.

Introduction Box 3

Looking at a chest X-ray

In the clinical sections of the book, cases are frequently illustrated with chest X-rays demonstrating a range of abnormalities. This section will introduce you to the appearance of a normal chest X-ray so that you can appreciate the abnormal chest X-ray appearances that are associated with some respiratory conditions.

Usually a chest X-ray is taken with the front of the patient's chest against a photographic plate. The patient's elbows are bent forward so that the shoulder blades move round to the side of the ribcage and X-rays pass through the patient. This sort of X-ray is called posteroanterior (PA) because the X-rays themselves travel from behind the patient (posterior) to in front (anterior). X-ray shadows of structures within the chest are cast onto the photographic plate; structures which are nearer to the plate (i.e. those in the front of the chest) appear clearer than those further away from the plate, which may appear distorted or blurred.

If a patient is too unwell to stand in front of the photographic plate – for example if they are too ill to leave his/her bed – the X-ray may be taken with the photographic plate behind the patient and with the X-rays administered from in front of the patient. This is a

anteroposterior chest X-ray; it is also possible to take a lateral chest X-ray from the side (see Fig. 1.5A).

It is important to remember the way an X-ray film is developed when you look at one for the first time. The film is equivalent to a black and white photographic negative. The darker areas of the film are the areas that have been exposed to X-rays. Structures such as bone, which block X-rays, appear white on the X-ray film. Structures such as the lungs, blood vessels and so on, which partially block the passage of X-rays, appear grey.

On the chest X-ray of a healthy person in Fig. 1.4 the following structures are visible:

① *Bones* The ribs, sternum and thoracic vertebrae can usually all be seen on a chest X-ray.

② *Heart* The outline of the heart is clearly visible. If the heart is enlarged, for example as a result of heart disease, this will be evident. The border of the heart may not appear sharp and distinct if the lung tissue around it is diseased.

③ *Aorta* The outline of the aorta is usually visible as it arises from the heart and arches round in the thorax.

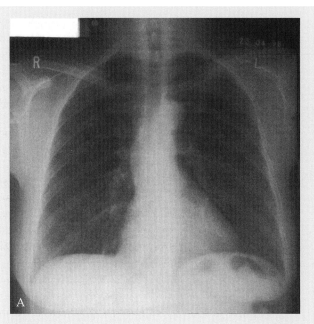
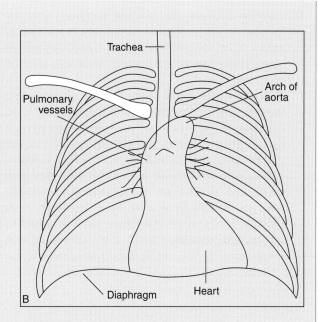

Fig. 1.4
Normal anteroposterior chest X-ray.

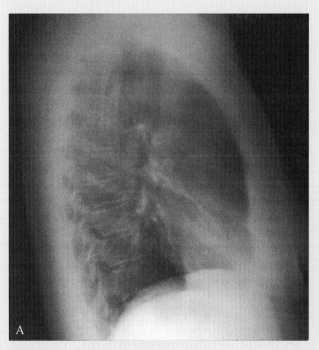
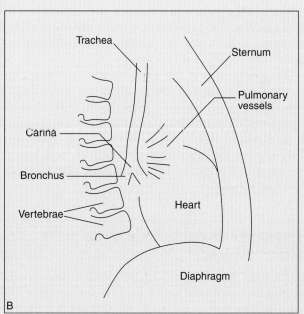

Fig. 1.5
Normal lateral chest X-ray.

④ *Trachea* Because the trachea is filled with air through which X-rays can pass easily, it appears as a dark structure in the midline. It is usually possible to see the carina, where the trachea divides into the two main bronchi.

⑤ *Pulmonary vessels* The pulmonary vessels are visible as they pass from the heart into the lungs.

⑥ *Diaphragm* The outline of the diaphragm is usually clearly visible. The right-hand side of the diaphragm is usually higher than the left. Collapse of the lung or damage to the phrenic nerve may cause the diaphragm to be shifted upwards, whereas emphysema and other diseases that increase lung volume may cause the diaphragm to be shifted downwards. If the outline of the diaphragm is not sharp, particularly where the shadows of the diaphragm and the ribs intersect (**the costophrenic angle**) this suggests that there is fluid in the intrapleural space adjacent to the diaphragm.

⑦ *Lungs* As the lungs are filled mainly with air, X-rays pass through them easily and they appear relatively dark on a chest X-ray. However, it is generally possible to make out the shadows of large blood vessels as they pass through the lung tissue. If there is fluid in the alveoli, for example as a result of oedema or infection, the lung fields will appear lighter as fewer X-rays will pass through them. If an area within the lungs appears darker than normal, this suggests that there is more air present than usual. This might be as a result of emphysema or as a result of a pneumothorax.

Taking examples from this list of phenomena we see that solids are elastic, and this **elasticity** of our respiratory system determines part of our work of breathing. Liquids exert a **vapour pressure** a property important in humidifying the air we breathe and in the administration of gaseous anaesthetics. Gases exert a **partial pressure**, the understanding of which is essential to the monitoring of how well the lungs are working. The volume of a mass of gas is described by laws relating it to temperature and pressure, and the resistance to flow of gases is related to the dimensions of the tube in which it is flowing.

These examples of the importance of the basic sciences in understanding the respiratory system do not mean that a great deal, or a great depth, of knowledge is required. The Appendix contains all that is required to understand the contents of this book. However, there is a vocabulary that is specific to the respiratory system, and it is probably helpful for you to be introduced to it here.

Respiratory symbols – the language of the respiratory system

Respiratory physiology and medicine contain some intimidating symbols which lead students to fear that some unpleasant mathematical exercises are immanent. Not so: the symbols used in respiratory physiology are assigned logically and make the description of processes and the identification of where measurements were made very much easier than using words.

Primary units are given capital letters:

V = volume, P = pressure, partial pressure, $\dot{V}$ = flow.

Locations in the gas phase are also given capital letters but smaller than the primary units:

A = alveolar, B = barometric, E = expired.

Locations in blood are identified by lower-case letters:

a = arterial, v = venous, c = capillary.

The primary symbol is written first, followed by the qualifying symbol at a lower level.

Table 1.1
The major respiratory symbols

Variable

P	Pressure, tension or partial pressure
V	Volume of gas
$\dot{V}$	Volume of gas per unit time (flow)
Q	Volume of blood
$\dot{Q}$	Volume of blood per unit time (flow)
F	Fractional concentration in dry gas
R	Resistance
G	Conductance

Location in blood		**Location in gas**		**Other suffixes**	
a	Arterial	A	Alveolar	pl	Pleural space
c	Capillary	I	Inspired	aw	Airway
v	Venous	E	Expired	w	Chest wall
v̄	Mixed venous	T	Tidal	el	Elastic
		L	Lung	res	Resistive
		B	Barometric	tot	Total
		D	Dead space		

Prefix	
s	Specific

Examples

V_T	Tidal volume
PaO_2	Oxygen tension in arterial blood
$\dot{V}_E$	Expired minute volume
$sRaw$	Specific airway resistance

NOTE: Sometimes S is used for saturation and C for content. These are not used here because of confusion with chemical names (e.g. SO_2, CO_2).

Drugs

Drugs are chemicals which change the natural functions of the body. Most prescribed drugs have therapeutic properties. Just as Fig. 1.2 demonstrates where specific physical phenomena have particular importance in the respiratory system, Table 1.2 gives examples of conditions where specific types of drugs are used therapeutically in treatment of specific conditions or for specific procedures.

CGS and SI units

The centimetre, gram, second system (CGS) of measurement, which has been in use in Europe since the French Revolution, is being displaced by Système International (SI), based on the kilogram, metre and second. The CGS system still receives considerable use in North America.

The SI unit of force is the newton and the unit of volume the cubic metre (m^3); as this is rather large, the cubic decimetre (dm^3), which is equivalent to a litre, is frequently used.

The unit of pressure in the SI system is the newton per square metre – the pascal (Pa). This is too small for practical use and so the kilopascal (kPa) is used with some surprisingly convenient results. 1 kPa = 7.5 mm Hg or 10 cm of water; equally usefully, barometric pressure at sea level is close to 100 kPa, which makes the arithmetic of calculating partial pressures easier (see p. 169).

In the SI system, concentration is measured in moles per litre, where a mole is 6.02×10^{23} molecules of the substance in solution. Measurement of blood pressure is still widely expressed in mm Hg, probably because it is usually measured using a mercury manometer.

Further reading

Arnold M. Essentials of general, organic and biochemistry. Brooks/Cole: 2001
Duncan G. Physics in the life sciences. Oxford: Blackwell Science: 1990
Lewis R, Evans W. Chemistry. Palgraves Foundation Series, 2001

Table 1.2
Drugs and the respiratory system

Drug Name	Type	Condition treated
Oxymetazoline	α-agonist	Nasal congestion
Atropine	Muscarinic cholinergic antagonist	Excess mucus secretion
Prednisolone	Corticosteroid	Allergic rhinitis
Chlorphenamine	Antihistamine	Rhinorrhea
Succinylcholine	Neuromuscular blocking	Facilitate tracheal intubation
Dextromethorphan	Synthetic narcotic analgesic	Non-productive cough (suppression)
Isoprenaline (Isoproterenol, USA)	β_2 agonist (bronchodilator)	Asthma
Cromoglicate	Inflammatory-cell stabilizer	Asthma
Beclometasone	Anti-inflammatory corticosteroid.	Asthma
Azathioprine	Cytotoxic immunosuppresant	Diffuse connective tissue
Aminopenicillin etc.	Antibiotic	Pneumonia and other infections
Amphotericin B	Antifungal	Fungal infections

This list is, of course, far from exhaustive. The examples are chosen to demonstrate that several approaches may be used to treat a specific disease (e.g. asthma). It also demonstrates that the UK and the USA are 'two nations separated by a common tongue' (Isoprenaline, UK = Isoproterenol, USA). This dichotomy extends to the units of measurement used in Europe and the USA and this sometimes causes problems.

Self-assessment questions (for help refer to Appendix, p. 167)

① Define homeostatis.

② Approximately how many times does your heart beat, and how much blood flows through your lungs during each breath when you are at rest?

③ What is the vapour pressure of water at body temperature?

④ Write the general gas equation.

⑤ What is the partial pressure of O_2 in air (21% O_2) at an altitude where the air pressure is 50 kPa?

⑥ What is the formula for the excess pressure inside a bubble?

⑦ What is the symbol for partial pressure of carbon dioxide in arterial blood?

Answers see page 174

STRUCTURE OF THE RESPIRATORY SYSTEM, RELATED TO FUNCTION

Chapter objectives

After studying this chapter you should be able to:

① Describe the structures of the upper airway which help it to protect the respiratory system against environmental agents of lung disease.

② Distinguish between the structure of conducting and respiratory airways and relate these structures to the aetiology of restrictive and obstructive lung disease.

③ Outline the structure of the bronchial tree and how this is disrupted in disease.

④ Describe the histology of the regions of the lung and relate it to function and pathology.

⑤ Explain the special features of the pulmonary circulation and pulmonary hypertension.

⑥ Outline the afferent and efferent innervation of the lungs.

⑦ Describe the gross structure of the chest and thoracic viscera, the way they bring about breathing, and how this is disrupted by pneumothorax.

⑧ Explain the embryological origins of the respiratory system and congenital abnormalities that may arise.

⑨ List the metabolic and non-respiratory functions of the respiratory system.

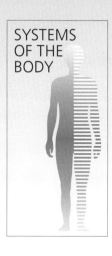

SYSTEMS
OF THE
BODY

2

STRUCTURE OF THE RESPIRATORY SYSTEM

Introduction

Just as each structural part of the respiratory system has its particular function, so each part has its particular pathologies. Respiratory structures are disrupted by disease, and the oft-repeated aphorism 'structure is related to function' is never more applicable than in the respiratory system in health and disease. Study of an outline of its structure considerably eases understanding of how the respiratory system functions.

We will first describe the airways of the lung and then the tissues that surround them.

The upper airways

> The neck is the part between the face and the trunk. The front part is of gristle and through it speech and respiration take place; it is known as the windpipe.
>
> Aristotle, *Historia animolium.*
> 4th century BC

The 'gristle' (cartilage) that Aristotle describes is of considerable importance in preventing the collapse of the upper airways, which in turn is of paramount importance to lung function because although the gas exchange we have defined as respiration takes place deep within the lungs, those parts of the respiratory system outside the chest, which may be referred to as the upper airways, allow and effect the process, and

are of such clinical importance that they must be considered.

The structures of the upper airways are best illustrated by a paramedial sagittal section of the head and neck (Fig. 2.1)

Mouth and nose – rhinitis, the common cold and obstructive sleep apnoea

It is unlikely that any of our readers have escaped the unpleasant obstruction to breathing associated with the common cold. The major discomfort of this condition is the result of an inflammation of the nose (rhinitis) and, if more severe, the paranasal sinuses. In about 50% of cases this rhinosinusitis is initially caused by rhinoviruses, 25% by corona viruses and the remainder by other viruses. A transient vasoconstriction of the mucous membrane (see below) is followed by vasodilatation, oedema and mucus production. With secondary bacterial infection the secretions become viscid, contain pus cells and bacteria, and contribute to the obstruction of breathing.

Rhinosinusitis may also be allergic in aetiology or idiopathic (i.e. intrinsic, of no external cause). Idiopathic rhinitis is thought to be a result of an imbalance of the activity of the sympathetic and parasympathetic nerves serving the mucosal blood vessels, and in this type of rhinitis anticholinergic medication often relieves symptoms.

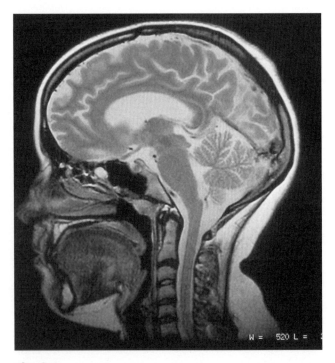

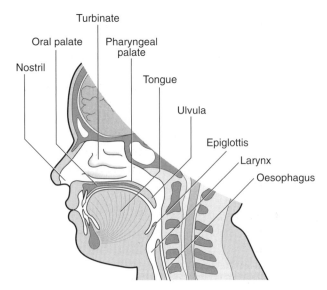

Fig. 2.1
Paramedial MRI scan of head and neck. The mouth is closed and the subject is breathing through his nose.

Allergic rhinitis may be seasonal in response to allergens such as pollen, or perennial, where a major cause is the allergen Der p1 in the faeces of the house-dust mite *Dermatophagoides pteronyssinus*.

The mite is just invisible to the unaided eye and lives on shed skin scales, particularly in human bedding. The allergen from this creature is also responsible for much asthma, but the rhinitis it provokes demonstrates the filtering action of the upper airways in trapping it in the nose.

Much more sinister and life-threatening than rhinitis is obstructive sleep apnoea (OSA; *apnoea = absence of breathing*). This should not be confused with central sleep apnoea, where the patient ceases to <u>make</u> respiratory efforts while they are sleeping. In OSA the patient's attempts to breathe are physically obstructed by anatomical and physiological peculiarities of the upper airways.

In Figure 2.1 the subject is breathing through his nose because the lips are closed and the tongue lies against the palate. When you breathe through the mouth – for example when you blow out a candle or suck through a straw – the soft palate is arched upward to form a seal against Passavant's ridge at the top of the pharynx. This form of airways obstruction is a normal function. Similarly, under normal circumstances, the genioglossus muscle of the tongue has a high resting tone in conscious subjects, and this holds the tongue forward, preventing it from obstructing the airway. During sleep, and particularly in those suffering from the dangerous condition of obstructive sleep apnoea, the tongue falls against the back wall of the pharynx and obstructs breathing. The muscle tone of the pharynx itself becomes reduced, particularly during REM (rapid eye movement) sleep and in OSA the pharynx collapses under the negative pressure of inspiration. Blocking of the airways by the tongue also and almost inevitably occurs during general anaesthesia and requires immediate attention from the anaesthetist.

Most, but not all, healthy persons breathe through the nose unless exercising. The resistance to breathing of the nose is about twice that of the mouth and nearly half the total resistance of the airways. The disadvantage of this is offset by the advantage obtained by the air-conditioning and filtering activities of the nose, which warm, moisten and filter the air before it comes in contact with the delicate respiratory regions of the lungs. Newborn babies have great difficulty breathing through their mouths: they are almost obligate nose breathers and become very distressed when their nose is blocked. Their predominantly nose breathing may be associated with their ability to suckle and breathe at the same time. On the other hand, many animal species, such as rabbits, manage to eat and breathe at

---

Structure of the respiratory system Box 1

Obstructive sleep apnoea

Mr Sinclair is 50 years old. He is rather overweight for his height: he is 168 cm tall but weighs 102 kg. He also drinks rather heavily and is a smoker.

For the past 2 years, Mrs Sinclair has slept in a different room from Mr Sinclair because of his very loud snoring and restlessness at night. Recently, Mr Sinclair has been feeling more and more tired during the day. For some time, he has been regularly falling asleep when he arrives home from work. Over the past month or so, he has found it increasingly difficult to concentrate at work and on one occasion recently, he was caught sleeping at his desk by his manager and he is facing disciplinary action. Mrs Sinclair eventually persuaded her husband to visit his doctor.

Mr Sinclair's doctor referred him to a specialist in sleep medicine. The doctor suggested that he may be suffering from obstructive sleep apnoea (OSA). He explained that during periods of deep sleep, Mr Sinclair's airway was becoming obstructed. During an episode of obstruction, Mr Sinclair's sleep becomes lighter until the obstruction is overcome. These episodes of obstruction and sleep interruption are responsible for Mr Sinclair's daytime sleepiness. The doctor went on to suggest that Mr Sinclair might be treated with a nasal continuous positive airway pressure device.

In this section we will consider:

① What causes obstructive sleep apnoea?
② What are the signs, symptoms and treatment of obstructive sleep apnoea?

---

the same time by having lateral food channels on either side of the larynx (see below) that bypass the airway. Marine mammals such as whales have completely separate air and food channels, with the airway ending at the back of the head.

In humans the nose extends from the nostrils (external nares) to the choanae (internal nares), which empty into the nasal part of the pharynx. Each nostril narrows to form its nasal valve, and at this level the total cross-sectional area of the airways is narrower (30 mm^2) than anywhere else in the system. This narrowing imposes the majority of the high resistance to airflow found in the nose (see Chapter 5) and, combined with the sharp turn the inspiratory air must make as it enters the wide (140 mm^2) lumen of the

STRUCTURE OF THE RESPIRATORY SYSTEM

cavum of the nose, causes turbulence. The walls of the nasal cavum are rigid bone projecting out into the airway from the lateral walls as the **turbinates**. These have a large surface area (150 cm²) covered by vascular mucosal erectile tissue important in the 'air-conditioning' activities of the nose. This mucosal tissue can swell considerably in conditions such as rhinitis (described above), and it is here that nasal decongestants such as oxymetazoline, an agonist of α adrenergic receptors on vascular smooth muscle, act to clear a blocked nose by causing the vascular smooth muscle to contract.

Normal physiological swelling of the mucosa and consequent restriction of airflow takes place asymmetrically over a period of time, so that one nasal passage is more constricted than the other. Thus both nasal passages are not uniformly constricted, with the major constriction, and therefore airflow, alternating between nostrils over a period of hours. This oscillation of airflow may help to sustain the nose in its air-conditioning activities by allowing one channel to rest while the other carries out most of the work.

The major function of the upper airway is to air-condition the inspirate. It is not essential to breathe through the nose to do this, and the mouth will make a fairly good job of warming and humidifying inhaled air before it reaches the larynx. However, the mouth has not evolved for that purpose and the unpleasant consequences of using it are well known to anyone who has had to breathe through their mouth because a cold has obstructed their nasal airways.

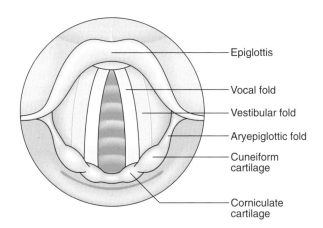

Fig. 2.2
The vocal folds, as might be seen by an anaesthetist about to intubate a patient.

larynx. Effective coughs depend on the closure and rapid opening of these 'curtains', which under less extreme circumstances are used to produce and modify the sounds that make up speech. The vocal folds can be drawn together so strongly that they are airtight against the greatest efforts to breathe the subject can make. This is clearly a 'bad thing' and can occur accidentally when an anaesthetist is trying to get an endotracheal tube into a patient's trachea. This dangerous closing of the larynx is called **laryngospasm**. A picture of what an anaesthetist would see when approaching the larynx is shown in Fig. 2.2.

The larynx – intubation of the airways

A common cause of accidental airway obstruction is the inhalation of food into the trachea. Normally, to prevent this during swallowing, the larynx, a box-like structure at the upper end of the trachea, is elevated by the muscles attached to it and the **epiglottis** folds backward, forming a very effective seal, like a 'trap-door' over the entrance to the larynx. Because a 'trap-door' can only open outwards, increased pressure in the pharynx makes the seal of the epiglottis on the larynx tighter and it can withstand considerable inward pressures of up to 100 kPa.

If this system of preventing solids entering the airways fails, powerful cough reflexes can be provoked by nerves in the lining of the larynx and trachea.

The larynx (see Fig. 2.1) is a rather complicated box made up of plates of cartilage. It can be closed off by drawing together the two curtains of muscle which make up the **vocal folds** across the lumen of the

Bronchoscopy

It is frequently useful to inspect the airways below the larynx. First the trachea (part of which is extrathoracic), and then the intrathoracic airways. The instrument used for this is called a bronchoscope and may be of the rigid 'open tube' type through which the airways are inspected, or the flexible fibreoptic variety (Fig. 2.3) which, as well as providing a view of the inside of the airways through its fibreoptic system, contains channels through which a variety of sampling and surgical instruments may be passed. Each type of bronchoscope has its advantages, but 95% of bronchoscopic procedures carried out these days are fibreoptic. Biopsy forceps, brushes and needles, balloon catheters and laser fibres can all now be passed through flexible bronchoscopes to carry out procedures after an initial inspection of even very small intrathoracic airways.

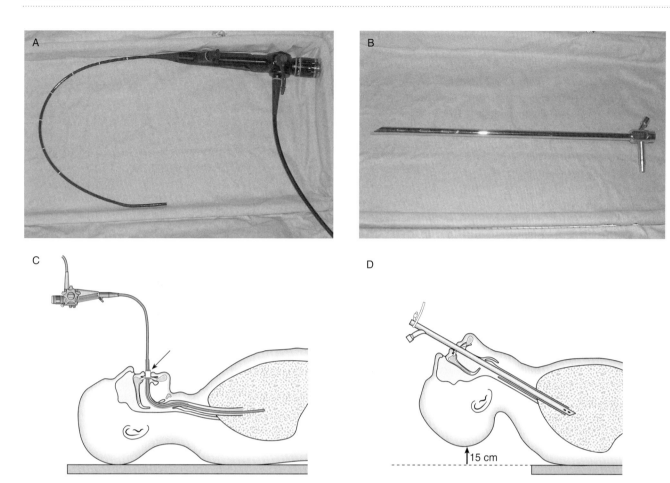

Fig. 2.3
Bronchoscopes. Both fibreoptic flexible (A & C) and rigid (B & D) types are shown. The vast majority of investigations these days are carried out with the flexible type.

The intrathoracic airways

The trachea is a single tube leading from the extrathoracic environment of the neck, where it is anchored at one end at the larynx, into the intrathoracic environment containing the lungs. It is the first of the **conducting airways** of the lungs. The conducting airways, as their name implies, conduct air to the **respiratory airways**, where the exchange of gas that makes up respiration takes place. The structure of these conducting airways differs from that of the respiratory region, mainly in having cartilage and smooth muscle in their relatively thick walls. This cartilage is particularly prominent in the trachea, where it forms horseshoe-shaped incomplete rings, with the two free ends facing backward and closed with a layer of smooth muscle (trachealis) with the oesophagus lying against it. (This arrangement can result in some interesting clinical conditions – see Self-assessment case study on Café coronary on p. 30.)

The airways of the lungs are often referred as the **bronchial tree**, and casts in which the airways are filled with plastic material and then the tissues dissolved away look like a deciduous tree in winter. The branches of this 'tree' can be represented in diagrammatic form as the 'generations' of a family tree (Fig. 2.4). In some bronchitic patients secretions sometimes fill small airways, solidify, and are coughed up as small 'casts'.

The trachea is the first and largest of about **23 generations** of airways. The airways of each generation arise from the previous one by a system of irregular dichotomous branching airways. Dichotomous because each 'mother' airway gives rise to two 'daughter' airways, and irregular because the daughters, although smaller than the mother, are not necessarily of equal size. The naming of these generations is illustrated in Figure 2.4, from which it may not be obvious that the number of airways (N) in a generation (Z), (counting the single trachea as generation 0) is:

$$N = Z^2.$$

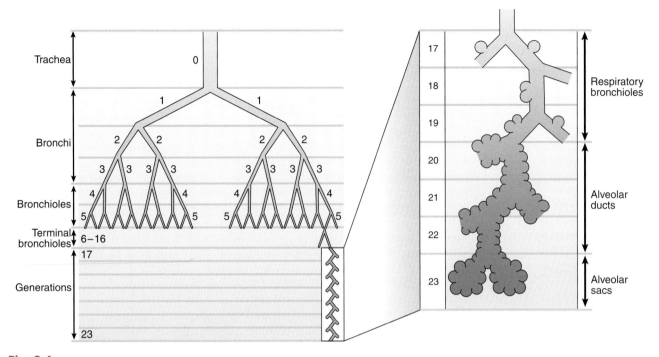

Fig. 2.4

The naming of airways. There is of course a gradual change in structure from one type of airway to another. One particular type of airway can occur at different distances into the lungs. (After Weibel, 1963.)

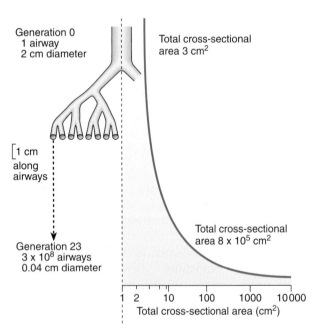

Fig. 2.5

Total cross-sectional area of the human airways. The total cross-sectional area at any level in the bronchial tree is the sum of the cross-sectional areas of all the airways at that level.

The effect of dichotomous branching of individual airways on the **total cross-sectional area** (the sum of the cross-sectional areas of all the airways at that level) at any level of the airways is remarkable and is shown in Figure 2.5. Notice that 'Total cross-sectional area' is measured on a log scale, and so this value increases much more than it appears to in the figure.

The functional consequences of this increase are profound because it causes the velocity of the air to fall rapidly as it moves into the lung. This effect is discussed in more detail in Chapter 5. The dimensions of some of the airways that make up the bronchial tree are given in Table 2.1.

As you go deeper into the lung the transitional and respiratory generations of the airways bear more and more **alveoli** until the **alveolar sacs** are totally made up of them. Alveoli do not look like the bunches of grapes or balloons stylistically represented in many textbooks, but rather pock-marked cavities with holes (pores of Kohn, K in Fig. 2.7C) between many adjacent alveoli and with macrophages wandering about over their surface ready to engulf and digest foreign particles (Figs 2.6 and 2.17).

It is a testament to the remarkable power of evolution that computer models which can analyse a branching system of tubes tell us that the branching angles and the changes in diameter of the airways of the human lungs are just right to cram the maximum alveolar surface into the minimum volume.

Table 2.1
Dimensions of some of the airways of the human tracheobronchial tree. Note the enormous increase in cross-section and percentage total volume in the last few generations

Generation	Name	Diameter (cm)	Total cross-section (cm²)	Cumulative volume (%)	Number
0	Trachea	1.80	2.5	1.7	1
10	Small bronchi	0.13	13.0	4.0	10^3
14	Bronchioles	0.08	45.0	7.0	10^4
18	Respiratory bronchioles	0.05	540.0	31.0	3×10^5
24	Alveoli	0.04	8×10^5	100.0	3×10^8

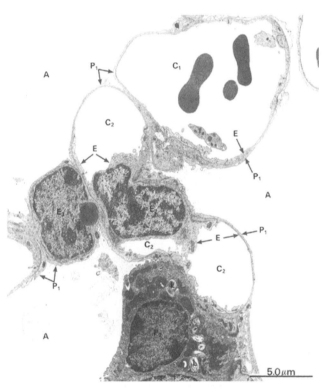

Fig. 2.6
Scanning electron micrograph of an alveolus.
A, alveolus; C_1, C_2, C_3, capillaries; E, endothelial cell; P_1, type I pneumocytes; P_2 type II pneumocyte; L, lamellar bodies. From Young and Heath 2000.

Histological structure of the airways

The microscopic structure of the wall of the airways changes as you go deeper into the lungs. Three 'snapshots' of airway wall structure are shown in Figure 2.7 but of course the structure changes gradually from generation to generation.

The conducting airways consist of three general layers which vary in proportion depending on airway type:

- The inner mucosal surface consists of ciliated epithelium and underlying mucus-secreting goblet cells. The activity of the cilia and the secretions of the globlet cells make up the **mucociliary escalator** (see Air-conditioning, below), which is important in removing inhaled particles in the lungs.
- Outside the mucosal layer comes a **smooth muscle** layer in which the fibres are in continuous bundles. This smooth muscle is found in decreasing amounts from the largest airways right down to the entrances to the alveoli.
- The outermost layer is of **connective tissue**, which in the large bronchi contains supporting cartilage. As the airways penetrate the lung they first lose their cartilage support and smooth muscle occupies a greater percentage of the airway wall. Then the ciliated epithelium becomes the squamous type, finally forming the respiratory region of the lung.

Bronchitis and the Reid Index

The arrangement representing bronchial structure illustrated in Figure 2.7 and described above is modified in chronic bronchitis in a way that provides a histopathological quantitative diagnosis of the disease. The **Reid Index** provides a measure of proportion of bronchial glands to total wall thickness (Fig. 2.8). In normal lungs mucous glands occupy less than 40% of total wall thickness. In chronic bronchitis this proportion is altered by hyperplasia of the glands. A characteristic of chronic bronchitis is an increase in the products of these glands.

The respiratory region

The respiratory regions of the lungs show a wonderful degree of adaptation. They carry out the functions of a respiratory surface while withstanding the assaults of a polluted atmosphere and the mechanical

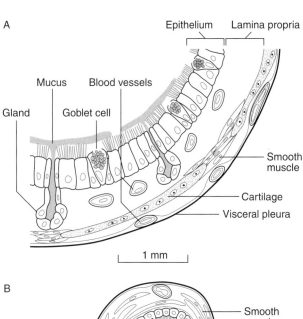

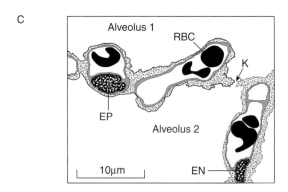

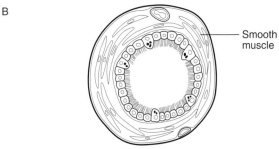

Fig. 2.7
Airways wall structure. The classification of airways would depend on the characteristics of structure illustrated here. (A) Bronchus; (B) bronchiole; (C) alveolus. RBC, red blood cell; K, pores of Kohn; EP, epithelial nucleus; EN, endothelial nucleus.

trauma of being stretched and then relaxed about 12 times a minute for the whole of your life owing to the movements of breathing. One of the characteristics of the respiratory surface of any animal is that it should be thin, offering minimal separation between the outside medium (air or water) and the blood. This is beautifully demonstrated in the lungs, which are the only place in our body where blood capillaries come into direct contact with the outside air, as a result of

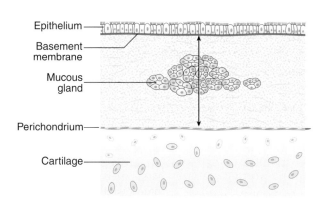

Fig. 2.8
The Reid Index. The percentage of bronchial wall thickness occupied by gland tissue is known as the Reid Index, and is used as a measure of chronic bronchitis.

the fusion of the **type I** epithelial cells (which make up about 95% of the lining of the respiratory zone; Fig. 2.6) with the pulmonary capillary endothelium. This fusion results in an ultrathin layer ideal for the diffusion of gas but not much good for support. Evolution has resulted in this thinning occurring on only one side of the pulmonary capillaries, whereas the cells on the other side remain separate and more robust, supporting the capillary in its place (Fig. 2.9).

The junctions between the endothelial cells of the capillaries are 'leaky' and allow an easy flux of water and solutes between the plasma and the interstitial space. The junctions between the epithelial cells, however, are sufficiently 'tight' to prevent the escape of large molecules such as albumen into the alveoli, which would result in pulmonary oedema. Macrophages can easily push their way through the epithe-

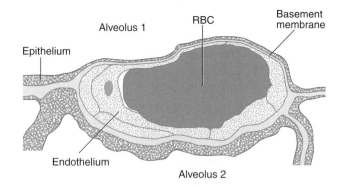

Fig. 2.9
The alveolar–capillary membrane. This diagram of an electron micrograph shows the way the alveolar and capillary cells on one side of the alveolar septum fuse to form an ultrathin layer which offers little barrier to diffusion. The other side of the septum is thicker and provides physical support. RBC, red blood cell.

lial junctions to carry out their scavenging activities on the air side of the alveolus.

The rounded **type II** cells, much less numerous than type I and found at the junctions of alveolar septa, are the stem cells from which type II epithelial cells are formed. They are also important in producing lung surfactant (see Chapter 3).

Blood vessels

The pulmonary circulation only offers one-sixth of the resistance to blood flow that the systemic circulation offers. It is therefore a **low-pressure** system and this is reflected in the thin walls of its arteries. These arteries follow the airways through the lungs in connective tissue sheaths. The pulmonary arterioles are also very different from systemic arterioles, having very little smooth muscle in their walls. This absence of smooth muscle in the arterioles, and of course the capillaries and venules, persuades many scientists to consider the microcirculation of the lungs as a whole, rather than making a special case of the capillaries, which snake along several alveolar walls, one after the other, before reaching the venules. Venules join to form veins which, unlike the arteries, do not travel with the airways but make their own way along the septa that separate the segments of the lung. The airways and pulmonary blood vessels down as far as the terminal bronchioles receive their nutrition from the **bronchial circulation** which, as part of the systemic circulation, is distinct from the **pulmonary circulation** of the lungs. Part of the bronchial circulation returns to the systemic venous system in the normal way, but part drains into the pulmonary veins, 'contaminating' their oxygenated blood with deoxygenated blood. This situation constitutes a '**shunt**' (see Chapter 7, p. 107).

Pulmonary hypertension

Hypertension (high blood pressure) can occur in the pulmonary circulation as well as in the systemic circulation. Pulmonary mean arterial pressure is normally about **15 mmHg**. This means that the limited smooth muscle in the pulmonary system is normally quite adequate to control flow. Pulmonary hypertension can arise for extrapulmonary reasons, such as mitral stenosis or left ventricular failure, both of which prevent the heart pumping away blood returning from the lungs. Congenital defects which allow blood to pass from the left (high-pressure) side of the heart to the pulmonary circulation also produce pulmonary hypertension.

By far the most common causes of pulmonary hypertension are changes in the pulmonary vessels themselves. They may be blocked by emboli, circulat-

ing fat, amniotic fluid or cancer cells. They may be obliterated by destruction of the architecture of the capillary beds by emphysema, or the smooth muscle in their walls may be provoked to contract by low oxygen tension, resulting from high altitude or diseases such as bronchitis and emphysema.

The clinical features of pulmonary hypertension are mainly the result of the increased pressure, producing oedema in the lung and imposing a pumping load on the right heart which it has not evolved to cope with. The patient complains of chest pain, dyspnoea and fatigue. Heart sounds are modified and the ECG demonstrates right ventricular hypertrophy.

The lymphatics

The perivascular spaces of the alveolar wall are drained by lymph vessels. The lymph system of the lungs begins as tiny blind-ended vessels just above the alveoli. These join to form lymphatics in close approximation to the blood vessels and airways. They are an important feature in the control of fluid balance in the lung and can contain considerable amounts of lymph, particularly during pulmonary oedema, when they produce the characteristic 'butterfly shadow' on the chest X-ray (Fig. 2.10).

As in other tissue the lymph system plays a key role in immune defence in the lungs. These reactions are more the province of a textbook of immunology, but can be classified in outline as:

- immediate hypersensitivity
- antibody-dependent cytotoxicity

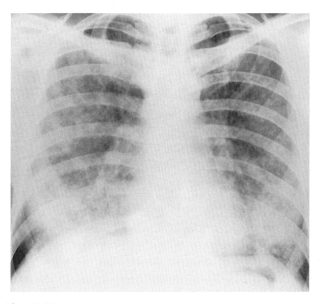

Fig. 2.10
X-ray of 'butterfly shadow' in pulmonary oedema.

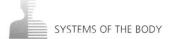
- immune complex reactions
- cell-mediated immune reactions.

Many immune disorders have the characteristics of asthma, whereas those causing interstitial lung disease are characterized by restrictive patterns (see Chapter 4).

The nerves

Innervation of the airways of the lungs is separate from that which brings about breathing (see below) and consists of afferent and efferent parts. The most dramatic efferent (motor) effects produced are on bronchomotor tone. The **parasympathetic** efferent supply is of most importance in this, and arrives at bronchial smooth muscle via preganglionic fibres which course through the jugular and then the nodose ganglia of the vagus nerves. As this is a parasympathetic outflow the fibres synapse in ganglia on the bronchi before sending short postganglionic fibres to the bronchial smooth muscle where

they release acetylcholine to produce bronchoconstriction (Fig. 2.11).

The **sympathetic** nervous system, which is anatomically represented, has yet to be proved to have functional importance. The **NANC** (non-adrenergic non-cholinergic) system, which runs in the vagus nerve, secretes a variety substances that contract and relax bronchial smooth muscle, depending on circumstances.

Afferent nerves from receptors near the alveoli (J receptors), in the smooth muscle of airways (stretch receptors), and free nerve endings between the epithelial cells of airways (rapidly adapting, irritant, receptors) conduct sensation and sensory reflex information from the lungs to the brain, where it influences patterns of breathing (see Chapter 11) and bronchomotor tone.

The pulmonary circulation is innervated by sympathetic and parasympathetic nerves, but unlike the situation in the airways the sympathetic supply is of greater functional importance than the parasympathetic, and

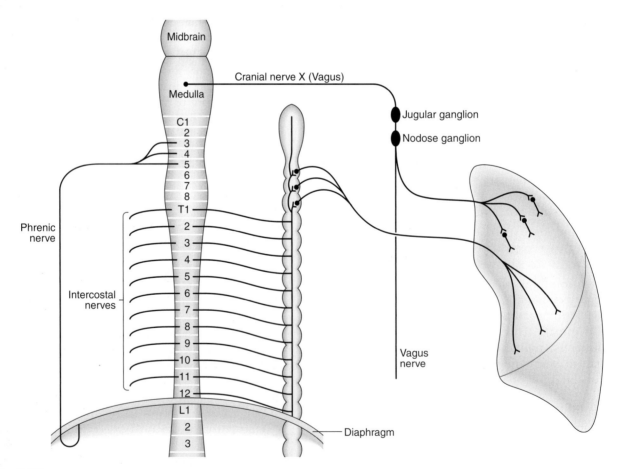

Fig. 2.11
Innervation of the diaphragm, intercostal musles and lungs. The efferent (motor) systems are shown. The afferent (sensory) system is mainly in the vagus nerves.

even then it only appears to exert a significant effect under conditions requiring 'fight or flight'.

The limited importance of all these nervous systems is demonstrated by the success of transplanted lungs which are in fact denervated!

Gross structure of the respiratory system

As with other organs the general name for the functional tissue of the lungs is **parenchyma**. The vast majority of the volume of what we see as the lungs when the chest is opened is in fact alveolar tissue surrounding air spaces (see Table 2.1). These air spaces make the lungs so insubstantial and light that they are the only organ that floats when placed in water, hence the Middle English name for lungs: *lights*.

Each lung is anatomically divided into **lobes**, made up of **segments** which are subdivided into **lobules** (Fig. 2.12).

The lungs lie on both sides of the **mediastinum** which contains the trachea, heart, major blood vessels, nerves and oesophagus. The trachea divides into the right and left main bronchi at the **carina**, which is close to the aortic arch and the division of the pulmonary artery into its left and right branches. The main bronchi, pulmonary arteries and veins penetrate each

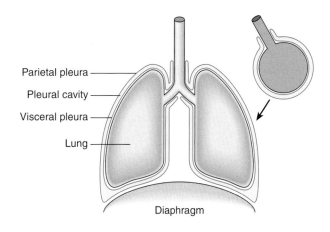

Fig. 2.13
Schematic diagram of the pleurae. It is important to remember that there is no real 'space' between the pleurae, just a few millilitres of slippery fluid.

lung at the **hila**. The lobes of the lungs are covered, except at their 'roots' at the medial surface, by a thin layer of tissue called the **visceral pleura**. The mediastinum and chest wall are lined by the **parietal pleura**. It helps some students to visualize the arrangement of the pleurae by thinking of a plastic bag, full of lungs, inside a second plastic bag, the two bags being the visceral and parietal pleurae, respectively (Fig. 2.13).

The pleurae secrete a few milliliters of viscous fluid which lubricates them as they rub against each other during breathing, this fluid constitutes a 'space' between the pleurae, but it is important to remember that this tiny space is fluid <u>not</u> air filled. Most animals have pleural space, although it is not essential for life. Elephants are said to lack one, and surgeons sometimes fix the lungs to the chest wall in patients with ruptured lungs, thereby obliterating the space.

Pleurisy

Inflammation of the pleura is called pleurisy and may be 'dry', where there is no appreciable effusion, or associated with an effusion, which may be of a variety of compositions. The pain of dry pleurisy is the result of the raw plurae moving over each other, and the patient complains of sharp localized pain associated with inspiration or coughing. Dry pleurisy occasionally accompanies pneumonia or carcinoma. Effusions of fluid into the pleural space result from a variety of conditions and can be of sufficient volume to collapse the lungs. If these effusions contain little protein they are known as transudates; if they contain much protein they are called exudates.

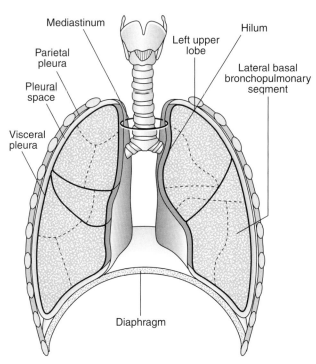

Fig. 2.12
Gross anatomy of the lungs. Each lung is divided into lobes made up of segments subdivided into lobules by fibrous tissue.

The diaphragm and chest wall

The base of the roughly cylindrical container which is the thorax is formed by the **diaphragm**. This is a sheet of muscle surrounding a large central tendon (Fig. 2.14).

The diaphragm lies surprisingly high in the thorax, the central tendon being about level with the eighth thoracic vertebra. Muscle fibres attached to the tendon run down obliquely to originate at the xiphisternum (see below), the lower margins of the ribcage and the upper lumbar vertebrae. Innervation of the diaphragm is by the right and left **phrenic nerves**, each of which serves its half of diaphragm. The phrenic nerves originate from cervical spinal cord segments C3–C5 ('C3, 4 and 5 keep the diaphragm alive'), with the major contribution being made by C4. Both nerves run through the thorax in contact with the mediastinum, penetrate the diaphragm, and innervate it from its inferior surface.

The walls of the thorax are made up of the ribcage (Fig. 2.15), which consists of the **sternum** anteriorly, to which ribs 1–6 are joined at about 45° by the costal cartilages. At the spinal column the ribs articulate by costovertebral joints which may involve more than one vertebra. Ribs 7–10 are joined by costal cartilage to the ribs above, and ribs 11 and 12 are free-'floating' at their anterior end.

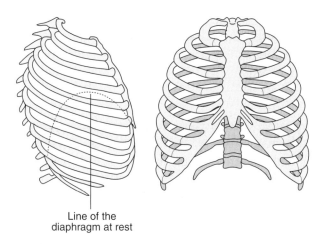

Line of the diaphragm at rest

Fig. 2.15

The ribcage. This 'cage' is much more flexible than prepared specimens or models sometimes suggest. The intercostal muscles stretch between the ribs.

Between the ribs are the three layers of the **intercostal muscles**:

1. External intercostals, running forward and downward
2. Internal intercostals, at right-angles to the externals, therefore running downward and posteriorly
3. Innermost intercostals, whose fibers run in the same direction as those of the internals.

These muscles are innervated by intercostal nerves from the anterior primary rami of spinal cord segments T1–T11.

Many muscles which do not have a primary role in respiration have their origins on the thorax. They move the head and neck and the upper limbs, for example. These muscles can be enlisted to aid breathing and are therefore called **accessory muscles of respiration**. The majority of these muscles aid inspiration, with only the flexors of the spine and the muscles of the anterior abdominal wall aiding expiration. Nevertheless, because of the mechanical advantage the accessory expiratory muscles have over the inspiratory muscles, we can blow out more powerfully than we can breathe in.

How breathing is brought about

Anyone who has sucked up fluid with a syringe has demonstrated how inspiration takes place. Before we go into the details of how the two processes are similar, we need to establish two very important facts:

1. The lungs do not have muscles that contribute to breathing: the small amount of muscle they contain controls the diameter of the airways.

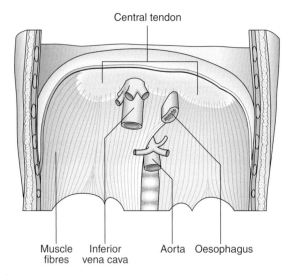

Central tendon

Muscle fibres   Inferior vena cava   Aorta   Oesophagus

Fig. 2.14

The diaphragm in coronal section. This figure illustrates how far into the chest the diaphragm bulges. This enables it to act very like the piston in a syringe as its muscle fibres shorten when stimulated by the bilateral phrenic nerves.

Structure of the respiratory system Box 2

Causes of OSA

In order for efficient gas flow to take place from the mouth to the alveoli, the airways that make up the respiratory system obviously need to be open and patent. The trachea and larger airways are held open by partial rings of cartilage within their walls. The smaller airways and the alveoli are held open by the tension in the lung tissue surrounding them. Above the larynx, the airway is held open by the actions of airway-dilating muscles, including genioglossus and palatopharyngeus. Were it not for the actions of these muscles, the upper airway would collapse, particularly in the supine position. During sleep, the tone in skeletal muscles throughout the body is reduced and this applies equally to the muscles which keep the upper airways patent. It is therefore normal for the upper airway to become narrowed during sleep.

In patients with OSA, this narrowing is greatly exaggerated and leads to periods of airway obstruction. There are a number of reasons why this happens, but obesity is the most important. It is thought that in obese patients, the pressure exerted by the fat in the neck tends to cause the airway to collapse. When the tone in the genioglossus and palatopharyngeus is reduced, as during sleep, airway obstruction may result.

The airway may remain obstructed for only a few seconds, or it may be well over a minute before the patient takes his next breath. During this time, the patient may become hypoxic and will begin to make vigorous efforts to try and breathe against the obstructed airway. Furthermore, he will become increasingly aroused from his sleep. Eventually, he regains the tone in his airway-dilating muscles and the airway obstruction is relieved. (Patients do not usually waken.) After the obstruction has been relieved, ventilation resumes and the patient's sleep deepens. This leads to a reduced tone in the airway-dilating muscles and the cycle starts to repeat itself.

Although obesity is probably the most important factor leading to OSA, there are other predisposing factors. These include anatomical variations predisposing to airway narrowing, such as enlarged tonsils, airway tumours and abnormalities of the mandible. Sedative drugs, including alcohol, may also predispose to sleep apnoea, probably by affecting sleep patterns and by reducing muscle tone. A small number of cases of OSA may be explained by abnormalities of neuromuscular function.

2. Air will only flow from a region of high pressure to a region of low pressure. In inspiration the pressure in the elastic alveoli is made low by stretching them by reducing the pressure around them by expanding the chest. Air is thus sucked into the lungs. During expiration pressure in the lungs is increased by decreasing the size of the chest, thereby compressing the gas in the lungs.

The reduction in pressure around the lungs which brings about inspiration is mainly the result of activity in the phrenic nerves, causing the diaphragm to flatten and descend in the chest like a plunger in a syringe. This draws air into the chest. In quiet breathing inspiration is the only *active* part of breathing; expiration is largely passive and is the result of the **elastic recoil** of the lungs pulling them and the diaphragm back into their resting position – something like a balloon deflating when its neck is released.

The central tendon of the diaphragm moves 1–2 cm during breathing at rest, but can move up to about 10 cm during vigorous breathing. Movement of the diaphragm normally accounts for about 75% of the volume of breathing, but is not essential for life: if the diaphragm is paralysed, other respiratory muscles can take over to a large degree. In quiet breathing only some (and not always the same) diaphragmatic muscle fibres contract with each inspiration. This may explain why we rarely suffer from fatigue of the diaphragm.

If we liken the diaphragm to the plunger of a syringe, the ribs can be likened to its walls. The action of the intercostal muscles on the ribs (mainly the second to the tenth) can, however, alter the diameter of the chest and so actively draw air into and expel it from the lungs. This is largely because the ribs are set at an angle, sloping down from the horizontal, and are capable of being raised and lowered (see Fig. 2.14).

The external intercostal muscles cause two types of movement during inspiration:

1. 'Pump-handle' movements, in which the anterior end of each rib is elevated like the action of an old-fashioned water pump.
2. 'Bucket-handle' movements, in which the diameter of the chest increases, each rib on either side acting like the raising of the handle of a bucket from the horizontal position.

Both these types of action increase the diameter of the chest and thus draw air into the lungs by reducing the pressure in the chest. Not only do the external intercostal muscles help to bring about this reduction in pressure, but by stiffening the chest wall during inspiration they prevent a 'sucking-in' of the chest (just as you can suck in your cheeks) that would take place if they did not contract. The action of the intercostal muscles accounts for about 25% of maximum voluntary ventilation. The importance of the ribs and intercostal muscles to breathing is seen in patients whose ribs are broken and who exhibit what is known as 'flail chest'.

Although expiration is largely passive during quiet breathing (resulting from the elastic recoil of the chest and lungs) expiratory muscles can contract actively during high levels of breathing or if the airways are obstructed by disease. The **abdominal muscles** are the most important muscles of expiration. By squeezing the contents of the abdomen up against the diaphragm they force it up into the chest, thereby expelling air from the lungs. These abdominal muscles are especially active during a cough or a sneeze, as will be apparent if you press your fingers into your abdomen and cough. The internal and innermost intercostal muscles, like the external intercostals, occupy the spaces between the ribs and are innervated by segmental nerves. They pull the ribs down, reduce the diameter of the chest, and so contribute to expiration. Like the external intercostals, they reinforce the spaces between the ribs and prevent the chest from bulging out during expiration. The changes in size and shape of the chest brought about by the activity of the diaphragm, intercostals and accessory muscles are transmitted to the outer surface of the lungs. Because the lungs are so flexible, any change in pressure on their surface is rapidly transmitted to the air within the alveoli. This does not mean that the actual pressure in the fluid between the layers of pleura that form the covering of the lungs and the lining of the chest is the same as the pressure in the alveoli (see Chapter 5): in fact, it is important for the student to realize that they are very different.

Embryology

A knowledge of the embryological origins of anatomical structures is often of use in understanding their physiological function, and many clinical situations. For example, the phenomenon of referred pain can be explained on the basis of common embryological origins of structures. Development of the fetal and neonatal lung can explain many differences in the function of the immature and the adult lung.

Prematurity, particularly with birthweights less than 2500 g, can result in respiratory distress in the infant because of the immaturity of type II pneumocytes, which produce surfactant (p. 38). This **respiratory distress syndrome**, also called hyaline membrane disease, develops within minutes or hours of birth and is characterized by high breathing rates requiring great effort owing to the reduced compliance of the lungs. When premature delivery of an infant is threatened its ability to secrete surfactant is estimated by measuring the ratio of lecithin to sphingomyelin in its amniotic fluid. If necessary, the activity of the type II pneumocytes can be enhanced by the administration of corticosteroids, and after birth exogenous surfactant can be administered as an aerosol. Nevertheless, mortality can be as high as 40%, which demonstrates how, even in the full-term baby, the development of the respiratory system is only just sufficiently complete.

In the 4-week-old human embryo the beginnings of the respiratory system are first seen as an outpouching, the **laryngotracheal bud**, on the ventral surface of the endoderm of the digestive tract (Fig. 2.16). As the bud elongates the proximal portion forms the trachea and the distal end bifurcates to form first the two main bronchi and then the more distal parts of the bronchial tree, eventually forming a limited number of alveoli. The whole of the epithelium lining the entire respiratory tract is therefore derived from **endoderm**. The cartilage, muscle and connective tissue which make up much of the structure of the lungs develop from

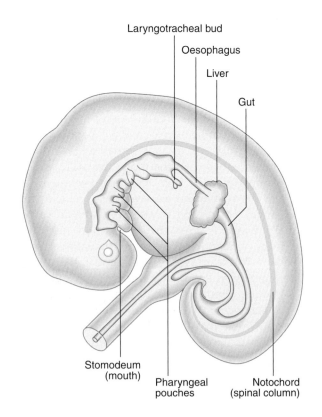

Fig. 2.16
Lateral view of a 4-week human embryo. The laryngotracheal bud is beginning to divide to form the two lungs.

embryonic **mesoderm** that becomes associated with the laryngotracheal bud.

The lung undergoes five overlapping phases of development:

- pseudoglandular
- canalicular
- saccular
- alveolar
- microvascular maturation.

In the **pseudoglandular** phase, which lasts from fifth to the 17th week, the lung resembles a primitive compound gland, with the airways down to terminal bronchioles becoming visible. From week 16 to week 26 is the **canalicular** stage, with the airway generations of the future respiratory regions being formed. At the same time the airways are pushing through the surrounding mesenchyme, picking up a sleeve of capillaries which forms a local network that grows with the airway. From week 25 to birth the future alveolar ducts and alveolar sacs are produced by growth and branching of the irregularly shaped saccules at the ends of the prospective respiratory bronchioles. Although alveolar formation has started as early as week 36 of gestation, at birth there are only 50 million alveoli present, compared with 300 million in the adult lung. Alveolization continues for about 2 years after birth. The maturation of the microvasculature of the lung parallels alveolization during the first 2 years of independent life. From then onwards, the lung compartments grow in proportion to each other and to body weight.

Air-conditioning

The characteristics of a respiratory surface do not lead to physical robustness (thin walls, vascular, moist). Therefore, it is of evolutionary advantage to have the respiratory surface of the lungs protected from damage by the air, or anything in the air, that must be moved over them during respiration. Even under the most congenial conditions the air around us is cold and dry compared with the respiratory surface of the lungs.

Heat and water

Because temperature and water vapour gradients between mucosa and inspired air are greatest in the nose and upper airways, these regions carry a large portion of the air-conditioning burden. This burden is, however, shared with the lower airways. During nose breathing at rest air transit through the nose takes

Structure of the respiratory system Box 3

Signs and symptoms of OSA

Often, the first person to complain about a patient's OSA is his or her spouse! OSA is invariably associated with loud snoring as the airway becomes narrowed and this combined with the cycles of obstruction and arousal can lead to a very poor night's sleep for anyone in the same room as the patient. By the time a patient presents for treatment, their spouse has often resorted to sleeping alone.

The main symptom that the patient complains of is daytime drowsiness. Because their sleep patterns are so disrupted by cycles of apnoea and arousal, these patients are very tired and sleepy during the day. This somnolence may begin to impinge upon the patient's work and home life as their ability to concentrate for long periods of time begins to diminish. At worst, the patient may have a tendency to lose concentration or even fall asleep at the wheel of their car – motor accidents are more common in patients with OSA.

Other symptoms that the patient may complain of include morning headaches and night sweating and relatives may notice personality changes. For reasons that are not fully understood, patients often complain of having to get up to urinate during the night, sometimes on a few occasions.

Treatment is aimed at reducing the incidence of airway obstruction. The patient is advised to lose weight and to limit alcohol consumption, particularly before retiring to bed.

The most effective form of treatment, and the one tried by Mr Sinclair, is nasal continuous positive airway pressure (NCPAP). The patient wears the small mask strapped over his nose at night. The mask forms an airtight seal around the patient's nose. A continuous positive pressure, generated by a small pump, is applied to the mask. This pressure is transmitted to the upper airways and tends to prevent them from collapsing.

Other treatments are available – a surgical treatment of the condition that was at one time popular is the uvulopalatopharyngoplasty (UPPP). This operation involves removing the uvula and part of the soft palate. It has only a limited success rate and is associated with complications including fluid refluxing into the nose during drinking. It is therefore infrequently performed today.

< 0.1 s. During that time temperature is raised (if in comfortable room air) from 20°C to 31°C by the time the air leaves the internal nares and to 35°C by the

time it reaches the mid trachea. Humidification takes place equally rapidly, inspired air being close to saturation by the time it reaches the pharynx. Humidification of inspired air places a thermal requirement on the body because of the high latent heat of vaporization of water. Five times as much heat is used to vaporize water to saturate inspired air than is used to warm that air. The air-conditioning process is a metabolic 'expense', and up to 40% of this cost is recovered from the expired air which warms and moistens the nasal mucosa as we breathe out. Desert animals such as camels and gerbils have highly developed turbinate systems in their noses which recover more heat and water than do ours.

This **countercurrent exchange** of heat and water in our nose is well demonstrated under cold conditions, when the mucosa of the nose is much colder than the exhaled air from deep in the lungs. Under these conditions sufficient water may condense to form a drop on the end of the nose. This is a purely natural physical phenomenon, not 'a cold' or other pathological condition.

At rest most people breathe through their nose, although 15% of the population are habitual mouth breathers. We all resort to mouth breathing during heavy exercise. The mouth is surprisingly good at air-conditioning, and by the time the air reaches the glottis conditions are very similar whether you are breathing through nose or mouth. The disadvantage of mouth breathing is in expiration, when much less heat and water is recovered. We have all experienced the discomfort of the dry mouth which often accompanies the nasal obstruction of a cold.

Particles and vapours

The respiratory system is threatened by many of the particles and chemical vapours in the air. The upper and conducting airways are much more robust than the respiratory surface, and they bear the brunt of protecting the respiratory surface by filtering these particles and vapours out of the inspired air.

Particles must be relatively small to penetrate the respiratory tract to any depth, and it is their size and shape that determine where they land. Where they land determines how they are dealt with.

An **aerosol** is a cloud of particles or droplets that remains stable and suspended in the air for some time. Because the volume (and hence the mass) of a drop is related to the cube of its diameter and its surface area is related to the square of its diameter, large drops fall faster than smaller ones. A shower of rain falls to the ground; a mist remains suspended for some time (Stoke's Law tells us that the terminal velocity of a

falling sphere is proportional to the square of its radius). Scientists interested in the way aerosols behave in the lungs often convert the weight and shape of the particles into the size of the aerodynamically equivalent spheres. The mass median diameter of an aerosol is the diameter about which 50% of the total particle mass resides. The mass median aerodynamic diameter (MMAD) is the product of the mass median diameter and the square root of the particle density. Using this system we see 95% of particles > 5 μm MMAD impact on the walls of the nose and pharynx, where they are trapped by the sticky mucus. This **impaction** is the result of turbulence and the particles' momentum throwing them out of the airstream, when they rapidly change direction. In our noses the mucus that has trapped the dust is wafted to the pharynx by cilia. It is then swallowed. In dogs the cilia beat toward the outside and this contributes to the wet nose of a healthy dog. Slightly smaller particles (1–5 μm) survive the twists and turbulence of the upper airways and are removed by **sedimentation** in the small airways. Sedimentation is the settling of particles' under gravity, and this slow process is only effective in the small airways because their diameter is so small that the particles have only a little way to fall. Small though they are, these particles are too massive to be much affected by the buffeting of the gas molecules around them that constitutes the phenomenon of diffusion. Particles which reach the wall of the small airways are trapped in the mucus there and travel up the **mucociliary escalator** at a rate of about 2 mm s^{-1} to the pharynx in considerable amounts, to be swallowed. The mucus blanket which traps the particles is 5–10 μm thick and in two layers. The outer gel layer rests on a less viscous layer in which the cilia beat toward the mouth at a frequency of about 20 Hz.

The smallest particles of all (< 0.1 μm) are deposited by **diffusion** of gas molecules producing Brownian motion. The particles are 'jostled' until they bump into the wall of a small airway or alveolus. In this region particles are stuck to the walls by surface tension because there is no secretion of mucus. They are also beyond the end of the ciliary escalator. In the alveolar region amoeboid **macrophages** (Fig. 2.17) engulf particles and carry them to the escalator, or take them into the blood or lymph. When the dust load is large the macrophages dump their load around the respiratory, bronchioles, and any pathologist from a coal-mining area will have seen the black 'halos' so formed. Bacteria are particularly susceptible to the attentions of macrophages, which kill them with enzymes and oxygen-based free radicals (see Metabolic activity, p. 28) or transport them out of the lungs. The activities of these phagocytic cells ensures that the alveolar region of the lung is effectively sterile.

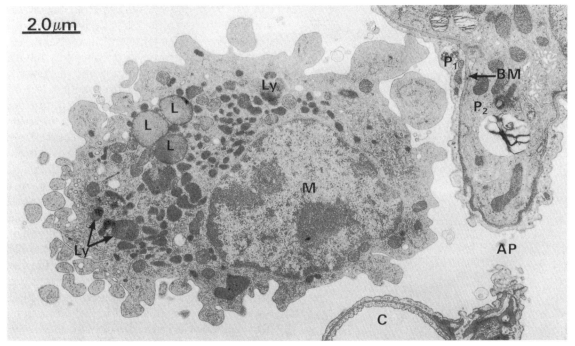

Fig. 2.17
Alveolar macrophage. Formed from monocytes produced in the bone marrow, these phagocytic cells contain enzymes destructive to microorganisms. These enzymes can produce emphysema in patients deficient in the protective protein α_1-antitrypsin. M, macrophage; C, septal capillary; P_1, type 1 pneumocyte; AP, alveolar pore; BM, basement membrane; Ly, lysosomes; L, lipid droplets. (Source: Young and Heath 2000.)

The free radicals and proteases produced by macrophages to deal with foreign material have the potential to damage the lung itself; how these dangerous substances are neutralized is described below (Metabolic activity, p. 28).

The influence of impaction, sedimentation and diffusion on particles of different aerodynamic diameters is illustrated in Figure 2.18.

The majority of particles of 0.5 μm aerodynamic diameter are not deposited: they ride the airflow into the lungs and back out again with expiration. Figure 2.18 represents the case during quiet breathing. Treatment of disease with therapeutic aerosols requires slow deep breathing to ensure deep penetration and sufficient time for diffusion. The increased ventilation of exercise enhances impaction and the danger of heavy work in dusty environments.

Particles account for only a small fraction by weight of the pollutants we breathe (Fig. 2.19).

Many gases and vapours also pose a serious threat, augmented by the self-abuse of tobacco smoking. Oxides of sulphur and nitrogen, hydrocarbons and chemicals produced by the action of sunlight on these substances inflame the respiratory tract. More than 1000 harmful constituents are inhaled in tobacco smoke. Smoking was identified by no less an authority than King James (VI of Scotland) I of England (1603–1625) as *'a custom loathsome to the eye, hateful to the nose, harmful to the brain and dangerous to the lungs'*. Little wonder he was known as 'the wisest fool in

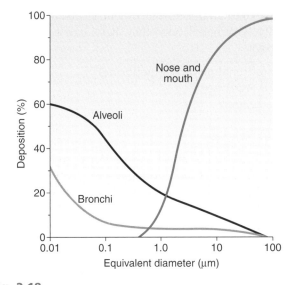

Fig. 2.18
Deposition of particles in the lung. Notice that the aerodynamic diameter is a log scale and that there is a point at about 0.5 μm diameter where deposition is minimal.

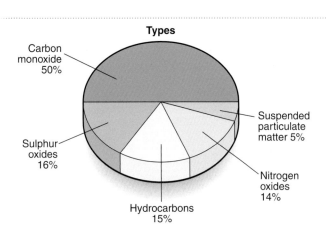

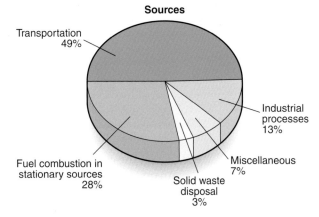

Fig. 2.19
Air pollutants and their sources. Note the contribution made by automobiles.

Christendom'. Many harmful substances are produced by internal combustion engines, but the introduction of catalytic converters has significantly reduced production of carbon monoxide which has a particularly deleterious effect on the carriage of oxygen by the blood (see Chapter 8).

Metabolic activity

The metabolism of the tissues of the lung itself is unremarkable, with a metabolic rate only slightly higher than average for the whole body. Although it is the major extrahepatic site for mixed function oxidation by the cytochrome P450 systems, gram for gram it is much less active than the liver and much less tissue is involved. The major role of the P450 system in the lungs may therefore be in **detoxification** of inhaled foreign substances. Bloodborne toxic substances are extensively sequestered or detoxified in the lungs, with basic substances being particularly well processed. This protective activity on the part of the lung

can be 'heroic' to a degree that causes fatal local damage: for example, the accumulation of oxygen-derived **free radicals** (useful in moderate concentrations to attack bacteria) is enhanced by the weedkiller paraquat (Weedol or Gramoxone), a dose of 1.5 g of which may be fatal because of its selective uptake by the lung. Although the initial clinical features of paraquat poisoning include dramatic ulceration of the mouth and oesophagus, diarrhoea and vomiting, it is usually the diffuse pulmonary fibrosis produced by the excess of free radicals that causes death. As well as free radicals the **proteases**, particularly elastase and trypsin, released by phagocytes in their normal defensive roles have to be neutralized or removed after they have carried out their function or they will attack the lung itself. Any of these substances caught up in the mucus of the mucociliary escalator will be carried out of the lung. In addition, their activity is terminated by conjugation with α_1-**antitrypsin** in the plasma. The importance of this mechanism is demonstrated by the high incidence and severity of pulmonary emphysema in people who lack antitrypsin because of a genetic deficiency.

Metabolism of circulating biologically active substances

As they are in series with the systemic circulation and receive the whole of cardiac output, the lungs are ideally situated to rapidly control levels of substances circulating in the blood. This they do by utilizing the enormous surface area of endothelium (100 m^2) to remove or degrade substances whose effects need to be rapidly terminated once they have carried out their function:

- Noradrenaline (norepinephrine)
- ATP, ADP, AMP
- Bradykinin
- 5HT
- Leukotrienes
- PGE_1, PGE_2, $PGF_{2\alpha}$.

Substances which are more generally active and sustained in their actions pass through the pulmonary circulation unchanged, and include:

- Adrenaline (epinephrine)
- Angiotensin II
- Dopamine
- Histamine
- Isoprenaline
- PGI_2, PGA_2.

Of particular interest, as the only example of activation of a bloodborne substance by the lung is the transformation of angiotensin I in the plasma to the powerful vasoconstrictor substance angiotensin II by **angiotension-converting enzyme** (ACE). Although this is not restricted to the lung, being found in plasma and endothelium, pulmonary vasculature does seem to be most plentifully supplied with this enzyme and 80% of plasma angiotensin I is converted in a single pass though the lungs. ACE is also responsible for the removal of bradykinin by the lung. The lung endothelium is also responsible for a tonic production of NO.

The vasoactive and bronchoactive **leukotrienes** and **prostaglandins**, which are released into the circulation under certain conditions, are metabolized from arachadonic acid by the pulmonary capillary endothelium.

As well as modifying the blood the lung also produces **mucopolysaccharides** as part of the production of bronchial mucus and secretes **immunoglobulins** (Ig) into the airways to defend against infection.

The production of **surfactant** by type II pneumocytes is discussed on p. 39.

Non-respiratory functions

Filtration

The blood filtering function of the lungs, protecting the vulnerable cerebral and coronary circulations, is frequently and justifiably mentioned. However, the capillary diameter of the pulmonary circulation (about 7 μm) can not be regarded as the overall pore size of the filter. Many studies have shown that particles up to 400 μm diameter can pass through the pulmonary circulation. The effective filter size depends, in part, on the level of exercise the subject is undertaking, and may be affected by normally closed arteries opening to 'shunt' blood across the lungs. The particles filtered by the lungs include agglutinated white and red blood cells, fat droplets, and droplets of amniotic fluid during pregnancy. Tumour cells may lodge and grow in the lungs, but it is blood clots from the systemic circulation that form the major filtered load and interfere with the fluidity of the blood.

Blood fluidity

As well as trapping blood clots the lung contributes to blood fluidity by being the richest source of factors that promote (thromboplastin) or inhibit (heparin) clotting. The balance between their effects maintains the fluidity of the blood. Any blood clots already formed are broken down by the proteolytic enzyme **plasmin**, activated from its inactive precursor in the plasma by factors found in large quantities in pulmonary endothelium.

Blood capacity

Pulmonary blood volume is about 500 mL in a recumbent man. This volume can be halved by increases in pressure within the chest, such as forced expiration against a closed larynx. On the other hand, the volume of blood in the chest can be doubled by a forced inspiration. This phenomenon allows the pulmonary circulation to act as a reservoir, for example at the start of exercise, when the output of the left ventricle rapidly increases. Activity of the sympathetic nervous system may influence the capacity of the system by triggering contraction of smooth muscle in the blood vessel walls.

Cooling

The high latent **heat of vaporization** of water makes its evaporation from the respiratory surface a useful mechanism for cooling in small furry animals. This mechanism is less evident in humans, perhaps because we use evaporation from our particularly hairless skin. However, a residue of this mechanism can be seen if you stay too long in a very hot bath, or if you have a fever – you will notice you begin reflexly to breathe through your mouth.

Behaviour

Breathing is unique among the major functions of the body in that it is both voluntarily and involuntarily controlled. For example, our hearts and kidneys pump and filter our blood without our being aware of it. We cannot, however, consciously control the rate at which they work. Breathing goes on unconsciously for most of the time (except for those unfortunate individuals suffering from Ondin's Curse, see p. 148), but in an instant we can take control of our breathing, for example to allow us to speak.

Our respiratory muscles help other systems of the body in many non-respiratory ways. When lifting a heavy weight our breathing stops, the muscles of the chest contract and it forms a rigid cage against which the muscles of the arms can act.

The diaphragm and abdominal muscles contract simultaneously to raise intra-abdominal pressure during vomiting, defecation and childbirth. Conversely,

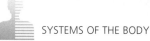
inspiration is switched off while you swallow food or drinks, to prevent their inhalation (have you noticed that each swallow is followed by an expiration?).

Changes in patterns of breathing can signal emotion, amicable or otherwise, and above all we use our respiratory system to power speech and vocalization.

Further reading

Horsfield K. Morphometry of the lungs. In: Macklem PT, Mead J, eds. Handbook of physiology. Section 3, The respiratory system. Vol III Mechanics of breathing, Part I, p. 75. Bethesda, MD: American Physiological Society, 1986

Murray JF. The normal lung, 2nd edn. Philadelphia: WB Saunders, 1986

Silverman ES, Gerritsen ME, Collins T. Metabolic function of the pulmonary endothelium. In: Crystal RG, West JB, Barnes PJ, Weibel ER, eds. The lung: scientific foundations, 2nd edn. New York: Raven Press, 1997

Weibel ER. Morphometry of the human lung. New York: Academic Press, 1963

Weibel ER. Design and morphometry of the pulmonary gas exchanger. In: Crystal RG, West JB, Barnes PJ, Weibel ER, eds. The lung: scientific foundations, 2nd edn. New York: Raven Press, 1997

Young B, Heath JW 2000 Wheater's Functional Histology: a text and colour atlas. Churchill Livingstone, Edinburgh

Self-assessment case study

A 30-year-old man is having lunch with his wife in a café. Suddenly the man starts choking. He stands up but is unable to breathe. He clutches his chest and starts to become cyanosed.

Fortunately, his wife is skilled in first aid. She strikes her husband five times, firmly between the shoulder blades. This causes the food to become dislodged, and happily her husband survives the ordeal.

From your knowledge of the structure of the respiratory tract you should be able to attempt the following questions:

① Why is food usually swallowed instead of being inhaled?

② Why does choking sometimes occur?

③ During choking, where in the respiratory tract would you expect the foreign body to lodge?

④ Why did the man in this case become cyanosed?

⑤ How did striking the man's back cause the foreign body to be dislodged?

⑥ Do you know another name for the syndrome of choking, based on the location where it often occurs and the appearance that the victim frequently has?

Answers see page 174

Self-assessment questions

① What are the three mechanisms by which particles are deposited in the lung, and to what size particles do they apply?

② What resistance to breathing resides in the nose, compared to the mouth and the total resistance of the respiratory system?

③ How does the diameter and number of airways at each level of the bronchial tree change as you move into the lung? What effect does this have on the velocity of the airflow?

④ Define the Reid Index and give its normal value.

⑤ What are the two circulations of the lungs, and what are their functions?

Answers see page 174

ELASTIC PROPERTIES OF THE RESPIRATORY SYSTEM

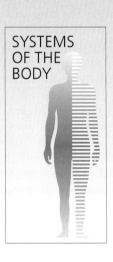

SYSTEMS
OF THE
BODY

Chapter objectives

After studying this chapter you should be able to:

① Define compliance and hysteresis.

② Describe why compliance changes in restrictive lung disease.

③ Explain why lung compliance is increased by filling the lungs with water.

④ Understand the relationship between diameter and pressure in bubbles.

⑤ Explain the problems that might arise because of different sizes of alveoli in the lungs and the development of atelectasis.

⑥ Explain the significance of the properties of the liquid lining of the lungs and their disturbance in prematurity.

⑦ Describe how the interaction between the lungs and chest wall produces negative intrapleural pressure.

⑧ Describe how compliance is measured.

Introduction

One of the properties of the respiratory system most often changed by disease is the ease with which it can be expanded and contracted in breathing.

The lungs and the chest wall that surrounds them are **elastic** structures, that is, they return to their original shape if a force that is distorting them is removed. The lungs have no muscles capable of changing their shape. The chest, on the other hand, is well supplied with internal and external intercostal muscles which can change its shape, and is separated from the abdomen by the most important inspiratory muscle, the diaphragm. Despite being closely pressed against it the lungs are not attached to the chest wall: there is a space of a few millimetres filled with a slippery plasma-like fluid. Because of this separation we can conveniently deal with the properties of the lungs and chest wall separately, but bearing in mind that in life they work together.

We can use a simple model to describe how changes in the volume of the elastic lungs are brought about by the changes in pressure around them.

The most commonly used model of lung inflation is a toy balloon. Many of the principles that follow can be demonstrated by this model. For example, if you inflate a balloon and prevent the air escaping by blocking the neck with your finger (Fig. 3.1A), the **elastic recoil** of the balloon will be proportional to its **elastance** (1/**compliance**, see below) and will produce a **recoil pressure**. The pressure inside the balloon will be the same throughout if no flow is taking place into or out of the balloon. These observations demonstrate important principles of lung function.

An even more physiological model of the respiratory system can be made by suspending a balloon in a jar with a piston at its base, like a large syringe (Fig. 3.1B). In this case the balloon represents the lungs, the jar represents the chest wall and the piston represents the diaphragm. Lowering the piston reduces the pressure round the balloon (**intrapleural pressure**) and causes it to inhale.

Intrapleural pressure (P_{pl})

For an object to be stretched or in some other way distorted it must be subjected to a force. In the case of a three-dimensional object this force may be pressure. In our simple model of breathing (Fig. 3.1A), inspiration would be inflation of the balloon and expiration deflation. The pressure that brings about inflation in Figure 3.1A would be applied to the inside. There is a pressure gradient from inside the balloon to outside. The other, more complicated, way for us to inflate the

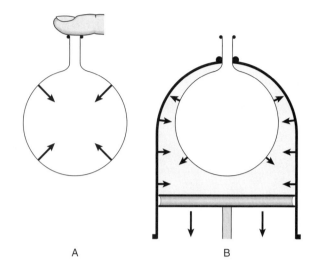

Fig. 3.1
(A) Balloon demonstrating elastic recoil. (B) Physiological model of the respiratory system.

balloon would be to reduce the pressure outside it using the jar and plunger (Fig. 3.1B): again there is a pressure gradient from inside to outside the balloon, and this is the way we inflate our lungs.

Even when we are completely relaxed, at the end of an expiration with no contraction of the respiratory muscles there is a tension in the thorax between the lungs, whose elasticity is causing them to collapse, and the chest wall whose elasticity is causing it to spring outward. These two structures are 'locked together' by the intrapleural fluid in the intrapleural space. Because it is a fluid and therefore not compressible or expandable, and the intrapleural space is airtight, the lungs are as firmly pressed to the chest wall as a suction cup attached to a window.

The tension between the lungs trying to collapse and the chest wall trying to spring out is most clearly seen in surgery, when the sternum is split to allow the surgeon to get at the heart, for example: the lungs collapse and the ribs spring out.

Another way of visualizing what is happening in the space between the lungs and chest wall is to imagine a syringe with two plungers being pulled in opposite directions (Fig. 3.2).

You can see from such a model that **intrapleural pressure** is negative with respect to atmospheric pressure. What is not immediately obvious is that intrapleural pressure is also negative with respect to air pressure within the alveoli, because the alveoli are connected to the atmosphere by a system of open tubes, the bronchial tree (Fig. 3.3).

This means a hole made between either the atmosphere or the alveoli and the intrapleural space will

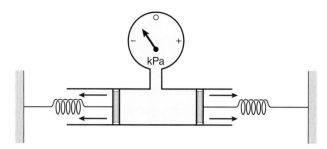

Fig. 3.2
How negative intrapleural pressure is generated.

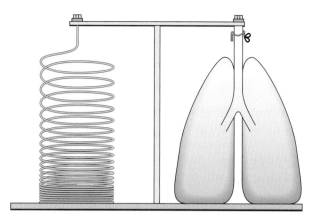

Fig. 3.4
How the lung behaves like a 'slinky'.

allow the pressure surrounding the lung to rise and the lung to collapse: this dangerous condition is called a **pneumothorax**.

Because the lungs are to some extent suspended from the trachea and rest on the diaphragm, they behave like a child's 'slinky' (a very soft spring), held at one end and supported from underneath. Gravity causes the spring or lungs to slump under their own weight (Fig. 3.4).

Because of this effect the chest behaves as if it is filled with a liquid of the average density of the lungs.

As you descend below the surface of any liquid gravity causes pressure to increase at a rate dependent on the density of the liquid. The intrapleural pressure

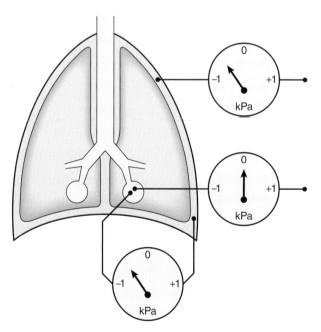

Fig. 3.3
Alveolar and intrapleural pressure compared to atmospheric pressure (100 kPa absolute) at the end of expiration. These lung pressures would become more negative during inspiration and be more negative at the apex than at the base of the lung.

therefore increases (in fact becomes less negative) as you move from the apex to the base of the lung. At the end of expiration the pressure is about –0.8 kPa at the top of the lungs and –0.2 kPa at the base. That this gradient of pressure depends on the effect of gravity on the contents of the thorax is clearly demonstrated by the fact that it reverses if the subject in which it is being measured stands on their head.

At any instant the negative pressures that surround the lung expand it to a given volume. If those pressures did not change lung volume would not change and we would not breathe. We cause our lungs to breathe by changing the negative pressure around them by making the diaphragm contract and, by acting like the plunger of a syringe, draw air into the chest.

Intrapleural pressure can be measured by inserting a hollow needle between the ribs into the intrapleural space. It is not easy to obtain volunteers to undergo this procedure, and as we are usually more interested in *changes* in intrapleural pressure than their absolute values, we frequently measure changes in pressure in the oesophagus, which forms a very flexible tube running through the thorax. Because the oesophagus is so flexible the changes of pressure within it closely follow changes in intrapleural pressure.

Static lung compliance (C$_L$)

We have seen that the lungs are elastic structures, i.e. they return to their original shape and size when distorting forces are removed. These distorting forces are usually those of intrapleural pressure, which becomes more negative to bring about inspiration and then becomes less negative, and the elasticity of the lungs leads to quiet expiration. This elasticity is a measure of how easily the lungs can be stretched and is

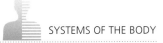

Elastic properties of the respiratory system Box 3

Respiratory distress syndrome of the newborn

Mrs Aldridge had been expecting her first child in about 12 weeks' time. Nevertheless, she had gone into labour and had given birth to a baby boy. The paediatrician examined Mrs Aldridge's son after he was born. It soon became apparent that the baby was breathing very rapidly and appeared to be having some difficulty: his chest was indrawing with each breath and he was making a grunting sound. The paediatrician made the diagnosis of respiratory distress syndrome (RDS) of the newborn.

In this chapter we will consider:

① The causes of respiratory distress syndrome of the newborn.
② Treatment and prevention of respiratory distress syndrome of the newborn.

---

conventionally expressed as **compliance**, the reciprocal of elastance. This 'stretchiness' of the lungs can be measured under static conditions, i.e. by measuring pressure and volume when there are no breathing movements taking place, or as **dynamic compliance** during breathing (see below).

The effect of disease

The compliance of the lungs is changed by most lung diseases. Such changes have a detrimental effect on lung function and increase the work of breathing. It seems that healthy lungs are at optimal compliance, and an increase or decrease from this norm is for the worse. For example, in lung fibrosis the lungs are stiffened by the laying down of collagen and fibrin bundles, so that compliance is reduced. In emphysema the parenchyma of the lungs is destroyed, there is less elastic recoil, and compliance is therefore increased. In infant respiratory distress syndrome it is the nature of the liquid lining the lungs that is at fault (see below), and this also reduces lung compliance. The origin of these changes becomes clear if we consider the two physical systems that contribute to the elasticity of the lungs and hence their compliance. One originates in the elasticity of lung tissues, the other depends on the nature of the liquid lining of the alveoli.

The physical basis of lung compliance

The elastic properties of the lungs, and hence their compliance, depends almost equally on the elastic properties of their tissues and on the elastic properties of their liquid lining.

Elastic properties of the respiratory system Box 2

Causes of RDS of the newborn

The principal cause of RDS of the newborn is a deficiency of lung surfactant related to prematurity, although the disease is also related to the general immaturity of a premature baby's respiratory system. The more premature an infant, the more likely it is to develop RDS.

The type II pneumocytes that produce surfactant develop at about 24 weeks' gestation, although most fetuses do not start producing large amounts of surfactant until about 34 weeks (babies are born, on average, at 40 weeks). Premature babies also have smaller lungs and alveoli than full-term babies. Remember the law of Laplace, which states that:

$$P = \frac{2T}{r}$$

where P is the pressure inside a bubble, T is the surface tension and r is the radius. In the alveoli of premature infants T is greater than normal because of the lack of surfactant, and r is less than normal because the premature infant has smaller alveoli. For both these reasons, a high pressure (P) is needed to keep the alveoli open. This means that the lungs tend to collapse during expiration, and the effort of inspiration is very much increased. Furthermore, the lack of surfactant means that fluid tends to be drawn from the blood into the alveoli, which therefore become oedematous. All these things mean that the dynamic compliance of the lungs is very much decreased.

Because it has not developed fully the compliance of a premature infant's chest wall is high, and this means that respiratory effort causes indrawing of the chest wall. Grunting in infants is thought to be an effort to increase airway pressure during expiration, which would tend to reduce airway collapse. Blood still flows through the collapsed areas of the lungs but remains deoxygenated. Without treatment, the baby's respiratory distress would become worse and would eventually lead to respiratory failure as the baby became increasingly exhausted and hypoxic by the effort of breathing.

The large number of collapsed alveoli lead to a characteristic chest X-ray appearance. Baby Aldridge's chest X-ray is shown in Figure 3.5. The collapsed alveoli give the chest X-ray a 'ground-glass' appearance. Against this are visible air bronchograms which are the shadows of the gas within the bronchi. These are only visible on a chest X-ray if the lung tissue around them is unusually dense.

The lungs of infants who have died from RDS have a characteristic appearance under the microscope. The alveoli are collapsed and they and the respiratory bronchioles appear to be lined with a membrane. This membrane is made up of a proteinaceous exudates from the airways and can, in fact, be caused by many types of lung injury, not only RDS. Because of its appearance with commonly used histological stains, the membrane is usually described as *hyaline*, meaning nearly transparent. For this reason, RDS is also called hyaline membrane disease.

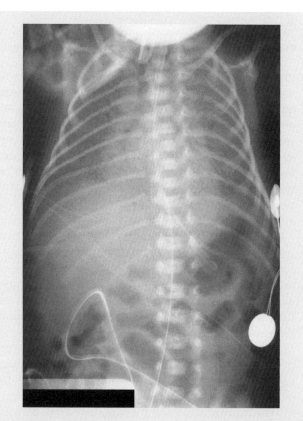

Fig. 3.5
X-ray of child with RDS. The 'ground glass' appearance of the lungs is clearly visible as is an air bronchogram. (Source: Haddad et al 2000.)

The elasticity of lung tissue

It might be reasonably assumed that the elastic properties of the lungs are due to the yellow **elastin** fibres of the lung parenchyma, the fibre type that gives most other organs their elasticity. In fact, only about half the elastic recoil of the lungs comes from the elastin fibres in the alveolar walls, bronchioles and capillaries. Also present in the lungs are collagen fibres, which are less easily stretched and limit overexpansion of the lung. The elastin fibres act in a rather complicated way to provide elasticity. The fibres are kinked and bent round each other, and during inspiration unfold and rearrange in a manner that has been likened to the straightening of the fibres of a nylon stocking when it is put on (Fig. 3.6).

In the lung disease emphysema the elastin fibres are degraded and therefore do not recoil so strongly. The lung is easier to inflate; it is more compliant.

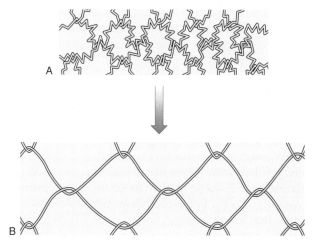

Fig. 3.6
How a nylon stocking stretches when put on.

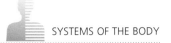
Elastic properties of the respiratory system Box 3

Treatment and prevention of RDS in the newborn

Baby Aldridge was initially given oxygen by the paediatrician. An endotracheal tube was then inserted into his trachea, he was placed on a mechanical ventilator and his lungs were ventilated artificially. Artificial surfactant was administered down the endotracheal tube in order to treat the deficiency of natural surfactant. Ventilation was continued for 1 week, during which time Baby Aldridge continued to improve. After this time, the endotracheal tube was removed and he was able to breathe for himself.

Mechanical ventilation is usually required in infants with RDS. Ventilation needs to be carried out very carefully, however. This is because of the low compliance of the infant's lungs, which means that relatively high airway pressures are needed to achieve an adequate tidal and hence minute volume. High airway pressure can cause trauma to immature lungs and airways and can cause a pneumothorax. Furthermore, high inspired oxygen concentrations (greater than 50% oxygen) can also cause lung damage. The damage is done by **oxygen free radicals**, which are toxic molecules, including the hydroxide ion and the superoxide ion, each of which has an unpaired electron, making it very reactive. High oxygen concentrations favour the produc-

tion of these molecules. The lung damage that can be caused by high airway pressure and high oxygen concentrations can lead to a chronic lung condition called **bronchopulmonary dysplasia**.

In addition to artificial ventilation of the lungs, RDS is treated with surfactant; indeed, it is common practice to administer surfactant to premature babies in order to try and prevent RDS from occurring. Both natural surfactant obtained from animal lungs and artificial surfactant containing dipalmitoyl phosphatidylcholine can be used. The administered surfactant acts in the same way as endogenous surfactant and reduces surface tension in the alveoli, stabilizing them and increasing lung compliance.

It is also possible to try and prevent RDS where a birth is expected to be premature, for example in the case of a fetus that is not growing adequately in the uterus and whose birth is to be induced. Administration of steroids to the mother increases the rate of maturation of the fetal lungs and reduces the likelihood of RDS occurring in the newborn infant.

With modern treatment survival rates in babies affected by RDS are good, particularly in older premature babies.

In the disease lung fibrosis there is an increase in the elastin and collagen of the interstitial tissues and the lung recoils more strongly, i.e. it is less compliant.

The liquid lining of the lungs

So, about half the elastic recoil of the lungs comes from the elastic properties of their tissues, just as there is recoil in an inflated rubber balloon. The remaining half of the elastic recoil of the lungs comes from their unique structure of millions of tiny bubble-like alveoli, lined with liquid and connected to the atmosphere by a series of tubes (the bronchial tree). The importance of this structure was demonstrated by von Neergaard, in 1929, when he showed that an isolated lung completely filled with water is about twice as easy to inflate as one filled with air. The cause of this change in ease of inflation lies in the removal of the air–liquid surface that lines the millions of spherical bubbles surrounded by lung tissue by filling the air space with water to form one single small air–liquid interface somewhere in the trachea (Fig. 3.7).

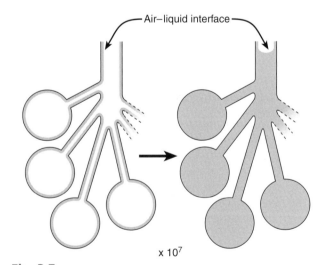

Fig. 3.7
Change in the area of the air–lung interface produced by filling the lungs with water.

To gain approximation of the change imagine an enormous bottle with a very narrow neck. When filled with air it has a large internal surface area exposed to

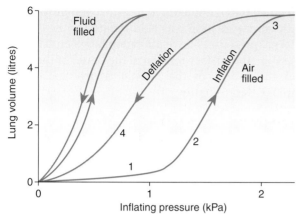

Fig. 3.8
The effect of filling a lung with water, so destroying the air–liquid interface. Pressure and volume were measured under static conditions. The air-filled lung required different pressures to hold it at a given volume, depending on whether it was being inflated or deflated (hysteresis). This effect is almost abolished by filling the lung with fluid. It is also much easier to inflate the fluid-filled lung. The air-filled lung does not begin to inflate until a 'critical opening pressure' of about 1 kPa is reached. At this pressure, alveoli begin to pop open.

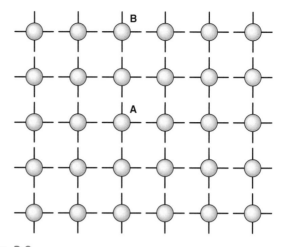

Fig. 3.9
How a surface arises in a liquid. Molecules of a liquid attract each other. The molecule at A is attracted on all sides and so is in a balanced situation. Molecule B, at the surface, has no molecules above it and is in tension with those on either side.

the air; when filled with water right up to its neck this surface area is greatly reduced. To complicate matters, the internal surface of the alveoli is curved, which has a significance we will deal with later.

Not only does filling a lung with fluid make it easier to inflate, it also abolishes the **hysteresis** seen in the normal lung. Hysteresis (Greek, *hysterion*, to lag behind) means that inflation of the lung follows a different pressure/volume relationship from deflation (Fig. 3.8). It requires a greater pressure to reach a particular lung volume when you are inflating it than to hold it at that volume when you are deflating it. Something is 'propping the lung alveoli open'. These peculiar changes are due to the nature of bubbles and the properties of the liquid that makes up the liquid lining of the lung. We need to consider the nature of the surface of liquids, the nature of bubbles and the very special properties of the liquid lining of the alveoli to understand static and dynamic compliance of the lungs.

The surface of liquids

That liquids form a clear boundary between themselves and the air above them could almost be a definition of a liquid. That this boundary is under tension or stress is clearly seen in the liquids we come

across in everyday life: the surface of a cup of coffee, if touched lightly with a spoon, seems to leap up to the spoon. This is the effect of **surface tension** (Fig. 3.9).

The 'skin' or surface of a liquid exists because at the surface there is an imbalance of the forces acting on the molecules at the surface, as explained in the Appendix (p. 173).

Just as mechanical and chemical systems move to a state of minimal energy (maximum entropy), so surfaces seek minimal energy and hence minimal area (this is why water droplets are spheres, the shape that has minimal surface for a given mass). The tendency to reduce in surface area produces tension in a liquid surface which can be measured by a surface balance (Fig. 3.10). In this, a bar of metal dips into the liquid and is exposed to the same forces as act on molecules at the surface of liquids, or the coffee spoon. These forces can be measured by a sensitive transducer. The total force will depend on the surface tension and the length of the bar, and the units of surface tension are therefore N m^{-1}. The surface balance was modified to produce the *Wilhelmi Balance* by the ingenious addition of a movable barrier that can compress the surface of the liquid in the balance trough. Under these circumstances the depth of the liquid alters as the barrier is moved, but this doesn't matter as it is the air–liquid interface that is important. If pure water is placed in a Wilhelmi Balance, moving the barrier to and fro, expanding and contracting the surface, has no effect on the measured surface tension. If, however, a phospholipid of the type found lining the alveoli of the lungs is placed on the surface of the liquid it spreads out to form a layer between water and air, and the

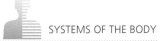

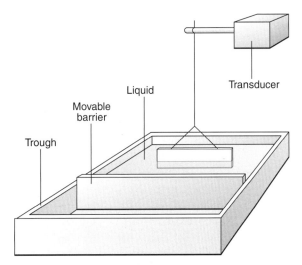

Fig. 3.10
The Wilhelmi Balance for measuring surface tension in a liquid while changing its surface area. The movable barrier compresses or expands the surface film. The tension in the surface is measured by the pull on the vertical plate suspended in the liquid.

surface tension changes as the barrier advances, forcing the phospholipid molecules closer together, or retreats allowing them to separate. The tension reaches a minimum when all the phospholipid molecules are neatly packed as a single layer on the surface. When the surface area is reduced further the molecules pile up on each other and the tension begins to rise again. It is possible to measure the size of the molecules of the phospholipid from the area of the surface at which the surface tension is minimal.

The nature of bubbles

Anyone who has indulged in the congenial occupation of blowing soap bubbles using a child's pipe or wire loop will have demonstrated most of the basic physical principles underlying elastic recoil of the lung due to its liquid lining.

They will have noticed that once a complete sphere has formed the bubble is stable. While there is a hole in the bubble, however, through the pipe or wire loop, if you stop blowing the bubble immediately collapses, returning to a flat layer of soap stretched across the pipe or loop. The molecular basis of this effect is explained in the Appendix (p. 170).

The same forces that produce this collapse are at work in the liquid lining the alveoli of the lung. The fact that the outer surface of the 'bubble' is in contact with lung tissue does not alter the tendency of this bubble to collapse, driving air out through the 'hole' which is its connection with the bronchial tree.

The stable, completely spherical, bubble you blew with your wire loop was held inflated by an excess of internal pressure. The relationship between this excess pressure, the surface tension of the liquid of the bubble and the radius of the bubble is described by the **Laplace Relationship**

$$P = \frac{4T}{R}$$

where P is the excess pressure (Pa), T is the surface tension (N m^{-1}) of the liquid making up the bubble, and R is the radius (m) of the bubble. The constant 4 appears in this equation because a bubble has two surfaces exposed to the air. For alveoli whose outer surface is in contact with the lung tissue it becomes:

$$P = \frac{2T}{R}.$$

Human alveoli are about 0.1 mm in diameter; if they were lined with **interstitial fluid** the pressure required to hold them open (the excess pressure inside them above the surrounding intrapleural pressure) would be 3 kPa. This is more than twice the pressure found in normal individuals. The liquid lining of the lungs must therefore be very different from interstitial fluid, with a significantly lower surface tension.

The nature of the liquid lining of alveoli

From the Laplace Relationship we can see, somewhat surprisingly, that the pressure in a small bubble can be expected to be greater than the pressure in a large one. This might lead us to anticipate problems in the lungs, as there exists a whole variety of sizes of alveoli, those at the top being larger than those at the bottom (see Chapter 5). Under these circumstances an unstable situation might be expected to arise, with small alveoli (containing higher pressure) emptying into large ones (containing lower pressure) (Fig. 3.11A). The nature of the liquid lining of the lungs provides an ingenious solution to this problem.

The liquid lining of the lungs can be extracted by washing them out with saline (bronchial lavage). The washed-out liquid can then be investigated in a Wilhelmi Balance, where it shows some interesting and useful properties. Adding the extract to water in the balance reduces the surface tension from 70 to 40×10^{-3} N m^{-1}. Surface tension falls even further when the surface is compressed, reaching a minimum below 10×10^{-2} N m^{-1} This effect is due to **surfactant** secreted by type II cells of the alveolar epithelium (Fig. 3.12).

The surfactant spreads over the inner surface of the alveoli and into the bronchioles. It is made up of dipalmitoyl phosphatidylcholine: the structure of this and the way it arranges itself at an air–liquid interface is shown in Figure 3.13.

A

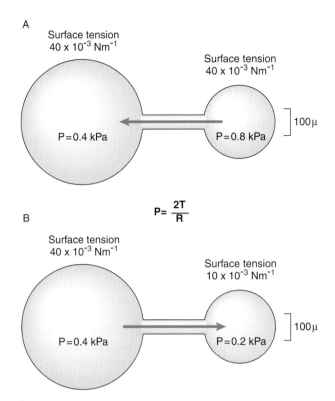

$$P = \frac{2T}{R}$$

Fig. 3.11
How the special properties of lung surfactant cope with the potential problem of differences in pressure arising in alveoli of different diameters.
(A) Two bubbles (alveoli) of different size but having the same surface tension are connected and the smaller empties into the larger. (B) The sort of change produced by inflation and deflation of the lung on the surface tension of its liquid lining. The change in tension compensates for the change in radius, and may even overcompensate and cause large alveoli to empty into small ones

The straight structure of these molecules enables them to pack more closely during expiration than would other shapes. This packing and unpacking during inspiration and expiration causes surface tension to decrease and increase in a manner that produces the characteristic hysteresis of the lungs. The change in surface tension also provides the solution to the problem posed earlier of the alveoli of different sizes containing different pressures, and the tendency for the small to empty into the large (Fig. 3.11A). If the surface tension in the large alveolus is sufficiently greater than the tension in the small the effect of the larger radius (R) in the Laplace Relationship

$$P = \frac{2T}{R}$$

will be matched or even overpowered by changes in tension (T).

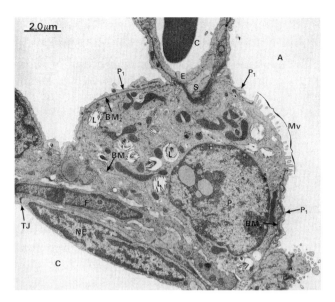

Fig. 3.12
Electron micrograph of an alveolar Type II pneumocyte (P_2). Most of the cell is surrounded by basement membrane (BM_2) and it is possible that surfactant from the lamellar bodies (L) is only secreted via the microvilli (Mv) into the alveolar space (A). P_1, type I pneumocyte; C, capillary; TJ, tight junction.

And this is what happens in the lung. The surface tension changes to match the radius, so that all alveoli contain about the same air pressure and the small do not tend to empty into the large (Fig. 3.11B).

The air pressure inside an alveolus not only resists the effects of surface tension causing the alveolus to collapse, but also resists exudation of fluid from pulmonary capillaries into the alveolar space. If surface tension is reduced at any particular air pressure within an alveolus more of that air pressure will be available to resist exudation and prevent pulmonary oedema.

The presence of surfactant is clearly important to normal lung function. It:

• reduces surface tension and therefore elastic recoil, making breathing easier
• reduces the tendency to pulmonary oedema

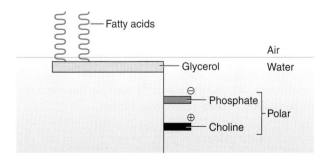

Fig. 3.13
The molecular structure of phosphatidylcholine, and the way it orientates itself at an air–water interface.

- equalizes pressure in large and small alveoli
- produces hysteresis, which 'props' alveoli open.

This important substance appears rather late in human embryological development, at about 30 weeks, and fetuses above that age which are not producing surfactant are stimulated to do so by the administration of corticosteroids.

The opening and closing of alveoli

Even in an isolated lung the relationship between pressure and volume is complicated by the interaction of the surface-active forces already dealt with and the elastic tissue of the lung. One of the most important aspects of this is the tendency for alveoli to close at low lung volumes despite the assistance from surfactant to stay open.

Range 1 of Figure 3.8 is the result of alveoli staying shut despite increased inflation pressure.

Range 2 begins at about 1 kPa, when alveoli begin to pop open and the lung inflates with very little increase in pressure.

Range 3 is where tissue elasticity, particularly from collagen fibres, stiffens the lung.

Range 4 is deflation, where hysteresis of surfactant 'props open' the alveoli.

Because of the pressure of overlying tissue the alveoli in the lower parts of the lung are always smaller than those at the top (except at total lung capacity), and therefore show a greater tendency to collapse. The lung volume at which the airways in the lower part of the lung begin to close (Range 1) is known as **closing volume**. This has considerable significance in life, as regions of the lung closed off from the atmosphere are functionally useless. In young people closing volume is less than functional residual capacity (FRC) and all is well, but by the average age of 66 closing volume equals FRC, with the unfortunate consequence of increased airway closure and reduced ventilation of the lower lung.

Static compliance

In respiratory physiology compliance is defined as the change in volume produced by a change in pressure across the wall of the structure being investigated: the lungs alone, the lungs and chest wall, or the chest wall alone (which is very rarely measured).

$$\text{Compliance} = \frac{\text{Change in volume}}{\text{Change in pressure}}$$

For the lungs alone, in life at least, the appropriate pressure measurement is from the alveoli to the intrapleural space. Change in volume can easily be measured using a spirometer, and as we are interested in measuring *change in pressure* we can use the change in pressure in the oesophagus within the chest as an indication of the change in pressure of the intrapleural space, which is difficult to measure in subjects or patients. Intraoesophagal pressure is usually measured by introducing a small air-filled balloon attached to a pressure transducer by a catheter into the oesophagus via the nose. Because intrapleural pressure varies with the position in the chest it is usual to standardize the position of measurement by pushing the balloon in 30–35 cm from the tip of the nose.

Measurement of total compliance (lungs + chest wall) is much easier because in this case the appropriate pressure measurement is from alveoli (or mouth pressure under static conditions) to atmosphere.

Neither pressure nor volume has the dimensions of time, and therefore these measurements can be made under static conditions where the subject breathes in slightly, relaxes his respiratory muscles while measuring mouth pressure with a transducer; he then breathes in a known volume and again relaxes against the transducer. The slope of the pressure–volume graph so formed is his total static compliance (Fig. 3.14).

The slope of the line that makes up the loop in Figure 3.15 is the compliance of the lungs, which in this case have been taken out of the body. This loop

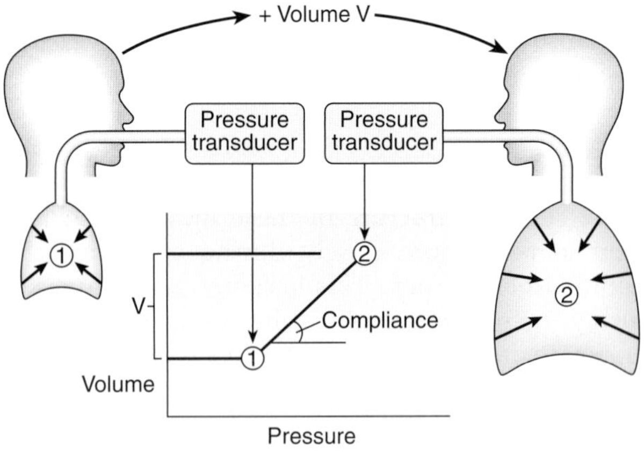

Fig. 3.14
Measuring total static compliance using only a spirometer and a pressure transducer.
The subject breathes in slightly and relaxes his respiratory system while holding a pressure transducer in his mouth. He breathes in a further known volume, holds it in his lungs, and again relaxes against the transducer. This provides a measure of increased lung recoil pressure for a known increase in volume.

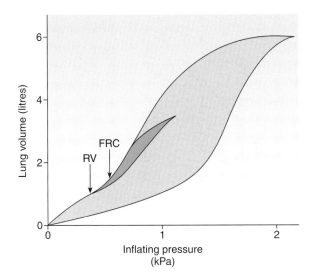

Fig. 3.15

The pressure–volume relationship of an excised lung (large loop) compared with that of quiet breathing in the intact situation (shaded small loop). In the intact situation the lungs start from a partially inflated state at FRC and there is little hysteresis. These curves were obtained under static conditions.

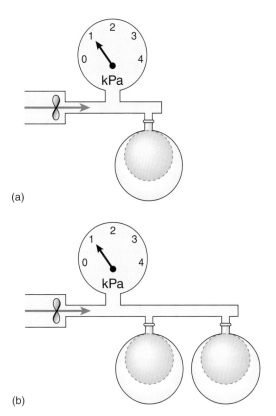

Fig. 3.16

The nature of specific compliance.

The pump with an unlimited supply of air but delivering a fixed pressure will inflate (a) one or (b) any number of identical balloons, each to the same volume. The compliance (change in volume/change in pressure) of these two systems is very different.

describes the condition of the lungs from total collapse to maximum volume.

In normal breathing there are about 3.0 L of air left in the lungs at the end of expiration (FRC), and we seldom inhale to total lung capacity (TLC). Most quiet breathing takes place within the shaded area of Figure 3.15, which shows less hysteresis than the total collapse to total volume manoeuvre, but still shows that compliance reduces due to airway collapse when residual volume (RV) is approached.

The lung compliance of an average healthy young male is about 2 L kPa^{-1}. That of a female is slightly greater, even taking into account the fact that lung compliance depends on lung size, and therefore body size. This effect is taken into account by measuring **specific lung compliance** (sC$_L$), which is compliance divided by maximal lung volume.

The nature of specific compliance can be visualized if you consider the inflation of one or more balloons by a pump that provides as much air as you like, but only to a maximum pressure of 1 kPa above atmospheric.

If you connect a single balloon to the pump and it inflates 2 L the balloon has a compliance (volume increase/pressure) of 2 L kPa^{-1} (Fig. 3.16a).

If two balloons are connected to the pump they will both be subjected to a pressure of 1 kPa and increase in volume by 2 L each (4 litres in all), which gives the system a compliance (volume increase/pressure) of 4 1 kPa^{-1} (Fig. 3.16b).

Dynamic compliance

The 'static conditions' referred to above and in Figure 3.14 consist of the lung neither inhaling or exhaling while pressure is being measured. These no-flow conditions only occur at two points during normal breathing: at the peak of inspiration and at the trough of expiration (Fig. 3.17).

This fact can be used to measure compliance while the subject is breathing – **dynamic compliance** – by measuring intrapleural pressure and lung volume at the same time (Fig. 3.17a). Alternatively, these two variables can be displayed as a loop (Fig. 3.17b), and in this case the angle of the long axis of the loop (volume/pressure) represents dynamic compliance. In this case the area of the loop represents the **work of breathing**.

In healthy lungs the ratio between dynamic compliance and static compliance is fairly constant at all frequencies of breathing. In obstructive lung diseases such as asthma the obstructed areas of the lung do not

ELASTIC PROPERTIES OF THE RESPIRATORY SYSTEM

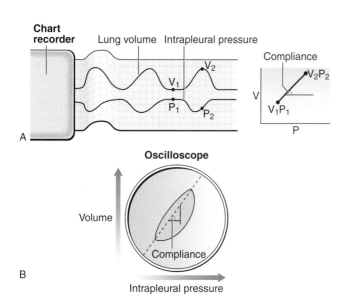

Fig. 3.17
Dynamic compliance.
As with static compliance we need to measure distending pressure and lung volume. The distending pressure is intrapleural pressure, and if this is displayed on a chart together with lung volume, points of zero flow can be detected at the peak of inspiration or the end of expiration (A). Compliance is worked out from these two states by the same method as with static compliance. Alternatively, intrapleural pressure (measured directly or using a balloon in the oesophagus) can be plotted against lung volume on what is known as a persistence oscilloscope; this draws a loop, the slope of which is proportional to compliance (B).

have sufficient time to fill or empty, a condition which worsens at high frequencies of breathing, resulting in a fall in the ratio as breathing frequency increases.

The thoracic cage

The term chest wall compliance (C_W) is frequently used to describe what should be called thoracic cage compliance, because the diaphragm and the abdominal contents pressing on it represent an important element of this component of respiratory mechanics which, unlike the lungs, contains no element of surface tension.

At the end of expiration the lungs do not collapse totally because the thoracic cage is holding them out in a slightly expanded condition. This means that the thorax is slightly pulled in. Because of this the elasticity of the thorax initially helps inspiration. The thorax reaches its neutral position at about two-thirds vital capacity, and after that the direction of its elastic forces is in favour of expiration (Fig. 3.18).

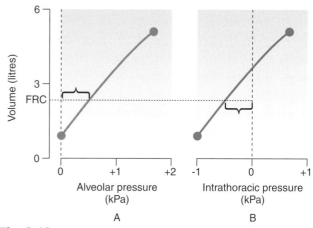

Fig. 3.18
The pressure–volume relationships of (A) excised lungs and (B) an empty thorax.
At FRC (functional residual capacity) the recoil pressures of both these structures are of the same magnitude but of opposite signs. Also, the slopes of these lines are about the same, showing that the lungs and chest wall have about the same compliance.

Perhaps surprisingly, considering their very different structures, the compliance of the thoracic cage is about the same as that of the lungs (2 litres kPa^{-1}). This truly elastic measurement is very difficult to make as it can only be properly measured when the respiratory muscles are totally relaxed – a very difficult thing for the conscious subject to do and best obtained in the anaesthetized patient.

Just like in the lungs, thoracic cage compliance is influenced by disease, and perhaps even more than the lungs by posture and position. Ossification of the costal cartilages, and scars resulting from burns of the chest, reduce compliance. The diaphragm passively transmits intra-abdominal pressure from obesity, venous congestion and pregnancy, and by this mechanism can reduce the static compliance of the total respiratory system by up to 60% as a result of changes in posture and changes from the supine to the prone position.

Total compliance (C_{tot})

Because the lungs fit inside the thorax, rather like the innertube inside a tyre, they must be treated as elements **in parallel** rather than in series when their properties are added together (Fig 3.19).

We can see that the pressure gradient for both the lungs and chest wall is from the intrapleural space to the atmosphere (or very nearly atmosphere, in the case of the lung alveoli). They are therefore in parallel with each other in terms of pressure gradients. In adding

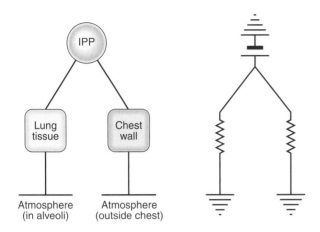

Fig. 3.19
How the lungs and chest wall behave like electrical components in parallel when summed together.

lung and chest wall compliance to give total compliance we must therefore use the relationship appropriate for parallel structures:

$$\frac{1}{C_{tot}} = \frac{1}{C_L} + \frac{1}{C_W}$$

Because the compliance of the lungs and that of the chest wall are about the same ($2 L kPa^{-1}$), an artificial ventilator needs to apply twice the normal change in intrapleural pressure to the air in the lungs of a paralysed patient to produce the normal volume change.

Factors affecting lung compliance

- *Lung size* The principles of calculating specific compliance (see above) tell us that although a man has a greater compliance than a mouse, this is due to the difference in the amount of lung being inflated.

The lung volume at which compliance is measured is a different effect from that of the amount of lung present, and also exerts an effect.

- *Recent pattern of breathing* Compliance is affected by breath-holding and recent pattern of breathing, probably owing to redistribution of air in the lungs, closing and opening of alveoli, stress relaxation and changes in circulation.
- *Age* Because a large part of lung compliance is due to a surface tension effect that does not age, there is little effect of healthy ageing on compliance.
- *Posture* The changes in lung compliance seen with posture are probably due to the effect of posture on lung volume.
- *Disease* Most diseases of the lung – congestion, fibrosis, consolidation, respiratory distress syndrome – decrease its compliance. Emphysema is unique in that static compliance is increased owing to the loss of lung tissue. Even in emphysema, however, dynamic compliance is decreased because of the disordered distribution of ventilation.

In asthma there is no change in compliance: the pressure–volume relationship of the lungs is moved bodily upward without any change in slope.

Further reading

Bangham AD. Lung surfactant: how it does and does not work. Lung 1987;165:17

Cotes JE. Lung function: assessment and application in medicine, 5th edn. Oxford: Blackwell Science, 1993

Haddad DF, Greene SA, Olver RE Core paediatrics and child health. Edinburgh: Churchill Livingstone, 2000

Macklem PT. Respiratory mechanics. Annual Reviews in Physiology 1978;40:157

Rahn H, Otis AB, Chadwick LE, Fenn WO. The pressure/volume diagram of the thorax and lung. American Journal of Physiology 1946; 146:161–178

De Troyer A. The respiratory muscles. In: Crystal RG, West JB, Barnes PJ, Weibel ER, eds. The lung: scientific foundations, 2nd edn. New York: Raven Press, 1997

Self-assessment case study

A 26-year-old man is in an intensive care unit being treated on a mechanical ventilator for acute respiratory distress syndrome (ARDS). This is a different condition from the infant respiratory distress syndrome that we have already looked at in this chapter, but the two conditions share a number of features.

ARDS is characterized by inflammation of both lungs that results in a failure of gas exchange and a reduction in lung compliance. It is a rare complication of a number of disparate conditions, including pneumonia, lung trauma and sepsis.

In order to ventilate this patient's lungs, his ventilator needs to deliver airway pressures that are much higher than normal. To ventilate the lungs of a healthy patient typically requires airway pressures in the order of 20 cmH$_2$O. The ventilator in this case was set to a maximum of 40 cmH$_2$O and it frequently occurred that this maximum pressure was reached. The high airway pressure was required because of the low compliance of the patient's lungs and was causing a great deal of concern to his doctors.

From your knowledge of lung compliance you should be able to attempt the following questions:

① What do you understand by the term 'low compliance'?

② Why is the pressure needed to inflate the patient's lungs higher than normal?

③ Why do you think there is a maximum pressure set on the ventilator?

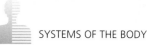
④ What effect do you think a low compliance will have on the tidal volume that a ventilator can deliver?

⑤ What effect will this have on gas exchange?

Answers see page 175

Self-assessment questions

① Describe the origins and nature of intrapleural pressure.

② Define lung compliance.

③ What is the origin and function of pulmonary surfactant?

④ To what and in what proportion is the elastic recoil of the lungs due?

⑤ A patient has one of his lungs removed. Assuming both lungs were the same volume and of the same mechanical properties, what would happen to his measured compliance? How does the concept of specific compliance address this problem?

Answers see page 175

AIRFLOW IN THE RESPIRATORY SYSTEM

4

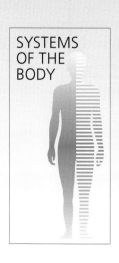

SYSTEMS
OF THE
BODY

Chapter objectives

After studying this chapter you should be able to:

① Define airway resistance.

② State the relationship between airway radius and airway resistance.

③ Describe the distribution of airway resistance throughout the respiratory tract.

④ Explain why airway resistance is a dynamic property.

⑤ Outline the physiological factors that determine airway resistance.

⑥ List factors influencing bronchial smooth muscle tone and their implications in asthma.

⑦ Relate the concept of an equal pressure point to the collapse of airways, particularly in emphysema.

⑧ Explain how pattern of breathing relates to work of breathing.

⑨ Differentiate between reversible and non-reversible obstructive disease.

⑩ Explain the basis of clinical tests to differentiate between these diseases.

AIRFLOW IN THE RESPIRATORY SYSTEM

Introduction

The lungs of mammals are structures which have evolved as part of the process of taking our delicate respiratory surface within the protection of our bodies. They are blind-ended structures with only one entrance or exit, the trachea.

This means that air must be moved into the lungs and then removed when the exchange of gas between air and blood is complete. Some of the most important diseases that interfere with this movement of air through the airways are known as **chronic obstructive pulmonary diseases (COPD)**. There are a variety of these diseases, which make up one of the major causes of morbidity and mortality in the industrialized world.

Although many patients present with a combination of more than one type of disease, making diagnosis difficult, obstruction of the airways, (other than by foreign bodies or neoplasms) can be generally attributed to:

- blocking of the airway by secretions, e.g. in bronchitis
- reduction in airways diameter due to contraction of smooth muscle in its walls or swelling due to inflammation, e.g. in asthma and bronchitis
- collapse of the airways due to disruption of the supporting parenchyma, e.g. in emphysema, or changes in intrapleural pressure, as in cough.

We saw in the previous chapter that negative intrapleural pressure holds the lungs 'stretched' against the chest wall. The degree of stretch, and hence lung volume, depends on the compliance of the lungs and the intrapleural pressure. If intrapleural pressure remained constant the lungs would remain at constant volume and breathing would not take place. To breathe we alter intrapleural pressure, making it more negative to bring about inspiration and allowing it to become less negative to allow expiration to take place.

During the dynamic process of breathing intrapleural pressure is to all intents and purposes made up of two parts, the part required to hold the lungs open (the static component) *plus* a component to move the air into or out of the lungs. The latter overcomes **airways resistance** to flow. Pressure to overcome the viscosity of the tissues is only a small part (less than 20%) of the total, and the inertia of the system need not be considered unless the system is moving very violently, as in sneezing or coughing.

How airflow is brought about

Our model from the previous chapter, which represents the respiratory system as a balloon inside a container like a syringe, is often used to illustrate the two components of intrapleural pressure mentioned above and illustrated in Figure 4.1. The plunger of the syringe represents the diaphragm, the walls of the syringe represent the chest wall, the balloon represents the alveoli, and the narrow tube represents the airways of the lung.

It is obvious that to hold the balloon inflated requires a certain effort; to draw air into the balloon (inspiration) requires more effort.

There are three further things that are not so obvious which can be deduced from this excellent model of breathing, and they all have clinical relevance:

1. The changes in **intrapleural pressure** that bring about breathing can be superimposed on a small lung volume (the balloon being only slightly inflated) or on a large lung volume (the balloon very inflated). Understandably, to hold the balloon at a large volume requires greater effort, and this is what happens, for example, in asthma, where the patient breathes at an increased lung volume to keep his airways open.

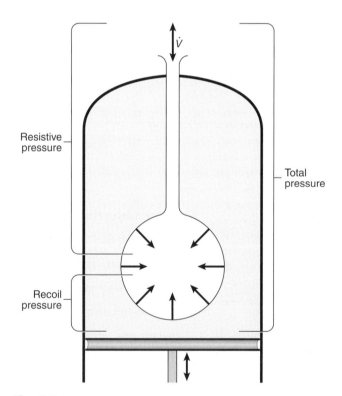

Fig. 4.1

A balloon inside a syringe is a good model of the human lungs and chest wall. To hold the 'lungs' stationary requires a certain negative pressure inside the syringe; to hold them at a larger volume requires a more negative pressure. These changes in intrapleural pressure bring about breathing, and are themselves brought about by movement of the diaphragm.

2. Airflow only takes place from a region of high pressure to a region of low pressure *along* the airway. Therefore, at two times in each respiratory cycle (when inspiration has just ceased and is about to become expiration, or when expiration has just ceased and is about to become inspiration) there is no flow, and pressure is the same all the way from the lips to the alveoli. This fact can be used to measure dynamic lung compliance (see Fig. 3.17). It should also be noted that under conditions of normal breathing the pressure in the airways is much closer to atmospheric pressure than the pressure in the intrapleural space.

3. Recoil of the lungs produces a pressure which resists inspiration but *assists* expiration. This is analogous to pushing a car up a hill: the weight of the car represents recoil pressure and resists going up (inspiration). The weight of the car would, however, assist going down (expiration). This effect of helping expiration and hindering inspiration is seen in flow/volume loops used to test lung function.

The nature of airflow

Gas flows from regions of high pressure to regions of lower pressure. This flow may be **laminar**, where the movement is orderly and streamlined, or **turbulent**, where movement is chaotic.

Flow in most, but not all, of the respiratory system can be considered laminar as a first approximation. Important exceptions include the nose, where turbulence causes inhaled particles to be thrown out of the airstream, and the larynx, where turbulence contributes to the production of sound.

Flow in a long straight smooth tube becomes turbulent when Reynolds' Number, which is calculated as 2rvd/n (r = radius of tube, v = velocity of flow, d = gas density, n = gas viscosity) exceeds 2000. Under turbulent conditions flow varies with the square root of the driving pressure, i.e. it is very much more difficult to produce the same flow when flow is turbulent (Fig. 4.2).

It is therefore important when designing breathing apparatus to avoid turbulence, which would increase the subject's work of breathing.

The major determinant of flow – radius

Laminar flow has been extensively investigated by scientists, one of whom, Poiseuille, defined the relationship between driving pressure (ΔP) and flow ($\dot{V}$) as:

$$\dot{V} = \frac{(\Delta P)\, \pi r^4}{8\eta l}$$

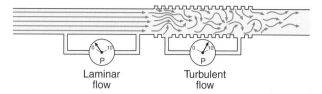

Fig. 4.2

Flow of gas in a tube, half of which is smooth and half of which is rough to produce turbulence. This demonstrates that the pressure gradient that exists when flow is turbulent is greater than when flow is laminar, although the flow in both tubes must be the same.

where r is the **radius** of the tube, η is the viscosity of the gas, and l is the length of the tube. This relationship applies to gas flow in the long straight smooth tubes under stable conditions – hardly conditions that apply to the lungs. However, it can be roughly applied to breathing, and you may notice that the most important factor affecting airflow in this equation is the radius of the tube, which is raised to the fourth power (r^4). This means that if you reduce the radius by half and keep everything else constant, the flow will be reduced to 1/16.

Laminar flow in a tube can be represented as a series of cylinders moving down the tube, with the central cylinder moving fastest. The outermost cylinder is stationary and is in fact a layer of the original gas in the tube left behind as the new gas moves forward, as shown in Figure 4.4.

These apparently esoteric considerations have important consequences in respiratory medicine. For example, adequate ventilation of the alveoli of the lungs can be achieved with a surprisingly small tidal volume, provided a high enough frequency of 'breathing' is used. This phenomenon is seen in clinical conditions when **high-frequency artificial ventilation** of the lungs is used where we want to avoid movements of the chest wall – in trauma victims with a crushed chest, for example. The patient is successfully artificially ventilated with a tidal volume less than his or her anatomical dead space (see p. 68) and frequencies up to 50 Hz. A 'spear' of fresh air in the centre of the airways penetrates deeper into the lungs than might be expected and provides adequate ventilation.

Airways resistance and obstructive pulmonary disease

We have established that it takes a greater pressure to inflate the lungs than simply to hold them in a steady inflated state. This extra pressure is required to

4

produce flow in the airways. We have also seen that the relationship between pressure and volume on slowly inflating and deflating the lungs is not a straight line, as you would get with a rubber balloon, but rather a loop, with a greater pressure needed to *inflate* the lungs to a given volume than that which exists at the same volume when they are being allowed to deflate (Fig. 4.3).

The small dotted loop in Figure 4.3 was produced by inflating and deflating the lungs extremely slowly, a situation that is called **pseudostatic**. If we were to carry out this inflation and deflation at a normal breathing rate (12 times per minute, say) the loop would be wider (the solid line), with inflation pressures required for a given volume being greater than under the static conditions and deflation pressures being less.

This situation arises because energy is used up to propel the air along the airways; the airways can be said to resist flow in a phenomenon known as **airways resistance**. This resistance during laminar flow can be

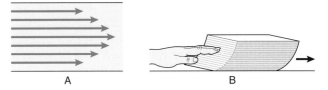

Fig. 4.4
A model of laminar flow.
Laminar flow of air in a tube (A) consist of very thin layers of air (laminae) sliding over each other, with the layer nearest the wall being stationary. It can be compared to a pile of paper on a surface being pushed along (B).

thought of as the friction between the layers of air as they are pushed down the airway. Pushing a pile of typing paper or a pack of cards across a table gives a good idea of what is happening (Fig. 4.4).

As its name implies, airways resistance is analogous to electrical resistance. To measure the electrical resistance of a length of wire you need to know two things, the potential difference (voltage) between the two ends of the wire, and the current flowing in the wire. Using reasonable currents (that do not overheat the wire) we find that the relationship between voltage (V) and current (I) is a straight line (Fig. 4.5).

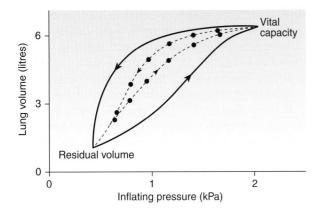

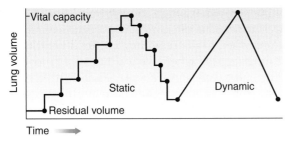

Fig. 4.3
Dynamic and pseudostatic lung inflation.
The different relationships between volume and inflating pressure in an excised lung when inflation is in a series of steps (with pressure measured under static conditions after each step), or dynamically, with air flowing continuously into or out of the lung. The pressure at any volume is greater than the static value when the lung is being inflated dynamically, and less when it is deflating dynamically.

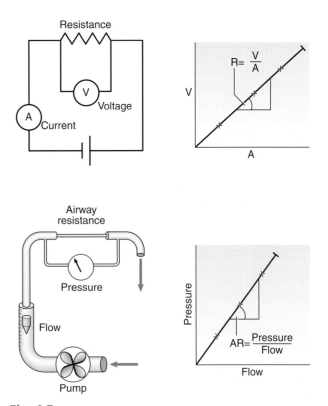

Fig. 4.5
The analogy between electrical and airway resistance, and how they are measured.

This is Ohm's Law, and the slope of the line (V/I) is the resistance of the wire in ohms.

Just as when describing the static properties of the lung we use the term compliance, rather than its reciprocal elastance, when considering airways resistance we frequently use its reciprocal, **conductance**. Airways conductance = 1/Airways resistance.

To measure the airways resistance of a tube you also need to know two things, the **driving pressure** (the difference in pressure) between the two ends of the tube, and the **airflow** of the tube. Using flows that do not produce turbulence, we find that the relationship between pressure (P) and flow ($\dot{V}$) is also a straight line, like electrical resistance.

The slope of the line is the airway resistance of the tube in kPa 1^{-1} s.

The airways resistance of an adult breathing quietly is about 0.2 kPa 1^{-1} s, which means that a normal sort of flow of 0.5 1^{-1} s is brought about by a pressure difference of 0.1 kPa between the lips and the alveoli.

Two important points arise from this apparently innocuous statement:

1. Airways resistance is a **dynamic** property and can only be measured when flow is taking place.
2. The figures used above to arrive at the figure of 0.2 kPa 1^{-1} apply equally well if flow is in an inspiratory *or* an expiratory direction: they are a property of the tube, not the direction of the flow.

The clinical situation

Airways resistance changes in disease and its measurement has been the focus of interest of doctors for many years. Measurement of airflow is not difficult and is usually accomplished using an instrument known as a **pneumotachograph**, which itself illustrates the principle of airways resistance. The pneumotachograph consists of a tube through which the subject breathes (Fig. 4.6).

The tube contains a resistance to flow. The pressure difference across the resistance is measured and is proportional to the flow.

Flow can then be instantaneously integrated (which is adding up moment by moment all the measurements of flow) to give volume.

Measurement of the driving pressure from alveoli to lips, or lips to alveoli, in a subject or patient is more difficult.

One way of getting round the problem of measuring the driving pressure is to use the fact that it is the *change* in alveolar pressure that brings about flow and stretches the lungs against recoil pressure. Consider the changes in intrapleural pressure and recoil pres-

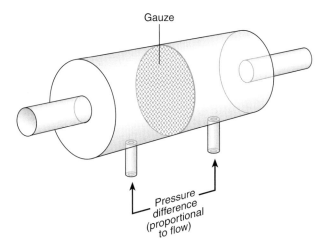

Gauze

Pressure difference (proportional to flow)

Fig. 4.6
The pneumatachograph, which is used to measure airflow, consists of a tube containing a gauze with low resistance to airflow through it. The pressure difference across the gauze can be measured and is proportional to the flow. In the direction shown $P_1 > P_2$ in reverse direction of flow $P_1 < P_2$.

sure due to the elasticity of the lungs in a single respiratory cycle (Fig. 4.7).

Subtract changes in recoil pressure from changes in intrapleural pressure and you are left with the changes in alveolar pressure that produce changes in airflow – the two variables we are interested in to measure resistance. This subtraction process can be done instantaneously electronically, and so we need to know the changes in **recoil pressure**, which can be worked out from lung compliance, and the changes in **intrapleural pressure**, which we obtain by measuring changes in the pressure inside the oesophagus passing through the intrapleural space.

Measuring pressure inside the oesophagus involves swallowing a pressure-measuring device, which initially goes down into the stomach and is then pulled back into the oesophagus. You can imagine that this is not very comfortable, and other techniques are generally used with patients.

The interrupter technique

This depends on interrupting the flow of air out of the lungs with a rapidly closing shutter in the tube through which the subject is breathing. The pressure at the lips very rapidly rises to equal alveolar pressure, and you can say that the pressure you measure at the lips is the pressure in the alveoli a fraction of a second before the shutter closes. This is the pressure that was

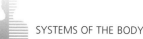
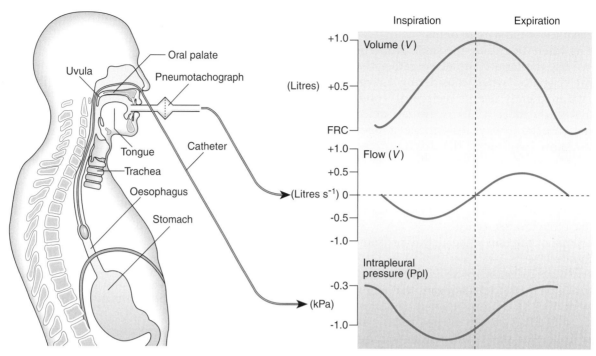

Fig. 4.7

Determination of airways resistance (Raw) by measurement of airflow and intrapleural pressure, which is measured by the rather unpleasant procedure of getting the subject to swallow a small air-filled balloon on the end of a catheter. The swallowed balloon is withdrawn from the stomach into the oesophagus, where it measures changes in pressure that match changes in intrapleural pressure.

producing flow just before the shutter closed. Using these values of pressure and flow, airways resistance is calculated.

The whole-body plethysmograph

This consists of an airtight box in which the subject sits. It depends on the principle that the total quantity of air in the box (inside the patient's lungs and around him in the box) is the same throughout the measurement – the box is airtight. The patient first pants against a closed shutter while the pressure changes in his mouth and the pressure changes in the box are measured simultaneously. The pressure changes at his mouth are assumed to be the same as those in the alveoli (by the same arguments as in the interrupter technique above). Pressure changes in the box while the patient is panting because he is compressing and decompressing the air in his lungs and therefore changing the volume of his chest in the closed box. (Consider him like the syringe in Figure 4.8: when he compresses the air in his chest he decompresses the air in the box, and when he decompresses the air in his chest he compresses the air in the box.)

The pressure changes in the box are therefore related to pressure changes in the alveoli, and so by

measuring box pressure change and flow while the patient breathes through a pneumotachograph, we can measure his airways resistance. Other uses of the whole-body plethysmograph are described in Chapter 11.

Sites of airways resistance

Total airways resistance becomes less during inspiration and greater during expiration owing to physical and reflex changes in almost all parts of the respiratory tract. Airways resistance is also not distributed uniformly along the respiratory tract: almost half the total resides in the *nose, pharynx* and *larynx*. The vocal folds of the larynx reflexly open during inspiration, reducing resistance, and come close together during expiration, forming an 'expiratory brake' preventing too-rapid collapse of the lungs. The significant resistance provided by the nose is a common experience, especially when the mucosa has become engorged because of the common cold. Even in health, where the resistance of breathing through the nose is approximately twice that of breathing through the mouth, we change to mouth breathing during exercise as a result of a reflex whose details are still not clear. An interesting point which may be raised here is that in babies the reverse

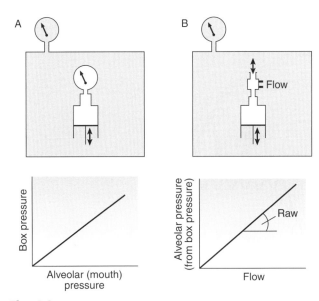

A

B

Flow

Box pressure

Alveolar (mouth)
pressure

Alveolar pressure
(from box pressure)

Raw

Flow

Fig. 4.8

Measurement of airways resistance using a whole-body plethysmograph (body box). Calibration of the relationship between the alveolar pressure and box pressure is being determined in (A), where the subject pants against a closed shutter. Because there is no airflow while the shutter is closed, changes in pressure measured at the mouth are the same as changes in pressure at the alveoli. (B) Airway resistance (Raw) is being measured while the subject breathes through a pneumotachograph which measures flow, while changes in box pressure are converted into changes in alveolar pressure.

distribution of resistance is the case, which is convenient as babies spend much of their time suckling.

Of the approximately half total airway resistance existing below the larynx 80% resides in the *trachea* and *bronchi*. This is difficult to reconcile with Poiseuilles's law (p. 170) that the airway resistance of a tube is proportional to the fourth power of its radius, as the trachea and main bronchi are the largest tubes in the bronchial tree. The explanation for this is that the number of airways doubles at each airway branching (each airway normally splits into two daughters), therefore the number (n) at each generation (g) (see p. 15) is $n = g^2$, starting with the two main bronchi as generation 1 (Fig. 4.9). This rapid increase in numbers more than offsets the decrease in diameter of the individual members of each generation, and the *total* cross-sectional area increases dramatically. The bronchi extend from generation 1 to 16, with the small bronchi (generations 5–11; 3.5–1 mm diameter) not being directly attached to the lung parenchyma. They are supported against collapse by cartilage and the transmural pressure gradient, which it is now believed

rarely reverses sufficiently to cause complete collapse of these airways.

The bronchi give rise to such an enormous number of **bronchioles** that less than 20% of the total resistance to flow resides in airways less than 2 mm diameter. For this reason a considerable number of these smaller airways must be damaged by disease before it has any effect on total airway resistance.

It is also very difficult to measure changes in their resistance, and so we are less informed about them than about the larger airways.

At the other extreme of the size range are the large airways, the trachea and main bronchi. Because these are few in number they form the narrowest part of the bronchial tree, but are well armoured against collapse by incomplete rings of **cartilage** in their walls. Even they can, however, be profoundly influenced by physiological conditions, such as cough, where positive pressure surrounding them squeezes them shut.

The most important part of the bronchial tree in terms of physiological control of airways resistance are the smaller bronchi and bronchioles. Not only do they contain virtually no supporting cartilage, but innervated **smooth muscle**, which can contract to reduce their diameter, makes up a large part of their walls. In addition, they are found at a level in the bronchial tree where the increase in number of airways has not yet exerted its effect (generations 7–14; Fig. 4.9), and therefore cross-sectional area is relatively small. If the airways resistance of each generation is compared the small bronchi are seen to have less resistance than the larger generations (Fig. 4.10). However, the important point is that the resistance of these smaller airways is *variable* (particularly in disease) and is under the influence of **bronchomotor tone**. Their content of smooth muscle and lack of support by cartilage makes these airways prone to influence by neural and hormonal factors that affect their muscle tone, and physical factors such as the pull of surrounding tissue (**radial traction**, see p. 57). Their position at a relatively narrow part of the bronchial tree makes them particularly important in terms of obstruction by inflammatory swelling or mucus.

Asthma and airways smooth muscle

Asthma affects more than 7% of the population of industrialized countries and its incidence is increasing. It can be described as a recurrent 'reversible' obstruction of the airways, an important component of which is spasm of bronchial smooth muscle. This is not the complete picture, however, because the characteristic features of asthma are bronchial hyperresponsiveness together with inflammatory changes in the airways,

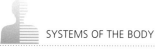
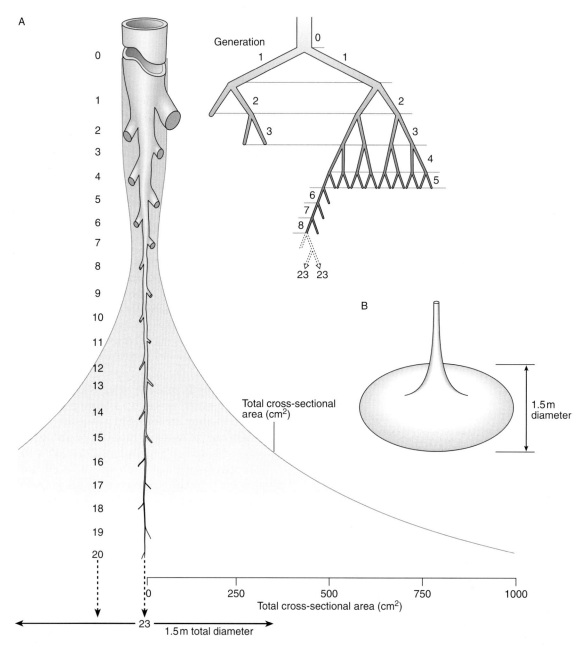

Fig. 4.9
Lung airway architecture. (A) How airway diameter and total cross-sectional area change with successive generations of the bronchial tree. (B) Change in total cross-sectional area represented three-dimensionally (from data of Weibel, 1964).

and it is becoming evident that the inflammatory changes may be causally related to the hyperresponsiveness. In all asthmatics the hyperresponsiveness of the airways extends to non-specific irritants such as cold air, smoke and exercise, which would not provoke a normal individual. Between attacks the patient frequently has no symptoms, although the inflammation persists.

A fall in FEV_1, $FEV_1/FVC\%$ and peak flow are all indicative of an asthma attack. The patient may be dyspnoeic, with breathing laboured and involving the accessory muscles of respiration. The picture the patient presents is clearly of someone labouring to breathe through a narrow tube. Any sputum produced is scant and viscid. Most asthma attacks can be divided into two phases:

- *The immediate phase* – due mainly to spasm of bronchial smooth muscle, and
- *The late phase* – an acute inflammatory reaction.

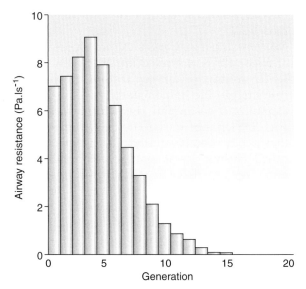

Fig 4.10
The resistance of airways making up individual generations. Note that the generations with the greatest resistance are not those made up of airways with the smallest diameter (from data of Pedley et al., 1970).

Asthma

Mr Graham is a 25-year-old man who suffers from asthma. He has had the condition since he was a boy. He finds that his asthma is brought on by domestic animals such as cats and dogs, as well as by cold or windy weather, or if he exercises too hard. However, his condition is kept under control with the inhalers that he takes. Twice a day he takes two inhaled doses of beclometasone, and he always keeps with him a salbutamol inhaler which he uses as and when he needs to, if he gets wheezy. The salbutamol inhaler nearly always relieves his asthma.

In this chapter we will consider:

① The pathaphysiology of asthma.
② What provokes an asthma attack.
③ The drug treatment of asthma.

Bronchomotor tone

The tension in the walls of the bronchi is the major determinant of their diameter. This tension is in turn determined by bronchial smooth muscle tone.

Physiological control of airways smooth muscle involves several mechanisms (Fig. 4.11).

Disordered physiological control of airway smooth muscle represents a major feature of asthma and other pathological conditions where the airways are hyperreactive. **Multiunit smooth muscle** is the motive force controlling the tension in the walls of the bronchi, and therefore in many cases their diameter. These muscle fibres are in turn controlled by:

- *Parasympathic nerves* Efferent preganglionic fibres of this most important system run in the vagus

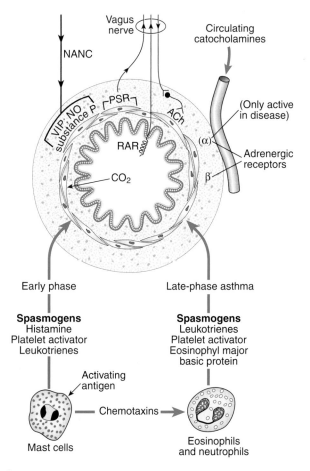

Fig. 4.11
Factors that affect bronchomotor tone. These are implicated in early- and late-phase asthma.
(NANC, non-adrenergic non-cholinergic nerve; VIP, vasoactive intestinal peptide; NO, nitric oxide; RAR, rapidly adapting pulmonary sensory receptor; PSR, slowly adapting pulmonary sensory receptor.)

Rational treatment of the condition addresses the aetiology of these phases (see Pharmacological treatment of asthma, p. 57) and must involve an understanding of the origins of bronchomotor tone.

nerve to ganglia located in the wall of the small bronchi. Postganglionic fibres release **acetyl-choline**, which stimulates muscarinic receptors on the smooth muscle fibres, causing them to contract. Atropine blocks these receptors, and injections of atropine in a normal individual can reduce airways resistance by about 30%. This limited response demonstrates that parasympathetic nerves, though important, are not the only method of broncho-motor control.

- *Sympathetic nerves* Most organs with a parasym-pathetic nerve supply also have a sympathetic input. In the case of the lungs this nerve supply does *not* extend as far as the bronchial smooth muscle. Any sympathetic effects seen in the lung are due to circulating catacholamines. The general lack of importance of nerves to lung function is demonstrated by the success of lung transplants, in which the donated lungs are completely denervated.

- *Circulating catecholamines* The membrane of airways smooth muscle carries β_2 receptors which, when stimulated by the naturally occurring catecho-lamine **adrenaline** (epinephrine), or drugs such as salbutamol, relax smooth muscle, inhibit the action of mast cells and improve mucociliary activity. They therefore form an important treatment for asthma. α-adrenergic agents only cause contraction of bronchial smooth muscle in diseased states.

- *Non-adrenergic non-cholinergic systems (NANC)* The airways are also provided with an autonomic nerve supply which is neither adrenergic nor cholinergic. The efferent fibres run in the vagus nerves and *mainly* release an inhibitory neurotransmitter which relaxes the airways. The identity of the transmitter is still open to question, although vasoactive intestinal peptide (**VIP**) and nitric oxide are strong candidates. This **NANC** inhibitory system is the main neurotransmitter-mediated relaxant system of the airways. However, bron-choconstrictor NANC mediators can also be released by this system. They included substance P and neurokinin A, which may have a role in the delayed phase of asthma.

- *Mast cell degranulation* Mast cells are plentiful in the walls of the airways. Allergens interact with IgE antibodies on their surface, causing them to undergo the process of **degranulation**, which is the rapid release (within 30 s) of preformed mediators, including histamine, heparin, serotonin, lysosomal enzymes and chemotactic factors. Prostaglandins and slow-reacting substances are synthesized and released some time later. It is now accepted that mast cell degranulation is responsible for less than 30% of the bronchoconstriction of asthma, let alone

the physiological control of bronchiolar smooth muscle.

- *Neutrophils and eosinophils* Although degranulation of mast cells is of limited importance in the *physio-logical* control of airway resistance, and its role restricted to the immediate phase of asthma, neu-trophil and eosinophil chemotactic factors are of such importance in the late (inflammatory) phase that is has been suggested that asthma should be called 'chronic desquamating eosinophilic bronchi-olitis', because of the degree of involvement of these cell types.

- *Rapidly adapting pulmonary receptors (irritant and cough receptors)* Stimulation of these receptors in the airways by inhalation of particles, chemicals, or by disease provokes contraction of airways smooth muscle by a reflex with both its arms in the **vagus nerves**. This contraction of the airways may improve the efficiency of coughing, but is not helpful in conditions of asthma.

- *Slowly adapting pulmonary receptors* These receptors also have their afferent nerves in the vagus. Their activity reduces bronchomotor tone. They are stim-ulated by stretching the lungs, so a large breath – a sigh, for example – dilates the airways both by passive stretch and by this reflex effect.

- *Carbon dioxide* This gas causes bronchodilation by direct relaxing action on the bronchial smooth muscle. In those parts of the lung that are under-ventilated carbon dioxide will build up, dilate the airways and improve ventilation locally.

The factors involved in the immediate and late phases of asthma which influence bronchomotor tone are illustrated in Figure 4.11.

Asthma and other hyperreactive airways diseases that change bronchomotor tone are said to be **reversible** – the physiological changes which are the manifestations of the disease can be reversed spon-taneously or as a result of treatment.

Pharmacological treatment of asthma

Although asthma is frequently referred to as 'reversible' obstruction of the airways, as opposed to the 'chronic' obstruction of bronchitis, acute severe asthma (status asthmaticus) may last for several days and in some cases be so irreversible as to be fatal.

The treatment of asthma may address the early (bronchoconstrictor) or late (inflammatory) phases of the disease frequently with drugs delivered directly to the airway, as droplets produced by a nebulizer. One of the many types used in hospitals in shown in Figure 4.12.

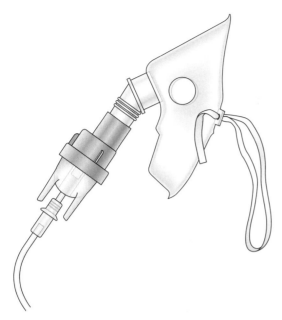

Fig. 4.12
A nebulizer. The flow of oxygen picks up droplets of the drug in the chamber of the nebulizer. Larger droplets are removed by directing the aerosol stream against a buffer. This leaves only fine droplets behind, which are able to reach the airways when inhaled from the mask.

Bronchodilators – early phase treatment

- *β₂ Adrenoreceptor agonists* – These include salbutamol and terbutaline, which are usually given as an aerosol. These drugs act directly to relax bronchial smooth muscle, and also inhibit degranulation of mast cells.
- *Xanthines* – Of these, theophylline is often the first choice of treatment for an acute attack. The mode of action of theophylline is still unclear, but may involve enzyme inhibition in bronchial smooth muscle.
- *Muscarinic receptor antagonists* – By blocking the activity of parasympathetic (vagal) nerves on the bronchial smooth muscle, drugs such as ipratropium bromide reduce any reflex component of an asthmatic attack.

Anti-inflammatories – late-phase treatment

- *Glucocorticoids* – given prophylactically as an aerosol, beclometasone, betamethasone or budesonide inhibit the late-phase response by inhibiting the generation of PAF (platelet-activating factor) and eicosanoids from mast cells, platelets, macrophages and eosinophils.

- *Sodium cromoglicate* – used prophylactically, cromoglicate appears to reduce hyperreactivity by depressing axon reflexes triggered by stimulation of rapidly adapting (irritant) receptors in the airways.
- *Histamine receptor antagonists* – H₁ antagonists such as azelastine and ketotifen are being used in mild asthma as a supplement for other drugs used in the early phase.

Clinical definitions

In the spectrum of obstructive pulmonary disease, between the 'reversible airway obstruction' of asthma and irreversible diseases such as emphysema, which are permanent – in the case of emphysema, as a result of loss of lung tissue – comes chronic bronchitis, which is almost inevitably associated with a greater or lesser degree of emphysema. The bronchitic element of this combination of diseases is fairly easily diagnosed by the chronic production of mucus. The emphysematous component is much more difficult to quantify during life and so, if for no other reason, the term **chronic obstructive pulmonary disease (COPD)** is useful to describe this combination, if only to cover our uncertainty.

Bronchitis and mucus

The airways are lined from nose to alveoli by a watery layer containing mucus. The normal mucus film within the lungs is approximately 5–10 μm thick and consists of two layers, the layer next to the airway wall is more watery to allow the cilia of the ciliary escalator to work, brushing the overlying more viscous layer, together with any foreign particles it contains, towards the mouth. Mucus is produced by ducted seromucous glands deep in the bronchial walls and goblet cells in the bronchial epithelium. The accumulation of mucus results from excess production, drying of the surface, failure of the ciliary escalator to clear it, or infection making it too viscous to be moved. This results effectively in a narrowing or total blockage of the airways (Fig. 4.14). The secretion of mucus is normally controlled by vagal reflexes and local chemical stimulation. Curry and other spicy foods provoke the vagal reflex, and tobacco smoke stimulates both mechanisms. In extreme cases of bronchitis mucus can solidify into tiny solid casts of the small airways, and chronic bronchitic patients cough up these casts.

Bronchitis, known to the French as 'the English disease', is defined clinically by the excessive production of lung mucus. A firm diagnosis is based on expectoration on most days for at least 3 months during 2 successive years. The pathology that produces this

Airflow in the respiratory system Box 2

The physiology of asthma

Asthma is a disease of the airways characterized by short-term episodes of bronchoconstriction. These can be so severe that the flow of gas along the airways is significantly reduced, leading to difficulty in breathing.

Airway narrowing, which is the principal feature of asthma, is brought about by the contraction of smooth muscle in the walls of the airways. Bronchial smooth muscle can contract in all individuals and hence the diameter of the airways changes, but the effect on ventilation is usually negligible. In asthmatics, the changes in airways diameter are exaggerated and the airways respond to stimuli which in non-asthmatics would be innocuous. These two effects are together called **bronchial hyperreactivity**.

In many asthmatics bronchial hyperreactivity is closely associated with an increased sensitivity of the immune system to everyday substances in the environment. This increased sensitivity is called **atopy**. Atopy is also associated with conditions such as eczema. Clinically, this sensitivity may be demonstrated by a characteristic skin-wheal reaction to common environmental substances.

Atopic individuals readily produce antibodies of the IgE class to a variety of environmental allergens. It is thought that these antibodies attach to mast cells in the airways. Mast cells are part of the immune system, and when an antigen binds to IgE on their surface they release a range of substances, including prostaglandins, leukotrienes and histamine. It is thought that these substances are responsible for triggering bronchoconstriction in susceptible individuals.

Asthma is not confined to atopic individuals and is not necessarily provoked by environmental antigens. This is particularly the case in asthmatics who are diagnosed later in life. Asthmatics who respond to environmental stimuli are sometimes referred to as having extrinsic asthma, whereas those who do not have intrinsic asthma.

Asthma is diagnosed on the basis of the symptoms of episodic wheeze, breathlessness, and often cough.

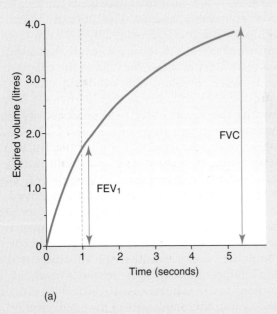

(a)

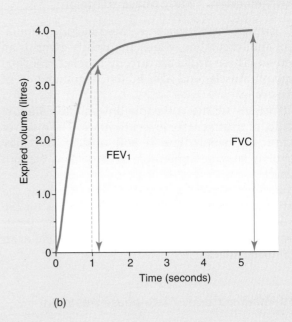

(b)

Fig. 4.13

Forced expiratory spirograms recorded from Mr Graham. Recording A was made while Mr Graham was feeling a bit wheezy. Recording B was made after Mr Graham had taken a dose of salbutamol from his inhaler. In recording A, the FEV_1 is very much reduced although the FVC is essentially little different from normal. This means that the FEV_1/FVC ratio is reduced, indicating an obstructive respiratory defect.

Airflow in the respiratory system Box 2 (continued)

These symptoms are often worse at night and may be brought on by trigger agents, as described above. Diagnosis is also helped by lung function tests, particularly forced expiration spirography and measurement of peak expiratory flow.

The principle behind measuring forced vital capacity (FVC) and forced expiratory volume in one second (FEV_1) is explained in Chapter 11. Figure 4.11A shows a forced expiratory spirogram which Mr Graham made one day at the clinic when he was feeling a little wheezy. After making the recording Mr Graham used his salbutamol inhaler, which relieved his wheeziness. He then made a second forced expiratory spirogram, shown in Figure 4.13B.

The spirogram in Figure 4.13A shows a reduced FEV_1, although the FVC is not particularly abnormal. In other words, the FEV_1/FVC ratio is reduced, indicating an obstructive abnormality. Following the administration of salbutamol the airway narrowing is reversed and the obstructive pattern on the spirogram improves. This reversibility of airway narrowing is characteristic of asthma.

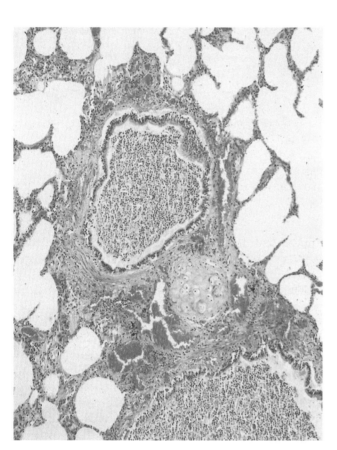

Fig. 4.14
Bronchitis with mucus totally blocking the airway lumen. (Source: Stevens et al 2002.)

excessive mucus is hypertrophy of the mucous glands of the large bronchi. The Reid Index (p. 17), which is normally 0.4, may exceed 0.7. The smaller airways, which some authorities believe undergo the initial pathological changes, are narrowed and inflamed and show oedematous changes in their walls. The pathogenesis of bronchitis is clearly linked to tobacco smoking. Air pollution plays a secondary role.

Emphysema and radial traction

The general connective tissue that surrounds the airways in the lungs is called the parenchyma. It forms a sort of scaffold round the airways, holding them open by what is called **radial traction**. As the lung expands during inspiration the traction increases as the fibres that make up the parenchyma are stretched. The importance of radial traction is grasped when you return to the concept of the airway resistance being inversely proportional to the fourth power of the radius of the airway. If the scaffold of the parenchyma was completely rigid (which of course it is not), doubling the length, breadth and height of a cube of lung tissue would increase its volume eight times, but this would theoretically (Poiseuille's Law) increase the conductance of an airway in that cube 2^4 times, i.e. 16 times.

The effect of radial traction is less profound than this at the lung volumes involved in normal breathing, with changes in resistance due to this effect being proportional to lung volume. The effect is, however, of great importance at low lung volumes, with the airways collapsing when radial support disappears. At this point airways resistance begins to increase dramatically (Fig. 4.15).

Because of the weight of overlying tissue this closure begins first in the lower lobes of the lungs at a volume known as **closing capacity** (CC). In young people closing capacity is less than FRC and so closing does not occur during normal breathing. At about 65 years it becomes equal to FRC in the upright position, and greater than FRC when supine. Under these conditions blood is shunted (see p. 107) through the lungs without coming into contact with air, and this is an important aspect of desaturation of arterial blood with increasing age. Closure of the airways can be prevented by increasing the pressure within them, and many patients whose airways are closing in this way

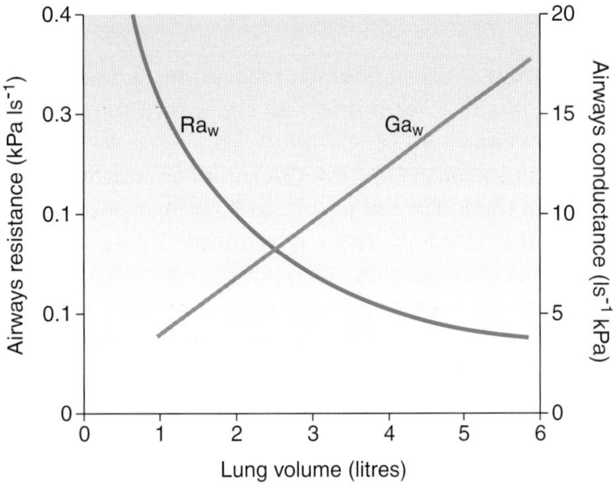

AIRFLOW IN THE RESPIRATORY SYSTEM

4

Fig. 4.15
The relationship between lung volume, airways resistance (Raw) and airways conductance (Gaw). Gaw, 1/Raw; Gaw is frequently used clinically in the form of specific conductance (Gaw. V_L), which takes into account the different lung sizes of different subjects.

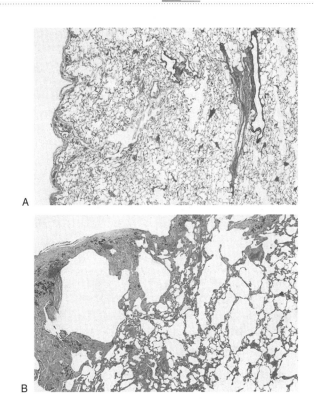

Fig. 4.16
Normal (A) and emphysematous lungs (B).
(Source: Stevens et al 2002)

intuitively exhale through pursed lips, the positive pressure within the airway produced by this 'pursed lip breathing' helping keep their airways open.

The support provided to the airway by radial traction is diminished in that important component of COPD, **emphysema** (bronchitis being the other component).

Emphysema is defined anatomically as an irreversible increase in the size of air spaces distal to the terminal bronchioles. The destruction of lung parenchyma that brings about this increase in size is now generally agreed to be due to uncontrolled action of proteolytic enzymes from leukocytes associated with pulmonary inflammation (Fig. 4.16). Cigarette smoke is again a major villain in the piece, stimulating elastase release from neutrophils. Lung elastase is normally inhibited by antiprotease enzymes, the most important of which is α_1-antitrypsin. About 1 in 4000 people has a genetic deficiency of **α_1-antitrypsin**, and therefore have a predisposition towards emphysema.

Airway collapse, owing to loss of radial traction, is exacerbated by changes in transmural pressure which brings about flow-related airway collapse, which we will consider next.

Intrapleural pressure and cough

During normal quiet breathing intrapleural pressure is always considerably negative relative to the atmosphere. In the airway, right down to the alveoli during quiet breathing, the pressure is only slightly below atmospheric during inspiration and only slightly above during expiration.

This means the **transmural pressure** (across the airway wall) always tends to keep the airway open. This of course applies only to the airways surrounded by the intrapleural pressure, the intrathoracic airways. Part of the trachea, for example, is extrathoracic and does not come into the following discussion.

When breathing becomes vigorous and expiration becomes active, conditions change. Passive expiration comes about because the elastic recoil of the lungs draws in the chest wall, which tends to spring out during normal tidal breathing. This action maintains a *negative* intrapleural pressure (see Fig. 3.2). When expiration is active, however, the internal intercostals and the abdominal muscles 'squash' the air out of the lungs by making intrapleural pressure positive with respect to the air in the airways. This can lead to **dynamic airway collapse**, with its associated **expiratory flow limitation**.

Under conditions of dynamic collapse the airways behave like a Starling Resistor (named after the physiologist who first described it). The Starling Resistor arises when air is being driven through a flexible tube by a pressure which is applied to the outside of the

Airflow in the respiratory system Box 3

What provokes an asthma attack in patients with extrinsic asthma?

One day, Mr Graham suffered a particularly bad attack of asthma. He had had a cold for a week or so, but apart from that there did not seem to be any particular trigger for his attack. However, he became increasingly wheezy and found it more and more difficult to breathe. He found it especially difficult to exhale. He used his salbutamol inhaler several times but did not get any relief from it. Mr Graham's wife became increasingly worried about him and decided to call an ambulance. In the ambulance, Mr Graham was given oxygen to breathe and he was taken to hospital, where he was examined by the emergency doctor. The doctor noted that Mr Graham's respiratory rate was over 30 breaths per minute and that his chest was very expanded. On auscultation, the air entry into Mr Graham's lungs was reduced and there were wheezes throughout his chest. The doctor asked Mr Graham to perform a peak expiratory flow test. Mr Graham's peak expiratory flow was about two-thirds of his normal value.

In most patients with asthma, a range of 'triggers' provokes attacks of bronchoconstriction. Such triggers include specific allergens, other non-specific substances, exercise and drugs.

Allergens

Allergens are foreign substances that are able to provoke an immune response in susceptible individuals. In patients with extrinsic asthma, an attack of broncho-constriction may be provoked by exposure either to a specific allergen or to a range of allergens. The commonest allergen responsible for provoking asthma is a protein derived from the faeces of the house-dust mite, which lives in warm locations such as bedding and feeds on scales of shed human skin. For many asthmatic patients the presence of animals, such as cats, dogs and birds, can provoke bronchoconstriction. In these cases, the allergen responsible is derived from animal skin, fur, feathers or excreta. Allergens derived from pollen, particularly grass pollen, can provoke asthma as well as causing hayfever. In such cases, asthma may be confined to certain seasons of the year. Although the allergen nor-

mally has to be inhaled to provoke bronchoconstriction, in a small number of patients an attack of asthma may be provoked by eating specific foods or chemicals.

Non-specific provokers of asthma

As well as reacting to specific allergens, the hyperreactive airways of asthmatic patients may also respond to a wide range of substances, including strong smells, dusts, vapours, smoke (including tobacco smoke) and airborne chemicals. These agents are thought to act directly on the airway itself, and an immune response is not provoked.

Exercise

In many patients, asthma may be provoked by exercise. The exact mechanism by which this occurs is not clear, but it is likely that cooling of hyperreactive airways may have an important role to play, as exercise-induced asthma often occurs more readily during cold weather. Drying of the airway mucosa may also play a role, as many asthmatics report that swimming is less likely to induce bronchospasm than other forms of exercise.

Drugs

A variety of drugs are known to induce asthma. Aspirin and other anti-inflammatory drugs can provoke bronchoconstriction in a small proportion of asthmatics. This action is probably brought about because these drugs interfere with the production of prostaglandins and leukotrienes, and an upset in the balance of these substances in the airway may cause bronchoconstriction. β-blocking drugs are also prone to producing bronchoconstriction in asthmatic patients, presumably by blocking β_2 receptors on the bronchial smooth muscle, although these drugs may also influence cells of the immune system.

Emotions

In many patients a strong emotional response may result in an attack of bronchoconstriction. This is presumably mediated by a central neural mechanism.

---

tube as well as the inside (Fig. 4.17). Inside the tube the pressure is being used up to drive the air along, and therefore pressure inside the tube falls from left to right. Outside the tube the pressure stays the same along the whole length of the tube. At a point somewhere along the tube the outside pressure exceeds the inside pressure and the tube collapses.

The concept of **equal pressure point**, where the pressures inside and outside the airway are equal, is frequently used to describe the state of the lungs in obstructive disease. At the equal pressure point the rigidity of the wall and surrounding parenchyma is the only factor holding the airway open. As lung volume decreases during expiration the equal pressure

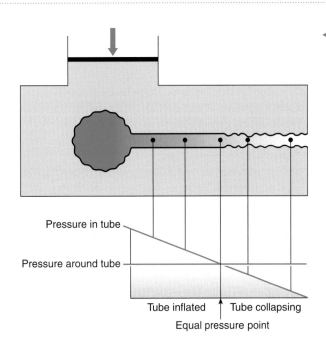

Fig. 4.17

A Starling Resistor. In this a flexible tube is surrounded by a uniform pressure. Pressure drives air along the tube. As this driving pressure is used up it falls until an equal pressure point is reached, where the internal and external pressures are equal. Downstream from that point the pressure around the wall of the tube is greater than the pressure inside, and causes it to collapse, frequently in an unstable vibrating manner.

point moves progressively toward the smaller airways as the contribution to the pressure within the airways from elastic recoil is reduced (Fig. 4.18).

Collapsed areas trap air behind them, within the lung. Extra expiratory effort does not relieve this trapping, as it simply presses the collapsed area more firmly shut. In healthy lungs these conditions do not occur above functional residual capacity. In lungs

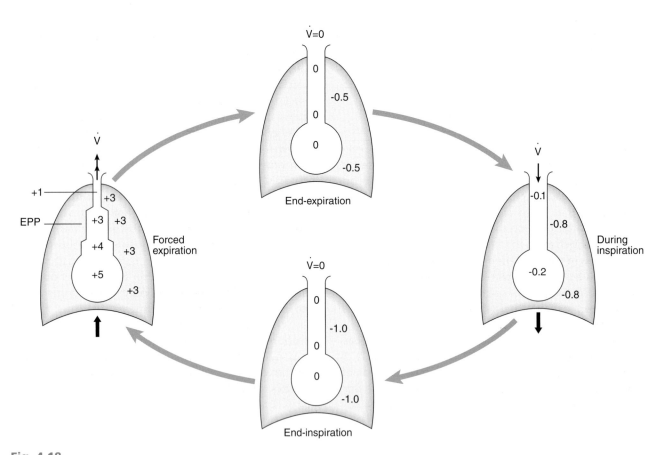

Fig. 4.18

Transmural pressure in intrathoracic airways. The pressure inside intrathoracic airways is usually not very far from atmospheric, which tends to keep them open because the pressure around the airways is usually negative (subatmospheric). During a forced expiration, however, the pressure may become positive and equal to that within the airway (an equal pressure point, EPP). The pressure within the airway downstream of the EPP is less than intrapleural pressure, and the airway there tends to collapse.

Airflow in the respiratory system Box 4

Treatment of asthma

After examining him, the emergency doctor gave Mr Graham some nebulized salbutamol, the same drug in Mr Graham's inhaler. However, whereas Mr Graham's inhaler administers a dose of 100 μg each time it is used, the doctor put 5 mg of salbutamol into the nebulizer. The nebulizer produces a fine aerosol of drug in a flow of oxygen. Mr Graham inhaled the aerosol, although only a very small proportion of it would have reached his lungs. Figure 4.13 shows a nebulizer of the type that might be used. In addition, the doctor administered some intravenous steroids to Mr Graham.

Fortunately, Mr Graham's condition began to improve with the nebulizer salbutamol. He was nevertheless admitted to hospital and received regular nebulized salbutamol. The next day he left hospital.

As we have already established there are a number of components to asthma. The airways are hyperreactive, resulting in constriction of the bronchial smooth muscle; there is a generalized inflammation of the airway mucosa, and in many cases the immune system is involved. Treatments for asthma are aimed at either:

① relieving bronchoconstriction
② reducing airway inflammation
③ influencing the immune system.

Relief of bronchoconstriction

Drugs that relieve bronchoconstriction act either to *stimulate* β2 adrenoceptors or to *block* cholinergic receptors on the membranes of bronchial smooth muscle cells.

β2-Adrenergic agonists

Activation of these receptors causes an increase in cyclic AMP in the cell cytoplasm, which triggers muscle relaxation. Drugs in this class include salbutamol and terbutaline, and they can be administered during attacks of bronchoconstriction or can be taken regularly to prevent attacks from occurring. They are generally administered with an inhaler or a nebulizer directly into the airways, although they may also be administered orally or intravenously. In severe asthma attacks they are regarded as the first line of treatment.

Anticholinergic drugs

These drugs act by blocking the muscarinic acetylcholine receptors on the bronchial smooth muscle, reversing the bronchoconstriction produced by activation of these receptors. They may also reduce bronchial secretions by blocking the parasympathetic innervation of submucosal glands in the bronchial tree. Drugs of this class include ipratropium. They are usually administered with an inhaler or a nebulizer and are usually regarded as being more effective in older patients with asthma.

Aminophylline/theophylline

These drugs act on the bronchial smooth muscle. They increase the levels of cyclic AMP in the cytoplasm by blocking the enzyme phosphodiesterase, which is responsible for breaking down cycle AMP. A rise in cyclic AMP in the smooth muscle cells causes them to relax.

Drugs that relieve airway inflammation
Corticosteroids

Steroids have a anti-inflammatory effect and are more effective in the prevention of asthma rather than in the treatment of an acute attack. They reduce the inflammation in the airways and also modulate the immune response to allergens. Steroids can be administered via an inhaler. In this way an effective dose is administered but many of the side effects of steroids can be avoided, as the blood concentration of the drug remains low. However, some patients require to take steroids orally. Whichever route is used, it is important that steroids are taken regularly to be effective. Although steroids are usually given during an acute attack, it probably takes some considerable time for them to have an acute effect.

Drugs that influence the immune system
Sodium cromoglicate

The exact mode of action of this drug is not known, but it is thought that one of its actions is to 'stabilize' mast cells and prevent them from releasing bronchoconstrictor mediators. Like steroids, cromoglicate must be taken regularly and is a drug which is used to prevent asthma rather than to treat an acute attack.

---

affected by damage to the airway wall, or when the supporting parenchyma has been destroyed, collapse takes place at higher volumes. During expiration the collapsing segment vibrates and is a major source of the **wheeze** heard in many lung diseases. In emphysema the destruction of the supporting parenchyma is clearly the cause of loss of support of the airways; in asthma it is the high bronchomotor tone and oedema of the airways that augments collapse and increases the rate of pressure drop along the airway.

Clinical tests for changes in resistance

Producing flow volume curves is rather the province of the specialized lung function laboratory, and tests used on a daily basis, either in the general practitioner's clinic or in the patient's home are usually Forced Expired Volume in 1 second (FEV_1) or 0.75 seconds, obtained from any one of a variety of types of spirometer, or Peak Expiratory Flow, where the patient's maximum expiratory effort blows a paddle along a tube – the higher the peak flow the further the paddle goes.

A most useful test for obstructive diseases is the flow/volume curve, or loop, which is obtained by a method described in Chapter 11. The peak flow obtained at large lung volumes depends largely on effort (Fig. 4.19), but toward the end of expiration there is an effort-independent segment of the loop where expiratory flow is determined by airway collapse below the equal pressure point. The alteration in this loop by disease is also dealt with in Chapter 11.

Work of breathing

Breathing requires work be done, mainly to overcome airway resistance and to stretch the lungs and chest wall. It is interesting but not obvious that part of the work of expanding the lungs and chest during inspiration is recovered as the elastic recoil during

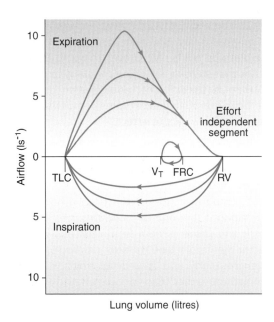

Fig. 4.19

Normal flow–volume loops. These were obtained using three different expiratory efforts. Note that all three loops meet in an effort-independent segment. Flow in this condition is being limited by airways collapse. A normal tidal volume breath is shown for comparison.

expiration, which is used to expel the inspired air from the lungs (rather as an archer stores up elastic energy in his bow by pulling back the arrow in one direction, and releases it by allowing the arrow to go in the other direction). At rest the work of breathing accounts for less than 5% of our metabolic rate. This small fraction is not due to the efficiency of our respiratory systems, which is low: only 10% of the energy used is converted into useful work.

Work is defined in the physical sciences as the product of a force × the distance it moves its point of application. In a three-dimensional system such as the respiratory system this translates into:

Work =
intrapleural pressure × change in lung volume.

This is illustrated in Figure 4.20, where work in a lung is the product of the volume change and the pressure change producing it.

In panel (a), if either volume or pressure does not change no useful work is done. In panel (b) a perfectly elastic lung is very slowly (pseudostatically) inflated. Here the work of inflation is the *area* of the figure ABC. In panels (c), (d) and (e) different patterns of breathing are seen to require different amounts of work to produce the same ventilation. This is because the work of breathing is made up of work against:

1. the elastic resistance of the tissues
2. airflow resistance.

Deep slow breathing (panel (e) in Fig. 4.20) requires the most work to be done against elastic resistance, whereas rapid shallow breathing (panel (d)) works largely against airways resistance.

So, if you begin breathing slowly and deeply and increase the frequency while reducing the volume, work against elastic resistance decreases and work to produce airflow increases (Fig. 4.21). We automatically choose the best pattern of breathing in terms of work, probably as a result of subliminal information received from mechanoreceptors in the lungs (see Chapter 11).

This system is quite efficient at minimizing the expenditure of energy by the respiratory muscles (as a fraction of our total energy use), and in healthy subjects the work done in breathing provides 'good value' in providing extra oxygen. For example, exercise is rarely limited by the respiratory system using too much energy. In diseased lungs, however, the airway resistance, elastic properties or the control system may be compromised, and the extra work done by the respiratory muscles to provide extra oxygen to the rest of the body during exercise demands more oxygen than it provides (Fig. 4.22), which of course is an untenable situation that limits the exercise.

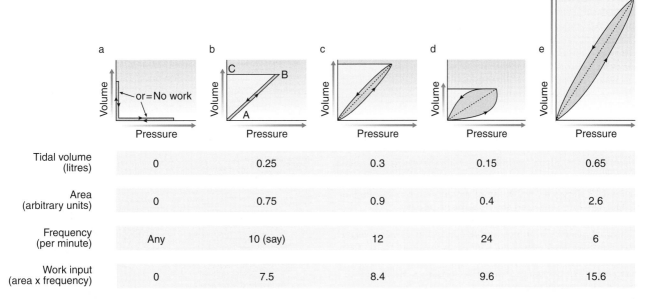

	a	b	c	d	e
Tidal volume (litres)	0	0.25	0.3	0.15	0.65
Area (arbitrary units)	0	0.75	0.9	0.4	2.6
Frequency (per minute)	Any	10 (say)	12	24	6
Work input (area x frequency)	0	7.5	8.4	9.6	15.6

Fig. 4.20
The work of breathing. This is the product of volume change × pressure change. If either of these remains the same (a), no work of breathing is done. Panel (b) is an artificial situation used to demonstrate how work of breathing is calculated: if the lung (or balloon, say) is completely non-elastic and is inflated from A to B it will stay there (like a piece of putty which has been stretched) and the work put into it will be the area ABC. If the lung or balloon is *perfectly* elastic, once the inflating pressure is released it will return from B to A, giving up all the energy that has been put into it. This straight diagonal line (shown dotted in subsequent panels) is the energy put into the compliance of the lung and is recovered in expiration. In normal quiet breathing (c), the work done in inspiration which is *not* recovered during expiration but is lost largely in overcoming airways resistance is to the right of the diagonal. If breathing is made deep and slow (e) or rapid and shallow (d), more work than normal is required to achieve the same ventilation as in (c).

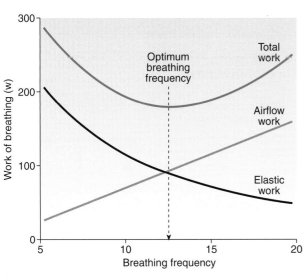

Fig. 4.21
Total work of breathing. This is effectively the sum of work done against the elastic recoil of tissue plus the work to produce airflow. These change with frequency of breathing, shown with the sum reaching a minimum at the frequency where the two lines intersect.

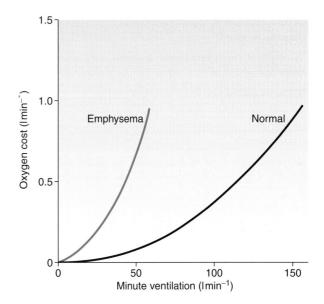

Fig. 4.22
Work of breathing at different ventilations. The work of breathing in a normal individual is low until high levels of ventilation are reached, and then begins to rise steeply. Diseased lungs consume more energy at low ventilation, and their requirement increases more rapidly than normal.

Further reading

Hoppin FG, Hildebrandt J. Mechanical properties of the lung. In: West JB, ed. Bioengineering aspects of the lung. New York: Marcel Dekker, 1977

Pedley TJ, Schroter RC, Sudlow MF. Gas flow and mixing in airways. In: West JB, ed. Bioengineering aspects of the lung. New York: Marcel Dekker, 1977

Rodarte JR, Rehder K. Dynamics of respiration. In: Macklem PT, Mead J, eds. Handbook of physiology, Section 3 The respiratory system. Vol III Mechanics of breathing, Part I, p. 131. Bethesda, MD: American Physiological Society, 1986

Orehek J. Neurohumoral control of airway calibre. In: Widdicombe JG. MTP International review of physiology, Vol 23, p. 1. Baltimore: University Park Press, 1981

Stevens A, Lowe JS, Young B, Weater's basic histopathology 4E. Edinburgh: Churchill Livingstone, 2002

Self-assessment case study

Figure 4.23 shows a chest X-ray of a man who has smoked all his life. The large mass on the right-hand side is a bronchogenic carcinoma – lung cancer.

The vast majority of tumours or neoplasms in the respiratory system are caused by smoking. Long-term exposure to tobacco smoke affects the epithelial cells lining the bronchi, causing changes in their nuclear proteins. These changes, which are beyond the scope of this book, cause cells to undergo repeated uncontrolled divisions, leading to a mass forming in the walls of the affected bronchus. Cells may enter the bloodstream and so the tumour may metastasize (spread) to other sites in the body.

Many of the signs and symptoms of bronchogenic carcinoma (e.g. weight loss) are related to body systems outside the lungs. Nevertheless, the mass of a primary tumour in the wall of a bronchus may produce effects of its own.

From your knowledge of gas flow in the respiratory system you should be able to attempt the following questions:

① As a bronchogenic carcinoma increases in size, what effect will it have on gas flow through the adjacent airway?

② What effect will this have on the ventilation of the regions of lung supplied by the affected bronchus? What symptoms may this produce?

③ What effect may a bronchogenic carcinoma have on gas exchange and why?

Answers see page 176

Self-assessment questions

① What will be the effect of doubling the radius and the length of a tube in which laminar flow is taking place?

② What is the most likely reason and consequences of flow being limited during a cough?

③ What is the significance of the total cross-sectional area of the airways of the lung?

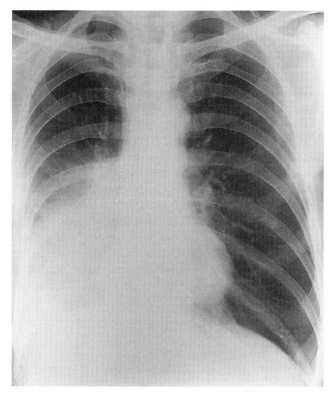

**Fig. 4.23
Bronchocarcinoma.**

④ When is intrapleural pressure positive with respect to atmospheric pressure?

⑤ Which branch of the nervous system is most important in producing bronchoconstriction?

⑥ What is the 'equal pressure point' in the airways, and what is its significance?

Answers see page 176

VENTILATION OF THE RESPIRATORY SYSTEM

THE IMPORTANCE OF ITS LACK OF UNIFORMITY IN DISEASE

5

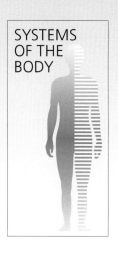

SYSTEMS OF THE BODY

Chapter objectives

After studying this chapter you should be able to:

① Define ventilation (differentiating it from lung volume).

② Define the common lung volumes and capacities and how they are changed in restrictive and obstructive diseases.

③ Explain the importance of respiratory tract structure (as blind-ended tracts in parallel) on ventilation.

④ Explain the alveolar gas equation.

⑤ Differentiate between physiological and anatomical dead space and relate increased dead space to emphysema.

⑥ Describe the physiological factors influencing the distribution of ventilation.

⑦ Explain the composition of the parts of a single expirate and why these are changed in disease.

Introduction

So far we have talked about breathing as if it simply consisted of a uniform repeated action of inhalation followed by exhalation. We now begin to explore the detail of this far from uniform phenomenon.

Normal breathing involves about 12 breaths per minute, each of about 0.5 L. The volume of air passing into the lungs per minute in this case (**minute ventilation**, $\dot{V}_I$) is:

$$12 \times 0.5 = 6.0 \text{ L min}^{-1}.$$

The symbol for ventilation, $\dot{V}$, has a dot over the V to show it is a *rate*. The volume breathed out is approximately equal to the volume breathed in (**tidal volume**, V_T), therefore the net flow over a complete cycle is zero. This is not a very helpful way of expressing ven-tilation if we want to express changes in breathing, as the result of exercise or disease, for example. We therefore measure the flow in one direction only – conventionally the volume breathed out per minute ($\dot{V}_E$) – to give us minute ventilation.

In respiratory medicine ventilation is the rate of flow of air into or out of the lungs, and results from the expanding and contracting of the lungs by the changes in intrapleural pressure described in Chapter 4 (p. 46) and illustrated in Figure 5.1.

The part of the air ventilating our lungs which is of paramount functional importance is that which forms **alveolar ventilation**. Insufficient (hypoventilation) or excess (hyperventilation) alveolar ventilation occurs in many lung pathologies.

We all know we can consciously alter the volume of our lungs, breathing in or breathing out more than

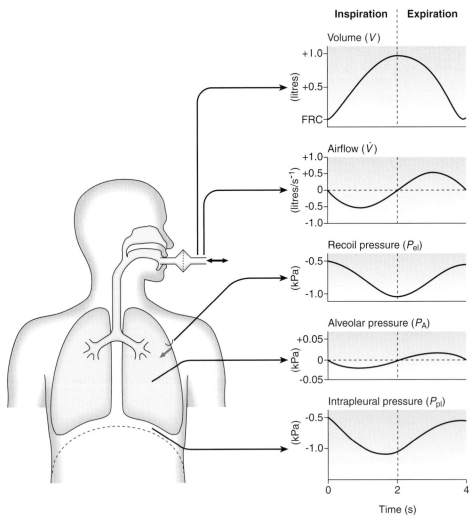

Fig. 5.1
A single respiratory cycle. Airflow would be measured using a pneumotachograph and integrated to give tidal volume. Recoil pressure has a negative sign because it is measured relative to intrapleural pressure.

normal: what is frequently not realized is that we cannot totally empty our lungs.

At the end of a normal quiet expiration average intrapleural pressure (P_{PL}) is approximately –0.5 kPa (below atmospheric pressure) and lung volume (V_L) 3 L. This volume is called the **functional residual capacity** (FRC). When you breathe in as hard as you can and hold your breath, P_{PL} decreases to –2 kPa and V_L increases to about 6 L.

Alternatively, if you breathe out as hard as possible P_{PL} will be –0.2 kPa and V_L 1.5 L. This **residual volume** (RV) cannot be expelled.

The anatomy (size) of an individual's chest, the elasticity of his lungs and chest wall and the strength of his respiratory muscles determine these static volumes. During dynamic breathing different volumes and values of intrapleural pressure are generated.

Changes in lung volume can easily be measured using a **spirometer**, as illustrated in Figure 5.2. This instrument, which comes in many forms, consists of a closed space from which the subject breathes. In the type illustrated a hollow bell is supported in a trough of water; as the subject breathes in, air is drawn from the bell and it sinks slightly; when he breathes out the bell rises. Movements of the bell are recorded as changes in lung volume on a moving chart.

Much information about lung properties and diagnosis of disease can be obtained by measuring changes in lung volume. When a maximum inspiration is taken the increase in lung volume (**inspiratory reserve volume**, IRV) to reach **total lung capacity** (TLC) is about 3 L. A maximal expiration from TLC will expel the IRV, V_T and the **expiratory reserve volume** (ERV), the total of all these volumes being the **vital capacity** (VC). In the vocabulary of lung volumes a capacity is the sum of two or more volumes.

Except for RV and FRC (which depends on RV), these volumes can be measured using a spirometer in the living subject. If the lungs are taken out of the body and allowed to collapse there will still be a little air left in them: the **minimal air**; these lungs will float (see

'lights' Ch. 2, p. 21). The lungs of a stillborn baby who has not taken a breath will not float because they contain no air; this test is important in forensic investigations.

The names of these volumes and their abbreviations are intimidating to students, but reference to Figure 5.2 should make all clear.

The changes in intrapleural pressure that bring about these volume changes do not vary much between individuals in health or disease in either humans or animals. The volumes themselves, however, do vary with:

- **body size** – all are larger in large people.
- **age** – all volumes are smaller in children, only partially due to their smaller body size. In old age VC is decreased and RV increased because of degenerative changes.
- **sex** – all volumes are smaller in women than in men the same size.
- **muscle training** – increases all the lung volumes and allows greater maximal ventilation during exercise.
- **disease** – changes in these lung volumes from the normal values, which have been measured in numerous extensive surveys, are used in the diagnosis of many diseases of the lungs and respiratory system.

Because RV cannot be breathed out, it and FRC (which is made up of RV + ERV) cannot be measured directly by a spirometer. They are measured by inhaling from RV a known volume of a non-absorbable tracer gas (e.g. helium) and measuring its dilution by the unknown volume of air in the lungs. Alternatively, the subject breathes out to RV and then breathes in and out a few times from a bag containing a known volume of pure oxygen. He then breathes out again to RV into the bag. The air in his RV was approximately 80% nitrogen, and the dilution of this by the known volume of pure oxygen in the bag enables RV to be calculated.

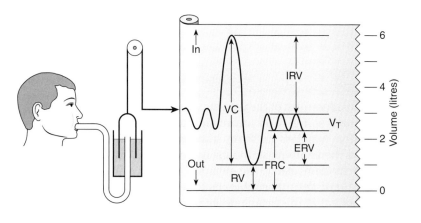

Fig. 5.2
A spirometer record of breathing. Average adult volumes are shown. Because the lungs cannot be completely emptied, residual volume (RV) and functional residual capacity (FRC) cannot be measured by direct spirometry.

Spirometric abnormalities in disease

Lung disease changes many of the lung volumes in Figure 5.2. It is usual, for diagnostic purposes, to exaggerate these changes by stressing the respiratory system by asking the patient to breathe in as deeply as he can and out as hard as he can for the single breath of a test. The forced expiratory volume in 1 second (FEV_1) is frequently abbreviated to forced expired volume (FEV), but is still the same creature: the volume of air forced out in the first second of such a test. Similarly, forced vital capacity is the total volume of air a patient can breathe out after a maximal inspiration. It is usual to express FEV as a percentage of FVC: this takes into account the fact that larger people normally have larger lungs and therefore a larger FVC.

Much careful work has gone into preparing tables that relate spirometric measurements to a normal subject's height and weight. Deviations from values predicted by these tables are diagnostic of lung disease.

Diseases of the thoracic cage, such as ankylosing spondylitis, diseases of the nerves and muscles of respiration, e.g. poliomyelitis, diseases that restrict expansion of the lungs, such as fibrosis, or diseases that cause airway collapse during expiration all limit these spirometric measurements. Examples of the modifications produced by diseases of the lungs on spirometric traces are shown in Chapter 11, and can be summarized in a very general way as follows:

Variable	Restrictive Disease	Obstructive disease
FVC	– –	–
FEV	– –	– –
FEV/FVC	0	– –
FRC	–	+
RV	–	+
TLC	–	+

0 = no change; + = increase; – = decrease.

NB: some of these changes are not seen to any degree until the disease is very advanced.

Uneven distribution

These considerations of the various volumes that make up breathing still give an impression of uniformity of distribution which is far from true. In Chapter 2 we described the anatomy of the bronchial tree as blind-ended sacks connected to the outside through a system of tubes. Some thought enables us to see that the composition of gas in this arrangement may be different at

Ventilation in the respiratory system Box 1

Pneumothorax: a failure of lung ventilation

Mr Price is a 21-year-old man who went to the Accident and Emergency department of his local hospital complaining of chest pain. The pain had come on suddenly while he was playing football. The pain was stabbing, on the right-hand side of his chest, and was very much worse when he took a breath in. He also felt rather short of breath.

After taking a history, performing a physical examination and taking a chest X-ray, the doctor in the emergency department made a diagnosis of pneumothorax.

In this chapter we will consider:

① What causes a pneumothorax.
② Diagnosis of a pneumothorax.
③ Treatment of a pneumothorax.
④ Tension pneumothorax – a rare medical emergency.

its entrance (the lips) from that at its ends (the alveoli) – differences in **series**; also, the composition in different alveoli may be different – differences in **parallel**; or a combination of both. Differences in the composition of air in different parts of the lung depend largely on how well that part is ventilated and how much gas exchange between air and blood and blood and air takes place there. In the ideal situation just the right amount of both air and blood are supplied to a particular region, so there is no 'waste' of either. One particular kind of inequality between air and blood supply is known as dead space.

Dead space

Essentially all exchange of gas between air and blood takes place at the alveolar surface. The system of tubes connecting this surface to the atmosphere can be considered anatomical dead space. These tubes are essential to bring air to the respiratory surface, but ventilating these connecting tubes is an inescapable waste of effort as far as gas exchange is concerned. To understand anatomical dead space you must understand that the lungs fill and empty in a sequential fashion (Fig. 5.3).

At the end of inspiration the contents of the alveoli have been diluted by inspired room air, which now also fills the anatomical dead space (Fig. 5.3C). As the lungs then empty during expiration, the rule of 'last in

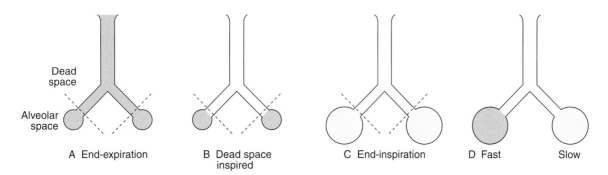

Fig. 5.3
Distribution of dead space gas. At the end of expiration dead space is filled with 'used' alveolar gas. When the lungs inspire a volume of fresh air equal to dead space, the alveolar region has expanded but the composition of the gas it contains is not changed, there is fresh air in the dead space and 'used' air in the alveoli. The alveolar air will be diluted by further inspiration, but the composition of the dead space air will remain that of fresh air. If alveoli fill at different rates they are said to have different time constants and receive different amounts of dead space gas. The alveoli that expand first will receive most dead space gas.

first out' applies and the dead space containing unmodified room air is exhaled first. At the end of expiration the anatomical dead space is filled with alveolar air, and this partly used air is inhaled first in the next inspiration (Fig. 5.3A, B). If some regions of the lung expand before others in the process of inspiration they will receive an inappropriately large part of this dead space gas, and the regions receiving air later in inspiration will receive more fresh air (Fig. 5.3C, D). So the timing of inflation of a part of the lung during inspiration will affect the composition of the gas it receives.

This type of dead space is called 'anatomical' because it measures the anatomical volume of the conducting airways. The strict definition of anatomical dead space is 'the volume of an inspired breath which has not mixed with the gas in the alveoli'. Because gas exchange effectively only takes place in the alveoli there is no CO_2 excreted into the dead space, and a scientist called Fowler pointed out that anatomical

dead space can be measured as the volume of expired gas leaving the mouth and nose before CO_2 appears at the lips (Fig. 5.4).

We will see in a little while that this 'cunning plan' for measuring anatomical dead space is fraught with difficulty, mainly because the alveolar gas appearing at the lips does not have the constant composition shown in Figure 5.4. More often there is a considerable slope, particularly when the subject is breathing vigorously, or when alveoli empty at different rates. This makes deciding where to draw the vertical line difficult.

In healthy subjects anatomical dead space is all the dead space there is, but as we get older or suffer from lung disease things become more difficult, as **alveolar dead space** begins to appear. By the same definition we used for anatomical dead space, alveolar dead space is contained in alveoli which have insufficient blood supply to act as effective respiratory membranes. These two types of dead space added together make up **physiological dead space**.

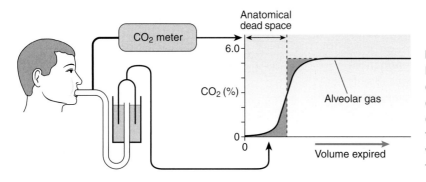

Fig. 5.4
Estimating dead space volume. Carbon dioxide concentration rises rapidly in the expired air when the dead space has been expired. The volume at the midpoint of this rapid rise is taken as dead space volume. The flat part of the curve is called the alveolar plateau.

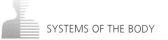
Physiological dead space =
Anatomical dead space + Alveolar dead space
(zero in healthy
subjects)

A 'rule of thumb' is that a healthy subject's weight in pounds (1 lb = 0.45 kg) is numerically equal to his dead space in millilitres.

Alveolar dead space in disease

It would be wrong to think of alveolar dead space as an absolute term, i.e. to imagine areas of the lung that are supplied with air by breathing but which have absolutely no blood supply to exchange O_2 and CO_2 with this air. We will see in Chapter 7 that most of the lung is

'on target', getting lots of blood to regions that are well ventilated and less blood to poorly ventilated regions. This '$\dot{V}/\dot{Q}$ matching' is of course very important, and it is the major defect in diseases as varied as emphysema and pulmonary fibrosis, in which areas of the lung may be expanded, but, because there is only a slow *change* of air within that space, are poorly ventilated.

The Bohr equation

The fact that we can measure partial pressures of gases in the expired air and the volume of air breathed in a minute has enabled those with an appetite for these things to calculate mathematically the way in which the lungs exchange gases between air and blood. These

Ventilation in the respiratory system Box 2

What causes a pneumothorax?

The pressure within the intrapleural space is negative with respect to the atmosphere and with respect to alveolar gas. If any connection is made between the alveoli and the pleura, gas will therefore flow into the intrapleural space. As gas flow takes place, the pressure in the intrapleural space approaches atmospheric. The lung partially collapses and the chest wall expands a little (see Fig. 5.5).

Pneumothoraces can be subdivided into two broad groups, **spontaneous** and **traumatic**. Most are spontaneous. It is thought that they arise as a result of the rupture of a small bulla on the surface of the lung. Bullae are small, thin-walled congenital abnormalities which are filled with air but do not normally affect ventilation. However, if a bulla ruptures through the pleura it may allow gas to enter the intrapleural space from the alveoli and the lung will start to collapse. As the lung collapses, the hole formed by the ruptured bulla is sealed, which prevents more gas from entering the intrapleural cavity. The gas within the intrapleural space is slowly reabsorbed into the blood and the pneumothorax resolves. The time that the pneumothorax takes to resolve depends upon its size, but a small one would be expected to resolve over 1–2 weeks. Larger pneumothoraces, although they would eventually resolve, usually require treatment in order to improve ventilation. Pneumothoraces usually occur in young adults and are about three times more common in men than in women. They also seem to be more common in tall individuals, possibly because in these people the intrapleural pressure at the lung apices is more negative than in smaller people.

As its name suggests, a traumatic pneumothorax is caused by trauma to the chest wall, for example following a stabbing to the chest. Gas may enter the intrapleural space either from the atmosphere through a hole in the chest wall, or from the alveoli through a hole in the lung. It is treated in essentially the same way as a spontaneous pneumothorax.

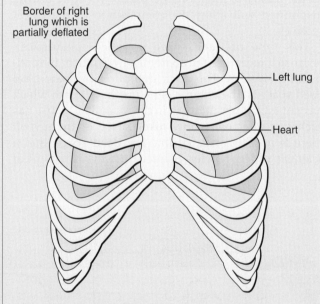

Border of right
lung which is
partially deflated

Left lung

Heart

Fig. 5.5
A right-sided pneumothorax. There is no space between the left lung and the chest wall whereas the right lung is partially collapsed and there is air in the interpleural space.

calculations are not popular with the general run of students, but were not devised deliberately to cause them pain; rather, they are an exact description of what is happening in the lungs, and in the days before medicine became the high-tech subject it is today enabled clinicians, using simple non-invasive techniques, to calculate how much of the lungs was not taking part in gas exchange (dead space), and partial pressures of O_2 and CO_2 in the alveolar gas, and hence in the arterial blood.

The definition of physiological dead space as 'the volume of inspired air which has not taken part in gas exchange' enables dead space to be calculated using a more analytical approach than that of Figure 5.4.

Carl Bohr, in 1891, developed an equation to calculate physiological dead space which is derived from the fact that the volume of gas expired in a single breath (V_T) is the sum of the volume from the physiological dead space (V_D) plus the volume from the alveoli (V_A):

$$V_T = V_D + V_A$$

The total amount of any gas (O_2, CO_2, N_2 or any other) in an expired breath is the volume of that breath (V_T) times the fractional concentration (%) of the gas (F_E) in the whole breath, i.e. ($V_T \times F_E$). This total is made up of the amount from the dead space ($V_D \times F_D$) plus the amount from the alveoli ($V_A \times F_A$):

$$V_T \times F_E = (V_D \times F_D) + (V_A \times F_A)$$

If there is none of the gas (e.g. CO_2) in the dead space, $F_D = 0$ and the equation becomes:

$$V_T \times F_E = V_A \times F_A$$

or
$$V_A = \frac{V_T \times F_E}{F_A}$$

since $V_A - V_T - V_D$
$$V_T - V_D = \frac{V_T \times F_E}{F_A}$$

or
$$V_D = V_T - \frac{V_T \times F_E}{F_A}$$

or
$$V_D = V_T \left(1 - \frac{F_E}{F_A}\right)$$

This is the simplified Bohr equation for CO_2.

Using this equation, and by knowing the volume of air expired, the concentration of CO_2 in it and the concentration of CO_2 in alveolar air, we can calculate dead space.

The volume of air expired and the concentration of CO_2 in it can easily be measured using a spirometer and CO_2 analyser. Figure 5.4 demonstrates the essentials of how to obtain a sample of end-tidal air. The subject breathes out as far as possible into the long thin tube; he then blocks the end of the tube with his tongue, and the gas in the tube nearest him is alveolar

air. Because conditions vary so much in different alveoli the air collected this way is not a very accurate average of alveolar air, and for CO_2 arterial P_{CO_2} is a better index of mixed alveolar CO_2, although obtaining arterial blood from a subject is a very different proposition from asking him to blow down a tube!

Because the fractional concentration (%) of a gas in a mixture is directly related to its partial pressure (P) the Bohr equation is more commonly, and perhaps usefully, expressed as follows:

$$\frac{V_D}{V_T} = \frac{P_{ACO_2} - P_{ECO_2}}{P_{ACO_2}}$$

which gives us the important information that the size of tidal volume influences dead space.

Factors affecting physiological dead space

Because alveolar dead space in healthy individuals is small, anatomical and physiological dead space are identical (about 150 mL in an adult). Like other lung volumes this varies with the size of the individual, and as age, sex and physical training all influence lung volumes they also influence dead space.

Lung volume changes with each breath, being about 3 L at FRC and increasing to up to about 6 L at vital capacity. Under these circumstances dead space will have doubled. Physiological dead space also varies with pattern of breathing. One might imagine that a tidal volume of less than 150 mL would not ventilate the alveoli at all, but during rapid breathing axial streaming causes the fresh air to form a 'needle' in the middle of the airways and this penetrates deep into the alveolar region. This is the principle by which **high-frequency artificial ventilation** is able to ventilate patients using a tidal volume smaller than their anatomical dead space and frequencies up to 10 Hz. This type of artificial ventilation is used when the lungs or chest have been damaged and normal breathing movement and intrapleural pressure changes would make things worse. On the other hand, breath-holding also reduces dead space by increasing the time available for diffusion in the airways and for the mixing action of the movements of the heart. Even if you breathe out immediately after inspiration, expiration is equivalent to breath-holding, with the last gas expelled being subjected to a longer 'breath-hold' than that expelled first.

Alveolar ventilation and respiratory exchange

We have made much of the effect of dead space on lung function, and this is because dead space increases in disease when regions of the lung receive too little blood

Ventilation in the respiratory system Box 3

Diagnosis of a pneumothorax

The diagnosis of a pneumothorax is made from the history, clinical examination and chest X-ray. The patient complains of pleuritic chest pain, and if there is a moderate or large pneumothorax the patient may complain of breathlessness as the affected lung is not well ventilated.

The usual clinical findings on examination are all predictable. Because the affected lung has partially collapsed away from the chest wall, the trachea may appear deviated towards the affected side. Air in the intrapleural space allows the ribcage to expand outwards. For this reason, the affected side of the chest may appear expanded and its movement during respiration may appear reduced compared to the normal side. On percussion the affected side of the chest sounds hyperresonant as a result of the air in the intrapleural space. On auscultation, breath sounds on the affected side are diminished. This is because less gas enters the collapsed lung during inspiration, and the air in the intrapleural space acts as a barrier to the transmission of sounds from the lungs to the chest wall.

The definitive diagnosis of a pneumothorax is made with a chest X-ray. On a chest X-ray of a healthy individual there is no gap between the lungs fields and the inside of the chest wall. Figure 5.6B is a chest X-ray of a patient with a left-sided pneumothorax. On the right, the lung field fills the space within the ribcage, but on the left-hand side the border of the partially collapsed lung is clearly visible and there is a dark area outside the lung caused by air in the intrapleural space.

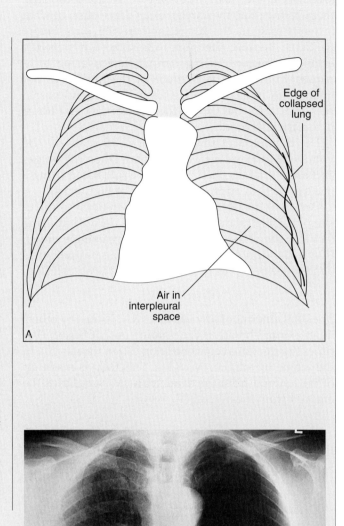

Fig. 5.6

Small left-sided pneumothorax. (A) Diagram showing that the left lung has partially collapsed and there is air between it and the inside of the right chest wall. (B) Chest X-ray of a patient with a left-sided pneumothorax. This chest X-ray is similar to the diagram in (A). The border of the left lung is clearly visible, and the air-filled space between the lung margin and the chest wall appears darker than the adjacent lung on the X-ray.

supply to do the job of gas exchange adequately. Remember, this exchange only takes place in the alveoli, and only in those alveoli that are ventilated and have a blood supply. The gas exchange is of course O_2 for CO_2.

Take, for example, a subject breathing with $V_T = 0.5$ L and $f = 12/\text{min}$: the flow of O_2 in and CO_2 out of the body is carried by a minute ventilation of 6 L min^{-1}. If $V_D = 0.15$ L, ventilation of the alveoli is:

$$6 - (12 \times 0.15) = 4.2 \text{ L min}^{-1}.$$

This is the effective ventilation that brings about the exchange of O_2 and CO_2.

Room air contains virtually no CO_2 and the alveolar gas contains 5.5%, giving an output of:

$$4.2 \times \frac{(5.5 - 0)}{100} = 231 \text{ mL min}^{-1}.$$

Oxygen, on the other hand, forms 21% of the atmosphere and alveolar gas contains about 14%; uptake of oxygen is therefore:

$$4.2 \times \frac{(21 - 14)}{100} = 294 \text{ mL min}^{-1}.$$

The ratio of CO_2 output divided by O_2 uptake is called the **respiratory exchange ratio** (or respiratory quotient, when used to describe the exchange in tissues or cells). It is usually given the symbol R and can range from 1, when only carbohydrates are being metabolized, to 0.7 when fats are being used. The ratio depends on the amount of oxygen already in the molecule being oxidized: the more oxygen the molecule contains the less has to be 'brought in' to complete the oxidation. For the figures above:

$$R = \frac{231}{294} = 0.79.$$

The partial pressure of O_2 or CO_2 in the alveoli depends on the rate at which it is being brought in (O_2) or removed (CO_2) by ventilation:

For CO_2:

$$P_{ACO_2} = \frac{\dot{V}_{CO_2}}{\dot{V}_A} \times K$$

where K is a constant which takes into account the air is being warmed and moistened within the lungs, P_{ACO_2} is partial pressure in the alveoli or arterial blood, $\dot{V}_{CO_2}$ is the rate of production of CO_2 by the body and $\dot{V}_A$ is alveolar ventilation.

The alveolar gas equation

Once P_{ACO_2} has been calculated P_{AO_2} can be calculated using what is known as the **alveolar gas equation**. If the respiratory exchange ratio was 1, then for each molecule of O_2 taken up one molecule of CO_2 would be released, and:

$$P_{AO_2} = P_{IO_2} - P_{ACO_2}$$

However, R is seldom 1, and P_{AO_2} is computed using the slightly intimidating alveolar gas equation:

$$P_{AO_2} = P_{IO_2} - P_{ACO_2} \times \left[\frac{\text{Fraction}_{IO_2} + 1 - \text{Fraction}_{IO_2}}{R} \right]$$

The correction factor in the square brackets is there to take care of R not being exactly 1 and its effect on the concentration of N_2 in the alveoli.

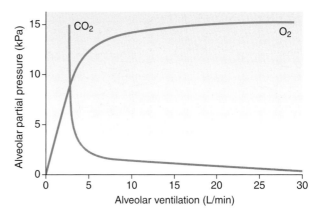

Fig. 5.7
The relationship between alveolar ventilation and alveolar P_{O_2} and P_{CO_2}. Alveolar P_{CO_2} varies inversely with ventilation in an asymptotic fashion. P_{O_2} rises with increasing ventilation and reaches a plateau.

A simplified form of this equation is:

$$P_{AO_2} = P_{IO_2} - \frac{P_{ACO_2}}{R} + \text{a correction for the concentration of } N_2$$

(usually < 3, which can be ignored)

The effect of changing alveolar ventilation on alveolar partial pressure of O_2 and CO_2 is shown graphically in Figure 5.7. It is clear that increased or decreased ventilation has opposite effects on the alveolar concentrations of these two gases. You will see later (Chapter 8, Gas transport) that this does not mean that the amount of O_2 carried into the circulation can increase or decrease in a linear fashion, as does CO_2, because in the case of O_2 the carriage is limited by the capacity of a carrier rather than the amount flowing into the lungs.

Distribution of inspired gas

Because the bronchial tree consists of a large number of paths in parallel, differences of composition can, and do, exist in **series** (along any path, from lips to alveoli for example or between **regions** (between right and left lung for example). These differences can become so large as to interfere with the functioning of the lungs and are due to the following effects.

Series differences

You can see from Figure 5.4 that the concentration of CO_2 in an expired breath does not rise as a sudden step to its alveolar value, as you might have expected from the series arrangement of anatomical dead space and alveolar space described so far. In other words, there

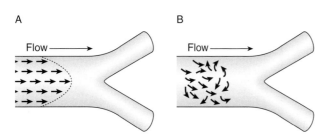

Fig. 5.8
Laminar and turbulent flow. Laminar flow moves in organized layers parallel to the sides of the airway, with the maximum velocity at the centre. Turbulent flow is disorganized and the velocity profile is flat.

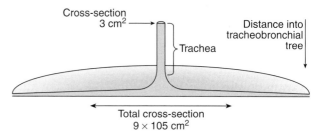

Fig. 5.9
Airways cross-sectional area. Total cross-sectional area increases as you penetrate deeper into the bronchial tree. The area of the alveolar respiratory surface, represented by the horizontal line, is 300 000 times greater than the cross-sectional area of the trachea.

is not a clear-cut boundary between the two spaces. This is due to several factors:

- The flow may be laminar or turbulent (Fig. 5.8) and both cause a gradient of concentration along the tube. In laminar flow the front is not square because of axial streaming, and in turbulent flow the square front mixes with the original air as it advances.
- Turbulent eddies at the points of branching of the airways and the churning action of the beating heart mix gas in the airways.
- Unequal pathway lengths from the respiratory surface to the lips mean alveolar gas has different distances to go to reach the lips.
- Differences in compliance and resistance of different regions mean they have different 'time constants' and take different lengths of time to fill and empty.

These considerations apply to both inspired and expired air flowing through the conducting airways of the lung.

As inspired air approaches the alveoli it moves into a region of rapidly increasing cross-sectional area and volume (see Fig. 2.5 and Fig. 5.9). The airways can be likened to a trumpet with a very wide mouth. The consequence of this is that the forward velocity of the gas slows down almost to a standstill, and the gas moves more by diffusion than by bulk flow. This slowing down of the advancing front allows concentration gradients to build up along the smaller airways. This **stratification** of inspired gas reduces the concentration of fresh air near the respiratory surface, but is not dangerously important in healthy lungs. However, in some lung diseases (e.g., emphysema) the geometry of the airways is changed, increasing the distance for diffusion and hence the effects of stratification to unacceptable levels.

Similarly, when direct pathways to the alveolar surface are blocked by disease the only ventilation may be by collateral channels (pores of Kohn) in the walls of adjacent normally ventilated alveoli.

Regional differences

Clinically more important differences in the composition of alveolar gas exist between **regions** of the lungs. These are due to:

1. differences in regional ventilation causing different dilutions of alveolar gas by inspired air, and
2. different blood flows exchanging O_2 and CO_2 with the alveolar gas at different rates (this effect is dealt with in Chapter 7).

The greatest difference in regional ventilation in a normal standing man is between the TOP and the BOTTOM of the lungs, ventilation in a horizontal plane being about the same in different regions.

To explain this vertical difference in regional ventilation we first must remember that:

- ventilation is the amount of gas moved into and out of a region, irrespective of the initial volume of that region;
- the motive force which brings about ventilation is change in the intrapleural pressure around the lungs, which becomes more negative (compared to the atmosphere) during inspiration, expanding the lungs (Chapter 3, p. 32);
- the effect of gravity on the contents of the chest is to cause intrapleural pressure to be less negative at the BOTTOM of the lungs than at the TOP. It increases (gets less negative) by about 0.025 kPa for every centimetre you move towards the base of the lung (see Chapter 3, p. 32).

The effect of this **gravity-induced** gradient of intrapleural pressure is clearly seen if the structure of the lungs of man or other mammal in the upright position at the end of expiration (FRC) is looked at under the microscope (Fig. 5.11). We see that the alveoli at the top are expanded to nearly their full size, whereas those at the bottom are only slightly expanded.

What happens when you breathe in from this situation was discovered in an ingenious series of experiments using the radioactive gas Xenon (^{133}Xe).

The radioactive gas was used to inflate isolated lungs suspended in a pressure gradient that mimicked that found in the upright human chest, i.e. increasing by 0.025 kPa for every centimetre moved towards the base. This can be achieved by placing the lungs in a foam of appropriate density. The amount of radioactive gas in a region at any time during the inflation can be measured by radioactivity counters placed over the surface of the lungs (Fig. 5.12).

Although these effects are exerted in a continuous fashion from top to bottom, for simplicity we can treat the lungs as if they were just two regions, upper and lower lobes, say.

The vertical axis of Figure 5.12 gives the volume of the upper and lower regions of the isolated lungs as a percentage of their ultimate volume when fully inflated. The horizontal axis gives the volume of the whole lungs, i.e. that of all regions. If the lungs were free of any gradient of pressure, both the upper and the lower regions would expand at the same rate and the points representing these volumes would fall along the same line, shown as a dotted line in Figure 5.12. With a pressure gradient applied over the lungs,

Ventilation in the respiratory system Box 4

Treatment of a pneumothorax

Mr Price's pneumothorax was treated using a **chest drain**. This consists of a length of plastic tubing inserted into the intrapleural space through a small incision made under local anaesthetic between two of Mr Price's ribs. The chest drain allows air to escape from the intrapleural space so that the underlying lung can reinflate.

So that the chest drain removes air from the intrapleural space rather than allowing more air to enter, it is necessary to place a one-way valve on the end of the drain. This usually takes the form of an **underwater seal** (Fig. 5.10). An underwater seal consists of a container of water with a tube extending below the surface of the water. Gas can pass from the tube into the atmosphere by forming bubbles in the water, but no gas can pass back up the tube and the water effectively acts as a one-way valve at the end of the tube.

As the pressure in the intrapleural space becomes positive, for example during coughing or forced expiration, air passes along the chest drain and out to the atmosphere through the underwater seal and the pneumothorax is drained. If additional air enters the intrapleural space from the defect in the visceral pleura, that air is drained from the pneumothorax too. Bubbles appear in the underwater seal until the hole in the pleura has sealed. After the hole has healed, the chest drain can be removed. As well as draining air from the intrapleural space, the underwater seal also collects blood and other secretions that pass along the chest drain and which would clog up a mechanical valve.

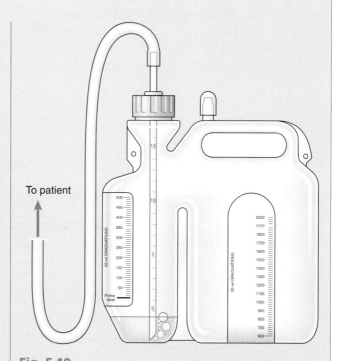

Fig. 5.10

An underwater seal. Gas from the pneumothorax passes from the chest drain and bubbles through the water in the seal. The water prevents gas passing from the atmosphere into the intrapleural space and also collects blood and other liquid secretions which might block a mechanical value.

Chest drains may also be used to drain blood that has accumulated in the intrapleural space (a haemothorax), for example as a result of chest trauma.

VENTILATION OF THE RESPIRATORY SYSTEM

5

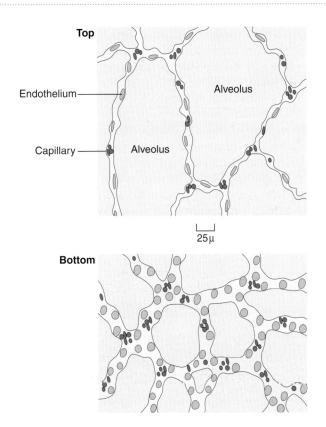

the two regions behave differently. The slope of the lines in Figure 5.12 represents the rate of change of volume: the steeper the slope the greater the rate of inflation. The cubes represent the fraction of its maximum achievable volume a cube of lung from top or bottom has achieved at that moment.

You can see:

- The lower lobe starts at a smaller percentage of maximal volume because it is compressed by the greater external pressure.
- It follows that the ventilatory capacity of the upper region is smaller than that of the lower, i.e. it operates in the range between 40% and 100% of its total volume range, whereas the lower lobe operates in

◀ **Fig. 5.11**
Alveolar dimensions at the top and bottom of the upright lung. These are images of the alveolar region of the top and bottom of a lung frozen in the upright position. In the top of the lung the alveoli are distended and the capillaries empty of blood compared with those in the bottom of the lung. This effect is due largely to gravity.

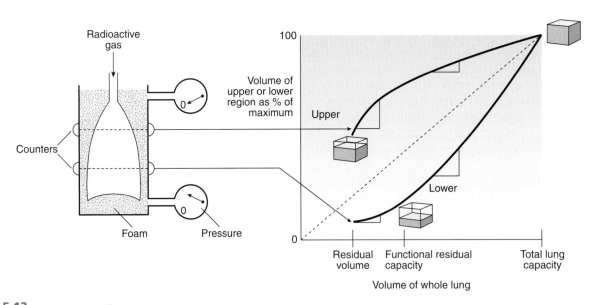

Fig. 5.12
The effect of gravity on ventilation. An excised lung is surrounded by foam to mimic the gradient of pleural pressure that exists due to gravity, and caused to 'breathe' radioactive gas. Ventilation in different areas is measured as the amount of radioactivity that goes to those areas with 'inspiration'. The graph shows the the volumes of the upper and lower parts of the lungs (ordinate) as total lung volume (abscissa) increases from residual volume to total lung capacity. The cubes illustrate what fraction of its potential volume unit lung volume at the top or bottom contains at different total lung volumes.

Ventilation in the respiratory system Box 5

Tension pneumothorax – a medical emergency

As we have seen, pneumothoraces are caused when gas enters the intrapleural space. In the majority of cases, gas flow stops when the pressure in the intrapleural space reaches atmospheric. Very rarely, the pressure within the intrapleural space continues to rise above atmospheric. This is usually because the defect in the lung wall behaves like a valve, allowing gas to enter the intrapleural space without allowing it to leave. Gas enters the intrapleural space when the pressure within the alveoli is positive: this is particularly a problem in patients whose lungs are being artificially ventilated, either in an intensive care unit or in an operating theatre.

As the pressure within the intrapleural space rises, the mediastinum is pushed *away* from the affected side. Pressure on the heart and the major vessels within the mediastinum results in cardiac output being reduced, and the displacement of the other lung may result in gas exchange being compromised. In severe cases, cardiovascular collapse occurs. Figure 5.13 shows an X-ray of a tension pneumothorax. The right lung is almost completely collapsed and the heart and mediastinum are deviated away from the affected side.

A tension pneumothorax is a medical emergency. Urgent release of the trapped gas is necessary. This is achieved by the prompt insertion of any available cannula through the chest wall into the intrapleural space. In most wards intravenous cannulas are readily available and are usually used for this purpose. Gas escapes under pressure with an audible hiss and the cardiorespiratory status rapidly improves. Once the patient has been stabilized, a formal chest drain can be inserted.

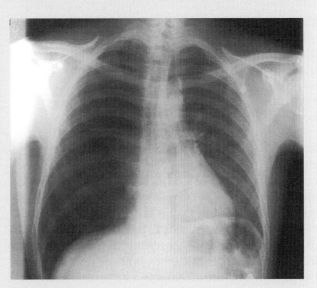

Fig. 5.13
Chest X-ray of a patient with a right tension pneumothorax. The air in the pneumothorax is under pressure and the heart and other structures are pushed *away* from the affected side.

the 15–100% range. This is because the upper region is more inflated initially.

- At volumes well below FRC there is proportionally more rapid inflation of the upper regions (compare the slopes of the lines in Figure 5.12). This is because at these volumes some of the airways to the lower lobes close, and it takes a critical pressure to re-expand them.
- At larger lung volumes the situation reverses and there is more ventilation of the lower region.

In deflation of the lungs the points in Figure 5.12 representing the volumes of the two lung regions move down the two curves, reversing the effects described.

It should be remembered that human lungs are roughly cone shaped, there being more tissue at the base than at the apex. This amplifies the effect of greater ventilation going to the base of the lung.

Other factors influencing distribution

Age

The degenerative changes of ageing produce differences in the mechanical properties of the lung regions. These cause ventilation to become increasingly non-uniform. The critical **closing volume** of the airways (the lung volume at which airways start to close) increases with age, and this becomes very important when some airways remain closed throughout the whole of a normal breath and make parts of the lung useless for gas exchange.

Airways muscle tone

Substances that increase airways smooth muscle **tone** and cause bronchoconstriction e.g. histamine, increase

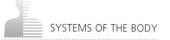
5

VENTILATION OF THE RESPIRATORY SYSTEM

non-uniform distribution of ventilation by non-uniformly changing the mechanical properties of regions of the lungs. Abolition of airways muscle tone also reduces uniformity of distribution. This suggests that normal muscle tone minimizes non-uniform distribution. The pharmalogical management of bronchoconstriction is dealt with in Chapter 4, p. 54.

Posture

Patterns of both lung ventilation and perfusion change with changes in posture, owing to changes in the direction in which **gravity** is acting. If the lung in Figure 5.12 were to be 'stood on its head', or if a subject stands on his head, the best-ventilated region of the lung now becomes what was the apex, because it has become the base.

This tidy explanation of distribution of ventilation in terms of the direction in which gravity is acting has recently received a blow. Astronauts under conditions of zero gravity would be expected to have uniform ventilation over the whole of their lungs. Not so. Although the differences in ventilation are markedly reduced, there still remains a slight top-to-bottom gradient of ventilation. This may be the result of the subjects spending most of their lives under normal gravity before they became astronauts. Gravity may have left a permanent mark on the regional mechanical properties of their lungs. We must wait until we can test the first individual to be born and spend his whole life in zero gravity before we can completely describe the effects of gravity on the lungs.

Pathological changes

Dramatic and acute changes, such as pneumothorax (see Boxes 1–5), can affect the distribution of ventilation between and within the lungs, in that case by limiting the expansion of one lung (Fig. 5.14A). Normal ageing, and less dramatic conditions, alters the distribution of ventilation and, to a greater or lesser extent, perfusion. Airway obstruction (Fig. 5.14B), found in asthma and bronchitis, restricts supply to the region served by the airway, and diseases such as emphysema change the compliance (Fig. 5.14C) and collapse of airways (Fig. 5.14D).

Ventilation in the respiratory system Box 6

Pneumonia

Mrs O'Donnell is a 70-year-old retired woman who lives alone. She has been troubled for some years with a chronic cough as a result of her smoking: she has smoked 20 cigarettes per day for over 50 years. She often finds that after a cold, for example, she develops a worsening cough, productive of green sputum.

On one occasion, however, after what seemed a relatively minor cold, she developed worsening respiratory symptoms. Her cough became much worse than usual and was productive of quite large volumes of sputum. She felt very unwell and was hot but shivery. She also felt quite breathless and tired, and was finding it increasingly difficult to cope at home.

She called her general practitioner, who came out to see her. He examined Mrs O'Donnell and decided that she should be admitted to the local hospital. In hospital, Mrs O'Donnell was examined by the doctors and a chest X-ray was performed and some blood taken. A sample of the sputum that Mrs O'Donnell was coughing up was also sent for analysis. A diagnosis of pneumonia was made on the basis of Mrs O'Donnell's symptoms, signs, chest X-ray appearance and laboratory results.

We will consider:

① The diagnosis of pneumonia and what causes it.
② How pneumonia is treated.

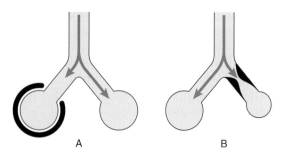
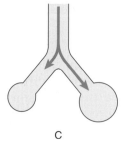
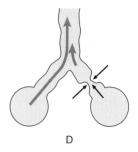

Fig. 5.14

Some pathological changes affecting distribution of ventilation. (A) Restriction, (B) obstruction, (C) change in compliance, (D) airway collapse.

Ventilation in the respiratory system Box 7

The diagnosis of pneumonia

Pneumonia essentially means an infection of the lung. It is not a rare condition and affects about two adults per 1000 in the community. It is responsible for far more deaths than all other types of infection put together. Pneumonia is usually caused by bacterial infections, and the most common bacterium to cause pneumonia outside hospitals is *Streptococcus pneumoniae*, which causes about half of all such pneumonias. Other bacteria that cause pneumonia include:

- *Haemophilus influenzae*, which is particularly common in patients with pre-existing lung disease such as chronic bronchitis
- *Staphylococcus aureus*, which is more common in children and intravenous drug abusers.

About one-fifth of pneumonias are caused by unusual agents such as:

- *Mycoplasma pneumoniae*, the second commonest bacterial cause of pneumonia
- *Chlamydia psittaci*, which causes **psittacosis**, a pneumonia caught from caged birds
- *Coxiella burnetti*, which causes **Q fever**, a pneumonia acquired from animal hides
- *Legionella pneumophila*, which causes **legionnaire's disease**, a pneumonia which was first identified in 1976. The disease was caught by several members of the American Legion (an ex-servicemen's association) who were attending a conference at a hotel in Philadelphia. *Legionella*, which had not previously been identified, had infected the water in the hotel's air-conditioning unit. Droplets of infected water in the air in the hotel were inhaled by the legionnaires, causing the disease.

Pneumonias caused by these agents are often known as **atypical pneumonias**.

Pneumonia may also be caused by viruses (most commonly by the influenza A virus) and of course by *Mycobacterium tuberculosis*, which is the agent that causes tuberculosis. A much wider spectrum of agents causes pneumonia in patients in hospital. Pneumonia acquired in hospital is sometimes called **nosocomial pneumonia**.

The term **lobar pneumonia** refers to the infection of one lobe of a lung, whereas **bronchopneumonia** refers to a more widespread infection. Infection causes the accumulation of fluid and pus in the alveoli and airways. This means that there is reduced or no ventilation to the affected areas. The blood that continues to flow through these areas therefore remains deoxygenated. Patients with pneumonia usually complain of

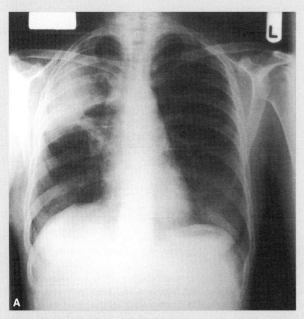

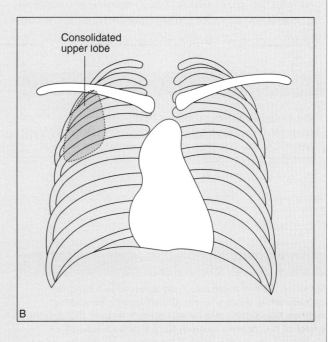

Consolidated upper lobe

Fig. 5.15

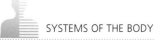
Ventilation in the respiratory system Box 7   (*continued*)

The diagnosis of pneumonia

fever and a cough, although the cough is not always productive at the start of the illness. If the area of infection extends to the pleura, then the patient may complain of pleuritic chest pain over the infected area.

On examination the patient usually has a fever, and may have reduced air entry on the affected side. If the patient is suffering from a lobar pneumonia, the chest wall over the area of infection may be dull to percussion and on auscultation may reveal bronchial breath sounds over the affected lobe. Bronchial breath sounds are harsher than normal because the fluid in the affected lobe conducts sound from the trachea better than does air.

Mrs O'Donnell's chest X-ray is shown in Figure 5.15 and shows an area of right upper lobe consolidation (fluid-filled lung) caused by her right upper lobe pneumonia. Note that the infection has a clearly defined lower border. This is because the area of infection lies completely within the upper lobe. The lower border of the opacification on the chest X-ray is the lower border of the upper lobe.

Blood tests often show a raised white cell count (often greater than 15×10^9 L^{-1}), and in the microbiology laboratory the causative agent may be identified from sputum samples and its sensitivity to a range of antibiotics can be ascertained.

Ventilation in the respiratory system Box 8

Treatment of pneumonia

After the diagnosis of pneumonia had been made, Mrs O'Donnell was given some oxygen and started on a course of penicillin. Laboratory tests confirmed that her pneumonia had been caused by *Streptococcus pneumoniae* and that it was sensitive to the penicillin she was being given. Her condition improved over the next few days and she was allowed home.

The mainstay of treatment for pneumonia is antibiotic therapy. Treatment can be tailored to the particular infective agent that is causing the pneumonia after it has been identified from sputum samples in the

microbiology laboratory; however, antibiotics are usually started before these results are available, on the basis of a 'best guess' as to the likely infective organism, as was done for Mrs O'Donnell. The choice of antibiotic can later be modified in the light of laboratory data.

Other supportive measures may include oxygen to help maintain oxygenation of the patients' blood, paracetamol to relieve the fever, fluids to keep the patient well hydrated, and analgesics to relieve pleuritic chest pain.

Further reading

Barnes PJ. The third nervous system in the lung: physiology and clinical perspectives. Thorax 1984;39:561

Hlastala MP. Ventilation. In: Crystal RG, West JB, Barnes PJ, Weibel ER, eds. The lung: scientific foundations, 2nd edn. New York: Raven Press, 1997

Paiva M. Uneven ventilation. In: Crystal RG, West JB, Barnes PJ, Weibel ER, eds. The lung: scientific foundations, 2nd edn. New York: Raven Press, 1997

West JB. Regional differences in gas exchange in the lung of erect man. J Appl Physiol 1962;17:893

Self-assessment case study

Mr Jones, a 35-year-old man, was involved in a head-on collision while driving his car. Unfortunately, he was not wearing his seatbelt and he was thrown against the steering wheel of his car with so much force that he fractured a number of ribs on the front of his ribcage. Luckily, he did not sustain any other major injuries. He was taken to hospital by

ambulance and was given oxygen to breathe during the journey.

He found breathing very difficult, each breath being very painful. On arrival at the Accident and Emergency department the casualty doctor noticed that part of Mr Jones' chest was moving in an abnormal manner during inspiration. An area over the front of the chest was moving *inwards* during inspiration, instead of *outwards* like the rest of the chest. Furthermore, Mr Jones was finding breathing increasingly difficult and painful. The casualty doctor diagnosed a *flail segment* in Mr Jones' chest. The doctor performed a chest X-ray to ensure that Mr Jones did not have a pneumothorax. This revealed that Mr Jones had fractured a number of ribs, but no pneumothorax was present.

As Mr Jones' condition was not improving an anaesthetist was called who gave Mr Jones a general anaesthetic and inserted a plastic tube into his trachea. He attached Mr Jones to a machine to ventilate his lungs. The machine periodically inflated Mr Jones' lungs with a fixed volume of oxygen and air. On the ventilator, the section of Mr Jones' chest that was previously moving *inwards* during inspiration was now moving *outwards* in the same manner as the rest of Mr Jones' chest.

Mr Jones was transferred to intensive care, where mechanical ventilation of his lungs could be continued until his condition improved.

After reading this chapter you should be able to answer the following questions:

① Why was a segment of Mr Jones' chest moving in the opposite direction to the rest of his chest?

② Why might Mr Jones have had a pneumothorax?

③ Why was Mr Jones finding breathing difficult?

④ Why, when he was on a ventilator, did the flail segment of Mr Jones' chest now move in the same direction as the rest of his chest during breathing?

Answers see page 176

Answers see page 176

Self-assessment questions

① Which of the following lung volumes cannot be measured with a spirometer alone, and why? (a) residual volume, (b) tidal volume, (c) functional residual capacity, (d) vital capacity, (e) total lung capacity?

② What is the relationship between anatomical dead space, physiological dead space and alveolar dead space? To what might the physiological dead space of a healthy subject be approximately numerically related?

③ What is the major type of inhomogeneity of ventilation in the healthy subject, and by what is it caused?

④ What is the value of alveolar dead space in healthy subjects?

⑤ What is FEV_1?

⑥ Define respiratory exchange ratio.

Answers see page 177

GAS EXCHANGE BETWEEN AIR AND BLOOD: DIFFUSION

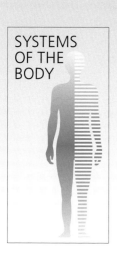

SYSTEMS
OF THE
BODY

Chapter objectives

After studying this chapter you should be able to:

① Explain the 'series' nature of diffusion in the lungs.

② State Fick's Law of Diffusion.

③ Define diffusing capacity and explain why the term transfer factor is preferred.

④ Relate the properties of O_2 and CO_2 to the influence of pathology on their transfer.

⑤ Explain why the equilibrium for O_2 is established at about the same rate as that for CO_2.

⑥ Outline the important components limiting rate of transfer in the lungs and how they are affected by disease.

⑦ Explain the selection of CO as a gas to measure transfer factor.

⑧ Explain why ventilation rather than diffusion is the most important factor in the transfer of CO_2.

The path from air to tissue

The lungs are so good at maintaining O_2 levels in the blood that it was until quite recently thought to be an active process, with the body actively extracting O_2 from the air. It is now known that the process is purely passive diffusion down concentration gradients. Diffusion is so important to our obtaining O_2 that the ability of the lungs to allow diffusion to happen is frequently measured, and is sometimes called the lung's **diffusing capacity**. This capacity is reduced in many diseases, including fibrosis, asbestosis, sarcoidosis and pneumonia.

In Chapter 5 we described the way in which ventilation of different regions of the lung results in different compositions of gas in the alveoli. In understanding the next step in the journey from air to blood or blood to air it is important to differentiate clearly between the *amount* of a gas present in a mixture at a site and the fraction or *concentration* of that gas, frequently expressed as **partial pressure** *(P)*. This concept is important because it is only the difference in partial pressure that drives diffusion from one place to another. To use an analogy: the pressure across the enormous lock gates holding the Atlantic Ocean out of a dock in which the water is 10 cm lower than the ocean is the same as that across the walls of a child's paddling pool containing water 10 cm deep. The amounts of water either side (or gas in the case of the lung) having nothing to do with the motive force (driving pressure): the difference in *depth* of water (or difference in *partial pressure of gas*) provides the motive force.

The partial pressure of a gas depends on its concentration, and so the partial pressure gradient across a membrane depends on the difference in concentration on either side. It is diffusion alone that transports gas between air and blood at the lungs, and between blood and cells at the tissues, and the circulation of blood effectively links the two sites. In the case of O_2 (Fig. 6.1) we can see that diffusion at the lungs is sufficient to reduce to virtually zero any difference in partial pressure (concentration) between alveolar air and pulmonary blood, whereas at the tissues a large difference in partial pressure between arterial blood and the mitochondria ensures a vigorous flow into these organelles of oxidative metabolism.

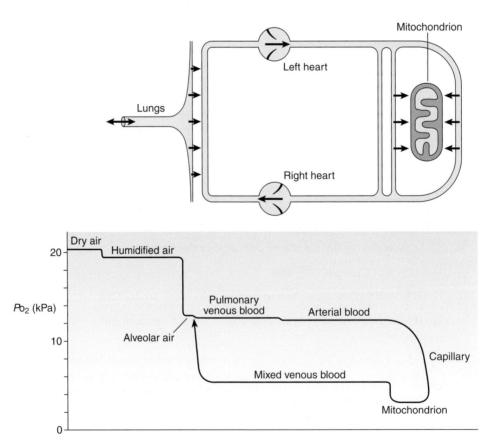

Fig. 6.1
The path of oxygen. The physical path is shown as a diagram above. The partial pressure of O_2 in air, blood and tissue fluid at the different points on its journey is shown below.

The single step of O_2 from air to blood in Figure 6.1 is in fact a series of steps through components which are in series and which will be considered in detail below. The important thing to remember is that they are **in series** (i.e. one after another), like the segments of a hosepipe made up of a number of bits joined together. *Constricting one segment reduces flow in all.*

Lung disease and diffusion

The lungs have such an enormous capacity for diffusion that there is some doubt in many diseases (e.g. emphysema) as to what part the impairment of diffusion plays in producing the characteristic hypoxia of the disease. In many cases a diffusional component can only be demonstrated when the patient is exercising. The destruction of the architecture of the respiratory regions in emphysema (Fig. 4.16) must impair diffusion, but the effect on distribution of ventilation and blood flow must be at least as important. Other diseases (e.g. interstitial pulmonary fibrosis) which produce profound thickening of the respiratory membranes reduce the lungs' capacity for diffusion to one-sixth of normal, and it is difficult to assume that this does not affect their function.

Fick's Law of Diffusion

The movement of gas into and out the blood is described by Fick's Law (Appendix, p. 170), which describes the rate of diffusion of a gas across a membrane as follows:

$$\text{Rate of diffusion} = \frac{A \times S (\Delta C)}{t \sqrt{MW}}$$

where A is the area of the membrane available for diffusion. S is the solubility of the gas in the membrane, ΔC is the concentration gradient – brought about by the differences in concentration (or partial pressure) either side of the membrane – t is the thickness of the membrane and MW is the molecular weight of the gas (Fig. 6.2).

The area available for diffusion is the area of the pulmonary capillaries that is in contact with alveolar air. This area can be changed by diseases which destroy alveolar septa, and by changes during exercise, when capillaries that were closed at rest open up and those already open become distended.

The solubility of a gas determines the rate of diffusion of a gas in solution. The gases we are particularly interested in are CO_2 and O_2. Carbon dioxide is 23 times more soluble in tissue fluid than is O_2 but has a higher molecular weight; it will therefore diffuse from blood to air 20 times more readily for the same partial pressure gradient than will O_2 moving in the opposite

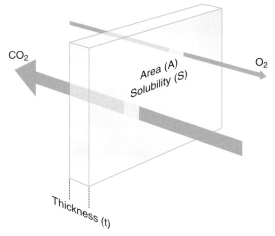

Fig. 6.2
Diffusion through a membrane. It is obvious that gas will diffuse more quickly if the area is great, the thickness is small and the concentration difference of the gas, which is highly soluble in the membrane, is high.

Gas exchange between air and blood: diffusion Box 1

Fibrosing alveolitis

Mr Paterson is 65 years old. Although he has never smoked, he has become increasingly breathless over the past few months, particularly when he exerts himself. He went to see his doctor, who examined him. He found that Mr Paterson was rather breathless and had finger-clubbing (see Fig. 1.3). He found that Mr Paterson's chest expansion was reduced on both sides and on auscultation he heard fine inspiratory crepitations (crackles) all over Mr Paterson's chest, but particularly over the bases of his lungs. He decided to refer Mr Paterson to a respiratory physician at the local hospital.

In this chapter we will consider:

① The clinical features of cryptogenic fibrosing alveolitis.
② The diagnosis and treatment of cryptogenic fibrosing alveolitis.

direction. However, equilibrium for CO_2 is established at about the same rate as for O_2 because:

1. the **reaction** releasing CO_2 from blood is relatively slow
2. the concentration **gradient** driving CO_2 from blood to alveolar air is only 0.8 kPa, whereas that driving O_2 in the opposite direction is 8 kPa.

Although the process of diffusion is a physical one, chemical reactions exert their influence on this process in the lungs. In particular, the rate at which O_2 can be taken up or released by haemoglobin in the red blood corpuscles (RBC) acts as a rate-limiting step, reducing its overall rate of transfer.

Although there are situations when the lung can be so damaged as to restrict the diffusion of CO_2 it is usually O_2 that is first affected by diffusional difficulties. The rate of removal of CO_2 is governed primarily by alveolar ventilation (Chapter 6; p. 90).

In Figure 6.1 we can see three places where diffusion is the major transport mechanism and where this transport can effectively be impeded by failure of diffusion:

1. Within the alveoli
2. From the alveolar air to the RBC
3. From the RBC to the tissue mitochondria.

As this is a textbook on the respiratory system we will concentrate on the first two. The anatomical sites of these two sources of impedance to diffusion are shown in Figure 6.3.

Within the alveoli

In healthy lungs the average diameter of the alveoli is about 200 µm. Any differences in the concentrations of the respiratory gases at different points

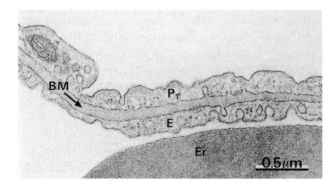

Fig. 6.3
The site of diffusion in the lungs. The distance involved in diffusion within the alveolar space is much greater than the distance within the lung tissue. However, diffusion within the alveolar space is in air and therefore much more rapid than in the tissue. The diffusional barrier between blood and alveolar air consists of attenuated cytoplasm of a Type 1 pneumocyte P_1, a common basement membrane BM, cytoplasm of a capillary endothelial cell E. Er is an erythrocyte in a capillary. Source: Stevens et al 2002.

within the alveolus will be obliterated by diffusion over these distances in less than 10 ms. It might be imagined, however, that in emphysema (where the air spaces are enlarged) increased distances for diffusion slow O_2 transport to unacceptable levels. Although it is true that these changes in geometry must have an effect, destruction of the alveolar septa, reducing surface area, together with ventilation/perfusion mismatching, exerts a malign influence in this disease well before diffusion problems need be considered.

Air to RBC

This step from air to blood or blood to air has a number of components of its own:

- Length of time blood is in the capillaries
- Crossing the alveolar/capillary membrane
- Diffusion in the blood plasma
- Reaction with haemoglobin.

Time in the capillaries
Although blood flow through the lungs is highly pulsatile (p. 95) it is legitimate when considering diffusion to consider blood flowing smoothly and taking on average 0.8 s to transit the pulmonary capillary. The way concentration and hence the partial pressure of O_2 in the blood changes during transit along the capillary is shown in Figure 6.4.

Consideration of this figure reveals a number of potential complications which can arise because:

- There are great differences in transit time through different regions of the lung. Transit times less than 0.2 s do not allow sufficient time for equilibration, and capillaries with these low transit times pass deoxygenated blood to the pulmonary veins. This is functionally equivalent to a spread of $\dot{V}/\dot{Q}$ (ventilation/perfusion) ratios, and this is 'a bad thing' (see Chapter 7).
- During heavy exercise cardiac output increases and all transit times are reduced.
- At altitude the partial pressure of ambient O_2 driving O_2 into the blood is reduced. This effect is shown as a dotted line in Figure 6.4. Clearly, exercise at altitude is the worst of all possible combinations, except for disease, and these effects account for much of the limitation of mountaineering achievement.

Crossing the alveolar membrane
The lining epithelium and basement membrane of the alveoli and the endothelium and basement membrane of the pulmonary capillaries are each about 0.2 µm

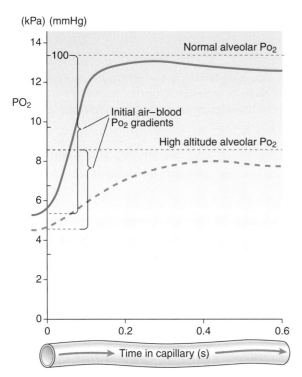

(kPa) (mmHg)

Fig. 6.4
Partial pressure of O$_2$ in blood during its transit through a pulmonary capillary. This example shows the mean transit time for a population which has an high degree of variation. The broken line represents reduced partial pressure of oxygen (as at altitude).

thick on *one side* of the capillary and somewhat thicker on the other, supporting, side (Fig. 6.3). The capillaries occupy most of the alveolar wall, generally being less than one capillary diameter apart, and with each capillary passing through up to three alveoli. It might be expected that diseases such as pulmonary fibrosis, sarcoidosis, asbestosis and pulmonary oedema, which affect the alveolar/capillary membrane, would interfere with diffusion. Remarkably, however, these problems seem to affect diffusion less than might be expected, because they are usually found on the inactive, supporting, side of the pulmonary capillary, leaving the functional side relatively undamaged. Their major effects are to reduce the surface area for diffusion by gross destruction of tissue and increased ventilation/perfusion mismatching.

Diffusion in blood plasma
Red blood corpuscles are about the same diameter as pulmonary capillaries: in fact, they have to be distorted to squeeze through many capillaries. This means there is very little plasma between the corpuscle and the capillary wall for gas to diffuse through. Also, the 'doughnut' shape of the corpuscles means that most of the

haemoglobin within is close to the wall, again shortening the distance for diffusion. The 'kneading' of the corpuscles as they squeeze through the capillaries probably causes mass movements of haemoglobin within the corpuscle, which also aids diffusion.

Reaction with haemoglobin
As the vast majority of O$_2$ in the blood is carried by haemoglobin, the rate at which they combine is an important limiting step in O$_2$ diffusion into the blood.

Because the transfer of O$_2$ into the blood is profoundly affected by such factors as reaction rates with haemoglobin and transit time through pulmonary capillaries, which have nothing to do with the physical process of diffusion, it has been suggested that 'diffusing capacity' is an inappropriate term to describe the process. In England, where both the language and the technique for measuring this transfer were developed, the term **transfer factor** is generally preferred.

Measuring transfer factor

It is important, clinically and scientifically, to be able to measure transfer factor (diffusing capacity). The physiology on which the technique of measuring transfer factor is based will repay study here.

Transfer factor is primarily to do with the rate at which the lungs allow O$_2$ to diffuse into the blood. We wish to measure this – or at least to compare this ability in people we know are normal with those suspected of having lung disease.

Frequently when we say we are measuring something we are in fact comparing it with a known standard. (When we carry out the simple act of measuring someone's height we are in fact comparing their length with 'the distance travelled by light in a vacuum in 1/299 792 458 seconds', which is the physicists' definition of the metre, but any other standard length would do. We could use the 'hand' (102 mm), normally used to measure the height of horses, so long as we define what we are using. Applying this principle to transfer factor means we do not have to actually measure the flow of O$_2$ into the body to compare transfer factor between people: we can measure the flux of another, more convenient, gas so long as it is influenced by the same things as those that influence O$_2$ transfer. This is fortunate because, as we will see, O$_2$ presents difficulties.

How do we choose a gas to measure transfer factor?

Transfer factor (diffusing capacity) =

Rate of transfer of the gas from lung to blood
───────────────────────────────────────
Driving partial pressure (alveolus–blood)

Gas exchange between air and blood: diffusion Box 2

Diagnosis and treatment of fibrosing alveolitis

At the local hospital, Mr Paterson was seen by the respiratory physician. The physician took a careful history from Mr Paterson, including details of all the occupations which Mr Paterson had had since he left school. His examination confirmed all the findings of Mr Paterson's GP. He performed pulmonary function tests on Mr Paterson, which showed a restrictive defect and a reduced carbon monoxide transfer factor. Mr Paterson also had a chest X-ray which looked like the one in Figure 6.5. In view of Mr Paterson's age and rather poor respiratory condition, the physician decided that further investigation of Mr Paterson's condition, which might have included lung biopsy, were not warranted, and he made a diagnosis of cryptogenic fibrosing alveolitis.

Patients with fibrosing alveolitis usually give a history of increasing breathlessness over a considerable period of time. A dry cough may be present, but wheeze is unusual. The history may also provide clues as to possible causes of fibrosing alveolitis such as exposure to metal dusts or asbestos. Clues in the history might also point to diseases or drugs that may be complicated by fibrosing alveolitis.

On examination, finger clubbing is present in the majority of patients. Fine crepitations at the end of inspiration are present throughout the lungs. In advanced cases, central cyanosis may be present.

Investigations include pulmonary function testing, which reveals a restrictive defect, and a chest X-ray which may demonstrate fine shadowing at the periphery of the lung fields (Fig. 6.5). A fine CT scan may provide more information than a chest X-ray in diagnosing the disease. Bronchoalveolar lavage, in which fluid is introduced into the airways through a bronchoscope and then sucked back up for histological analysis is sometimes used for diagnosis and a lung biopsy provides a definitive diagnosis of the condition.

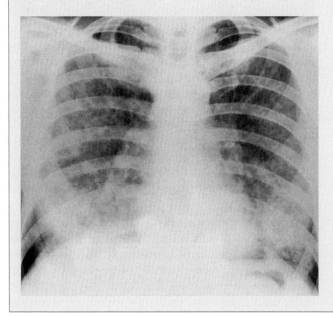

Fig. 6.5

Chest X-ray of a patient with cryptogenic fibrosing alveolitis. This shows fine reticular shadowing, which appears more pronounced towards the outer parts of the lung fields. The shadowing is also more pronounced near the bases of the lungs because there is a reduction in lung volume, and it is the bases of the lungs which tend to collapse first.

We therefore need to know the *rate* at which our chosen gas is taken up and the *pressure* which is driving it into the body.

If the blood in the pulmonary capillaries is very quickly saturated with the gas we are using it cannot take up any more, and this 'puts a stop' to the movement of the gas into the body. In this case, the rate at which blood flows through the lungs, and not diffusion, determines the rate of transfer and we are measuring pulmonary **blood flow** not transfer factor. Nitrous oxide behaves in this way and is used to measure pulmonary blood flow, but it is useless for measuring transfer factor (Fig. 6.6a).

As we are interested in the transfer of O_2 why not use O_2? We can certainly measure the rate at which O_2 is taken up by a subject, but the problem comes with having to measure the '**driving partial pressure** (air-to-blood)'. Blood enters the lung capillaries already carrying some O_2. Venous blood, which contains variable amounts of O_2 is beginning to be oxygenated in the pulmonary arterioles even before it reaches the capillaries, and so it is very difficult to know the exact driving pressure between alveolar air and this variable capillary blood. Also, except at low inhaled Po_2 blood is almost totally saturated with O_2 when it leaves the lungs, producing the same difficulties as with nitrous oxide, where uptake is governed by blood flow rather than transfer factor (Fig. 6.6b).

The gas that turns out to be most suitable for measuring transfer factor is the poisonous gas **carbon monoxide** (CO). This is poisonous because it competes with O_2 for binding sites on haemoglobin, and binds 250 times more strongly than O_2, thereby denying O_2 access to the haemoglobin – the victim of CO poisoning therefore dies of O_2 lack. (For this reason only very low concentrations of CO are used in measuring transfer factor.) Because it binds so strongly CO is 'locked up' in the haemoglobin and to all intents and purposes disappears from the blood. In other words, its partial pressure in the blood is zero. Knowing the rate at which CO disappears from a gas mixture the subject holds in his lungs for 10 seconds, and the partial pressures of CO in that mixture before and after inhalation, transfer factor can be calculated (Fig. 6.6c).

Treating diffusion difficulties

Bearing in mind that a large part of the problems of patients who might be suspected of having diffusional difficulties may be due to ventilation or $\dot{V}/\dot{Q}$ abnormalities, the rational treatment of patients whose lung diffusion problems lead to hypoxaemia depends on understanding the properties of the lung membrane illustrated in Figure 6.2. In these patients diffusion may have been reduced by thickening of the membrane (fibrosis) or loss of surface area (emphysema). These conditions are usually irreversible, and so we are left with only the option of increasing the partial pressure driving O_2 into the blood. Fortunately this is very effective, and increasing the inspired fraction of O_2 from the normal 21% in room air to 30% doubles the O_2 flux into the blood. In appropriate cases of progressive lung disease O_2 supplied via a nasal cannula or mask can much improve the quality of life of the unfortunate patient who requires O_2 to relieve his breathlessness at rest. These patients, perhaps realizing how precarious their existence is, were once thought to become dependent on O_2 administration. This dependency is usually

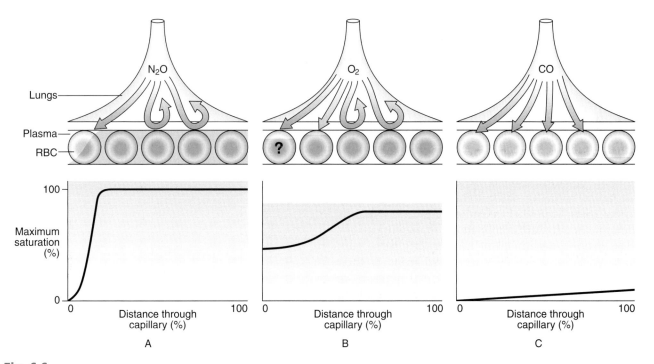

Fig. 6.6
Measuring transfer factor.
Nitrous oxide immediately saturates pulmonary capillary blood and so prevents any further transfer. Its uptake is therefore limited by pulmonary blood flow, not transfer factor. Oxygen partial pressure in the pulmonary capillary is impossible to measure accurately along the capillary, and so driving pressure into the blood cannot be calculated. Carbon monoxide is so tightly bound to haemoglobin in the blood that it exerts no partial pressure there. Driving partial pressure is the partial pressure in the inhaled air.

Gas exchange between air and blood: diffusion Box 3

Clinical features of fibrosing alveolitis

Cryptogenic fibrosing alveolitis is a rare condition that affects middle-aged and elderly patients. Its cause is unknown, but it has been suggested that it may be linked to the Epstein Barr virus and it is more common in smokers.

In its early stages, the disease is characterized by thickening of the alveolar walls. There is an increase in type II pneumocytes in the alveolar wall at the expense of type I pneumocytes. The type II cells have much more cytoplasm than the very thin type I cells and therefore represent more of a barrier to gaseous diffusion. Furthermore, the alveolar walls become infiltrated with cells of the immune system including neutrophils and lymphocytes and with time fibrin is laid down there. Because it is the tissue between the alveoli that is initially affected, pulmonary fibrosis is sometimes known as interstitial pneumonia, to distinguish it from inflammation involving the airways and the alveoli themselves.

The effect of fibrosis on gaseous diffusion is only part of the reason for the hypoxia that accompanies fibrosing alveolitis. Probably as important is the effect that fibrosis has on the ventilation–perfusion matching of the lungs, in other words it causes a mismatch of gas flow and blood flow between different areas of the lungs.

Cryptogenic fibrosing alveolitis has no known specific trigger, although it may be associated with rheumatoid arthritis. Fibrosing alveolitis is also associated with hypersensitivity to dusts, when it is known as extrinsic allergic alveolitis. The hypersensitivity is to very fine dusts containing particles of diameter of $0.5-5\,\mu m$. Dusts containing particles of a larger diameter would be deposited higher in the respiratory system and would not reach the alveoli. The dust may be associated with a particular occupation, which has led to specific names for particular types of the disease. Hence there is a farmer's lung, bird fancier's lung, mushroom worker's lung, wood worker's lung and even a sewerage worker's lung and a maple bark stripper's lung! In these cases, the dust may be from microorganism spores, from animal proteins or from chemicals.

---

psychological and is best avoided by giving the gas only to patients who obtain relief, and then only when needed and at the minimum effective dose.

Carbon dioxide and other gases

Gases such as nitrous oxide, helium or carbon monoxide may be administered experimentally to those unfortunate enough to fall into the hands of respiratory physiologists. Vapours of volatile anaesthetics such as halothane or ether are administered therapeutically.

The major determinant of how readily these substances diffuse across the lung membrane is their solubility in water. Ether is almost 600 times more soluble in water than O_2, and diffuses into the blood almost 400 times more readily. Nitrogen, on the other hand, is about half as soluble and diffuses at half the rate.

Carbon dioxide is a special case. We have seen that it is 24 times more soluble than O_2 and diffuses 20 times as readily. Returning to the series nature of transfer of gases, we know that rate of diffusion depends on the rate of supply of CO_2, which in turn

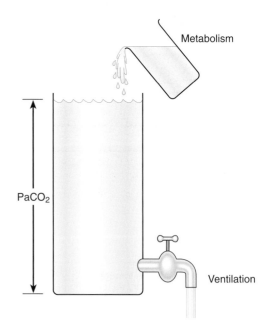

Fig. 6.7
The factors determining arterial P_{CO_2}. In this analogy $PaCO_2$ is the height of water in the cylinder which is added to by metabolism and removed by ventilation.

depends on the chemical reactions that release CO_2 from carbamino compounds and bicarbonate in the blood. The only time hypercapnia occurs other than as a result of hypoventilation is when the enzyme that accelerates the equilibrium of bicarbonate and CO_2 in the blood (carbonic anhydrase; see p. 120) is inhibited. So, the rate of CO_2 removal from the body is determined primarily by alveolar **ventilation**.

Carbon dioxide diffuses so readily that its arterial partial pressure is almost entirely the result of a balance between CO_2 production by metabolism and CO_2 removal by ventilation (Fig. 6.7).

Further reading

Forster RE, Crandall ED. Pulmonary gas exchange. Annual Reviews of Physiology 1976;38:69.

Krogh M. The diffusion of gases through the lungs of man. Journal of Physiology (Lond) 1914–1915;49:271–300

Roughton FJW, Forster RE. Relative importance of diffusion and chemical reaction rates in determining rate of exchange of gases in the human lung, with special reference to true diffusing capacity of pulmonary membrane and volume of blood in the lung capillaries. Journal of Applied Physiology 1957;11:290–302

Scheid P, Piiper J. Diffusion. In: Crystal RG, West JB, Barnes PJ, Weibel ER, eds. The lung: scientific foundations, 2nd edn. New York: Raven Press, 1997

Stevens A, Lowe JS, Young B. Wheater's basic histopathology, 4th edn. Edinburgh: Churchill Livingstone, 2002.

West JB. Ventilation blood flow and gas exchange, 5th edn. Oxford: Blackwell Science, 1990

Self-assessment case study

A 60-year-old woman is being treated for pulmonary oedema. As a result of her poor cardiac function, the pressure in her pulmonary capillaries is higher than normal. This leads to an imbalance of fluid entering and leaving these vessels, and fluid tends to collect in the walls of the alveoli, eventually leaking into the alveoli themselves.

As a result of her pulmonary oedema the patient feels breathless and her breathing is very rapid and shallow. She also starts to become cyanosed. Her chest X-ray looks like the one in Figure 6.8, which shows an enlarged heart and prominent blood vessels in the lung fields.

She is treated with oxygen and is given a diuretic, and her condition improves.

From your knowledge of the diffusion of gases across the alveolar membrane, you should be able to attempt the following questions:

① Why do you think that the pressure in this patient's alveolar capillaries is high?

② What effect do you think the build-up of fluid in the alveolar walls will have on gas exchange, and why?

③ What do you think is the rationale for the treatment that this patient was given?

Answers see page 177

Self-assessment questions

① Write the equation for diffusion of a gas across a membrane and define the terms used.

② Would it be reasonable to measure transfer factor in a patient with lung disease using CO in 100% O_2 to help his difficulties with breathing?

③ What factors determine Pa_{CO_2}?

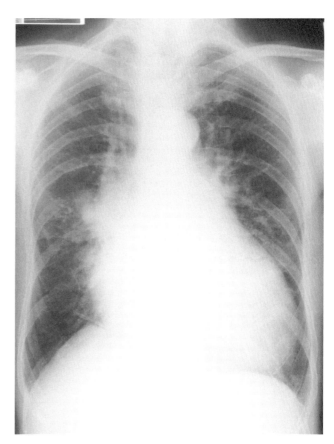

Fig. 6.8

④ What is the single physical phenomenon that moves gas from alveolar air into the blood, and vice versa?

Answers see page 177

THE PULMONARY CIRCULATION
BRINGING BLOOD AND GAS TOGETHER

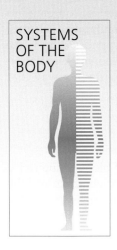

SYSTEMS OF THE BODY

Chapter objectives

After studying this chapter you should be able to:

① Describe the anatomy of the pulmonary circulation and compare its structure and function with that of the systemic circulation.

② Describe the pressures within the pulmonary circulation and how they are raised in pulmonary hypertension.

③ Describe the mechanisms affecting the distribution of blood within the lungs.

④ Describe ventilation/perfusion matching and discuss how this is achieved.

⑤ Discuss mechanisms by which lung disease may affect the pulmonary circulation.

The functions of the pulmonary circulation

So far, we have considered how the respiratory system transports gas between the atmosphere and the alveoli. In this chapter we will consider how blood and gas are brought together so that gas exchange can take place between them. This is a complex process: in order for all the blood to undergo gas exchange, virtually the entire cardiac output is directed through the lungs, and blood is brought close to gas within the alveoli. Furthermore, it is very important that **ventilation** (gas flow) and **perfusion** (blood flow) to a given area of the lung are matched. There is no point in directing air to areas of the lung that have little blood flow, and conversely there is no point in perfusing an area of lung with little or no ventilation. This matching of ventilation and perfusion is vital in maintaining adequate oxygenation and carbon dioxide removal from the blood.

In this chapter we will consider the anatomy of the pulmonary circulation, and in particular compare it to the systemic circulation. We will then consider the factors that influence the flow of blood to different regions of the lungs. Finally, we will consider the very important issue of ventilation/perfusion matching: the way in which air and blood are brought together in order to achieve optimal gas exchange of oxygen and carbon dioxide.

The anatomy of the pulmonary circulation

In humans the circulation behaves in many ways as if it consisted of two parts. In the systemic circulation the left ventricle pumps oxygenated blood through the organs and tissues of the body, where oxygen is removed and carbon dioxide added before the blood returns to the right atrium. In the **pulmonary circulation** the right ventricle pumps deoxygenated blood through the lungs, where oxygen is added and carbon dioxide is removed (Fig. 7.1). Of course, the two parts of the circulation work in series to form a single circuit of blood, but there are a number of differences between the pulmonary and systemic circulations which reflect their different functions.

First, virtually the entire cardiac output is directed through the pulmonary circulation. This means that, at any one time, there is as much blood flowing through the lungs as through all the other organs and tissues in the body put together.

Second, the purpose of the pulmonary circulation is to bring blood and air into very close contact in order to allow gas exchange to take place. This requires a very thin separating membrane and for this reason the pressure in the pulmonary circulation needs to be very

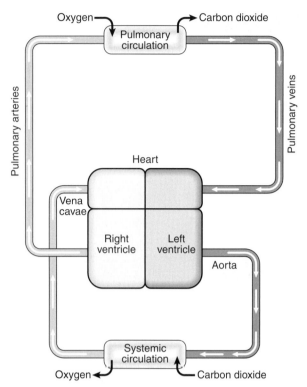

Fig. 7.1
Diagrammatic representation of the circulation. In humans the circulation behaves as if it consisted of two parts, the systemic circulation and the pulmonary circulation. The blood flow through the two parts is the same. In both circulations *arteries* carry blood away from the heart and *veins* carry blood to the heart. For this reason, the pulmonary artery carries *deoxygenated* blood and the pulmonary vein carries *oxygenated* blood.

low compared to the systemic circulation. If the pressure in the pulmonary circulation were higher, it could cause fluid to leak from the pulmonary capillaries into alveoli. In fact, the pressure in the pulmonary artery is about 25/10 mmHg, compared to 120/70 mmHg in the systemic circulation. The pulmonary circulation is therefore a *low-pressure, high-flow system*. The components of the pulmonary circulation differ from their systemic counterparts in a way that reflects this.

The right ventricle

Every minute, the same volume of blood – about 5 L at rest – flows through both the right ventricle and the left ventricle. However, the two ventricles look very different (Fig. 7.2). The left ventricle has a thick, muscular wall that takes up most of the cross-section of the

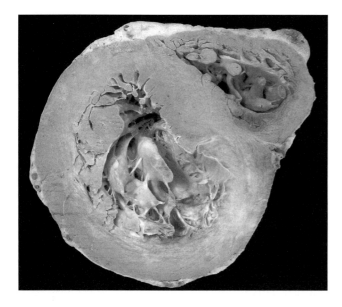

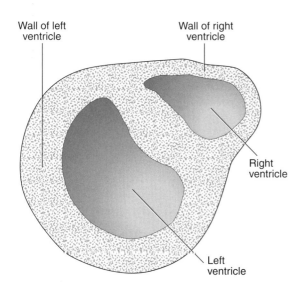

Fig. 7.2
Cross-section of the heart. Note that the left ventricle has a thick wall, reflecting the high pressures it generates. At rest, the systolic pressure in the left ventricle is about 120 mmHg, but during exercise, for example, the pressure can be much higher. In contrast, the right ventricle has a much thinner wall. The systolic pressure in the right ventricle is only about 25 mmHg, and in health does not increase much above this, even during exercise.

heart. The right ventricle has a much thinner wall, about one-third of the thickness of the left, and to accommodate the muscle of the left ventricle the right almost seems to be 'wrapped around' the left. Why is there such a difference between the two?

The reason is that the left ventricle pumps blood into the systemic circulation, which has a high resistance and which operates at a relatively high pressure. If cardiac output increases, for example during exercise, this pressure can increase even more, which means that the left ventricle needs a thick, muscular wall to produce these high pressures. On the other hand, the right ventricle pumps blood into the pulmonary circulation, which has a very low resistance and which operates at a low pressure, always less than that in the systemic circulation. Furthermore, as we shall see later, if cardiac output increases the pulmonary artery pressure does not increase very much. For this reason, the right ventricle needs only a relatively thin muscular wall in comparison to the left.

Pulmonary blood vessels

Pulmonary blood vessels are very different from their systemic counterparts. The larger vessels have much thinner walls, reflecting the lower blood pressure that they need to withstand: for example, the thickness of the wall of the pulmonary artery is only about one-third of the thickness of the aorta.

As well as having thinner walls, the pulmonary vessels are much more distensible than systemic arteries, which is important in keeping pulmonary blood pressure low in the face of increases in cardiac output. In circumstances such as exercise, cardiac output can increase from its normal 5 L per minute to as much as 25 L per minute. In order to keep pulmonary blood pressure low, the pulmonary circulation is able to reduce its resistance to even lower values than normal. It does so by two mechanisms, illustrated in Figure 7.3.

1. Pulmonary blood vessels are able to dilate or **distend**. A small increase in the diameter of a vessel decreases the resistance of that vessel substantially (Poiseuille's Law p. 170).
2. During normal conditions, some blood vessels in the lungs are closed. During periods of high cardiac output these vessels open up and blood is able to flow through them. The increase in number of blood vessels able to carry blood is called **recruitment**. However, it is likely that very few vessels are completely collapsed under normal conditions, and distension is probably much more important than recruitment in reducing vascular resistance.

The anatomical position of the capillaries and their function in gas exchange means that they are different from their systemic counterparts. The density of the capillary network in the alveolar walls is extremely high so that efficient gas exchange can take place. In fact, there are so few cells between the capillaries in

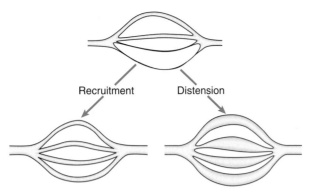

Fig. 7.3
Recruitment and distension of pulmonary blood vessels. If cardiac output increases the resistance of the pulmonary circulation decreases, meaning that the pulmonary artery pressure remains relatively low. This occurs because some pulmonary vessels increase in diameter (distension, lower right of diagram) and because some vessels which were virtually closed begin to open and blood can flow along them (recruitment, lower left of diagram).

the alveolar walls that the alveolar circulation behaves almost like a film of blood flowing around the alveoli. At rest, blood flows through an alveolar capillary in about 0.8 seconds, which is about three times longer than the time needed for oxygenation of mixed venous blood.

There is very little space between the blood in the pulmonary capillaries and the air in the alveoli. In fact, for the most part, the only cells separating blood from air are the endothelial cells of the pulmonary capillary

and the epithelial type I cells of the alveolar wall. This is clearly very important in allowing the most efficient transfer of gases between the alveoli and the blood (see Chapter 6).

However, because the pulmonary capillaries are very thin-walled and lie in the alveolar walls they can be readily influenced by changes in the gas pressure within the alveoli. Increased alveolar gas pressure can compress the capillaries, with a consequent increase in capillary resistance and reduction in blood flow, which can affect the **distribution** of blood flow within the lungs (see below). This is very different from the conditions affecting systemic capillaries, which are supported by surrounding tissues.

In contrast to the situation in the systemic circulation, the pressure in the pulmonary **veins** exerts a considerable influence over the pressure in the pulmonary arteries. This is another consequence of the low pressures in the pulmonary circulation.

In the systemic circulation, the pressure at the precapillary sphincters, which regulate the blood flow through the capillary beds, is about 90 mmHg, very much higher than the pressure at the venous end of the capillary beds. The difference in pressure between the arterial and venous ends of a capillary bed is called the **driving pressure** and flow is dependent on this. Because the venous pressure in the systemic circulation is so much less than the arterial pressure, changes in venous pressure do not make large changes to the driving pressure.

However, in the pulmonary circulation the difference between pulmonary arterial and venous pressures is much less, and a relatively small change in venous pressure can make a considerable change to the driving

---

The pulmonary circulation: bringing blood and gas together Box 1

Pulmonary embolus

Mrs Dodds is an 80-year-old woman who unfortunately tripped and fell at home, fracturing her right hip. She was taken to hospital and the next day she went to the operating theatre where her hip was fixed surgically. Postoperatively she was initially doing well, although she was quite slow to mobilize. However, on the third day after her operation she developed left-sided chest pain. The pain was pleuritic (it was sharp in nature and was made worse with breathing) and was associated with breathlessness.

The doctor who came to see Mrs Dodds examined her. He thought she looked a little cyanosed, but the examination of her chest did not reveal anything remarkable. Her trachea was not deviated, the expansion of her

chest was normal, and there was no abnormality on percussion or auscultation of her chest. The doctor examined Mrs Dodds' legs but found no abnormality.

The doctor felt that the most likely diagnosis was that of a pulmonary embolus and he sent Mrs Dodds to undergo a CT pulmonary angiogram (Fig. 7.5A). This confirmed the diagnosis of pulmonary embolus, and Mrs Dodds was started on intravenous heparin.

In this chapter we will consider:

① What causes a pulmonary embolus and how it can be diagnosed.
② How a pulmonary embolus can be treated.
③ Massive pulmonary embolus.

pressure. To keep a constant driving pressure the pulmonary artery pressure has to increase. In certain pathological situations this can eventually lead to failure of the right ventricle (**cor pulmonale**; see below).

The bronchial circulation

Not all of the blood flowing into the lungs does so via the pulmonary artery – a small volume of arterial blood flows through the **bronchial circulation** (Fig. 7.4). The bronchial circulation supplies blood to the airways and to the lung parenchyma, although it is not essential to their survival; during a lung transplant the bronchial circulation is not reconnected, and this apparently does not produce any serious ill effects. Blood flowing through the bronchial circulation does not pass through the alveolar capillaries and therefore does not take part in gas exchange.

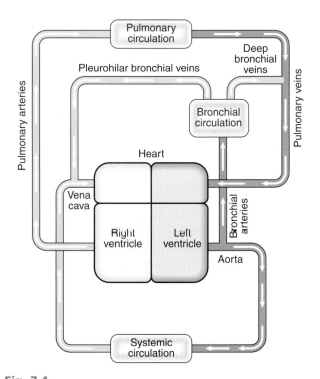

Fig. 7.4
The bronchial circulation. The bronchial arteries arise from the aorta and therefore carry oxygenated blood. The blood in the bronchial circulation supplies tissues within the lung but does not take part in gas exchange, and the blood in the bronchial veins is therefore deoxygenated. Some of the blood from the bronchial circulation drains via the pleurohilar bronchial veins into the azygous vein or the vena cava, whereas blood draining the deep bronchial veins drains into the pulmonary veins.

The bronchial arteries arise from the aorta. Bronchial vessels supply blood to the lower trachea, the bronchi, and to the smaller airways as far as the respiratory bronchioles. Blood from the proximal part of the bronchial circulation around the bronchi drains via the pleurohilar bronchial veins into the azygous vein and into the superior vena cava. This blood is effectively part of the systemic circulation in that it flows from the aorta to the vena cava.

However, the blood from the more distal parts of the bronchial circulation drains via the deep bronchial veins into the pulmonary circulation. This blood therefore forms a **shunt** (see below). In other words, the blood arises from the aorta, but instead of draining into the right-hand side of the circulation, the partly deoxygenated blood of the deep bronchial veins drains into the oxygenated blood that has passed through the alveolar capillaries. The resulting mixture of blood therefore has an oxygen content less than that of the original pulmonary artery blood. The significance of this will be discussed later in the chapter.

Matching ventilation and perfusion

In an ideal pair of lungs all the alveoli would be supplied with equal volumes of air of uniform gas composition during inspiration. Also, all the alveoli would be ideally supplied with the same flow of mixed venous blood. The ventilation and perfusion of all parts of these ideal lungs would therefore be optimally **matched**, and optimal gas exchange between the blood and the alveoli would take place.

However, in real lungs this is not the case. Per unit of lung volume, ventilation and perfusion both tend to be greater at the bases of the lungs compared to the apices. Nevertheless, for most of the lung tissue the two tend to be fairly optimally matched. This means that the ratio of ventilation to blood flow, the **ventilation/perfusion ratio**, or $\dot{V}/\dot{Q}$ **ratio**, varies by a relatively small amount throughout the lungs.

In order to see how ventilation/perfusion matching takes place we will first look at the way in which the blood flow is distributed throughout the lungs, then we will see how this is matched with ventilation before looking at how regional variations in the $\dot{V}/\dot{Q}$ ratio in the lungs affects arterial blood gases.

Distribution of blood flow through the lungs

As we have just seen, the distribution of blood to different regions of the lungs is not uniform but varies considerably. Furthermore, the blood flow to different

The pulmonary circulation: bringing blood and gas together Box 2

What causes a pulmonary embolus and how can it be diagnosed?

A pulmonary embolus occurs when something, usually a thrombus (blood clot), occludes part of the pulmonary artery tree. Generally the thrombus forms in the veins of the pelvis or lower limb, and part of that thrombus or the whole thrombus may dislodge and pass through the vena cava, through the right atrium and ventricle and into the pulmonary artery. The thrombus finally lodges in a branch of the pulmonary artery, occluding it. The segment of lung tissue supplied by the obstructed artery has a reduced blood supply (although it often receives some blood – remember the bronchial circulation) and may finally infarct.

In a small number of cases (probably less than 10% of the total number of pulmonary emboli) the thrombus does not form in the veins of the pelvis or leg but forms in the heart. This may be as a result of atrial fibrillation, in which the atria of the heart do not beat properly, or thrombus may form on a part of the myocardium which has infarcted. Very occasionally the embolus is not formed from thrombus but from other substances, such as fat or amniotic fluid.

Conditions that lead to the formation of thrombus in the pelvic and lower limb veins include prolonged immobility, lower limb or pelvic fractures, abdominal surgery, pregnancy, the presence of cancer and clotting abnormalities. Mrs Dodds had two of these risk factors, including immobility (she was bedridden) and a lower limb fracture. If the thrombus forms in the lower limb it may become swollen and painful, which is why the doctor examined Mrs Dodds' legs. If thrombus occurs in the lower limbs it usually occurs in the deep veins in the muscle, rather than the veins near the skin. Hence the condition is usually called **deep venous thrombosis (DVT)**. Several cases have been reported of patients suffering DVTs and pulmonary emboli following the prolonged immobility that occurs during a long-distance flight, sometimes in rather cramped conditions. The true incidence of this so-called 'economy class syndrome' is yet to be established, however.

Small emboli in the lungs cause no symptoms and no haemodynamic problems and go unnoticed. Larger emboli, particularly if they result in pulmonary infarction, can cause clinical symptoms, including pleuritic chest pain and sometimes haemoptysis.

Very large emboli are a medical emergency (see Box 4).

Usually there is very little to find on clinical examination of a patient who has suffered a pulmonary embolus – occasionally there may be a few crackles on auscultation. Occasionally, though, a pleural rub may be heard over an area of infarcted lung. A plain chest X-ray is not generally very helpful in diagnosing a pulmonary embolus: if there is quite a large embolus it is said that the affected lung fields can appear 'oligaemic': in other words, they appear darker on the chest X-ray as those areas of lung contain less blood. This is not always easy to see, however. Larger pulmonary emboli increase the amount of work that the right ventricle has to do, as it has to pump blood into a partially obstructed pulmonary circulation. This can result in changes in the ECG. Classically these changes consist of S waves in lead I and Q waves and inverted T waves in lead III (hence the mnemonic: 'S1 Q3 T3'), but these changes are rarely seen in practice.

Diagnosis of a pulmonary embolus can be made using a radioisotope scan of the blood flow in the lungs, but nowadays is often made with a CT pulmonary angiogram. In this test, X-ray contrast is injected into a vein and its flow through the lungs is monitored with a fast CT scanner. Clot in the pulmonary vessels can then be identified.

A CT pulmonary angiogram of a patient with a large pulmonary embolus is shown in Figure 7.5A. The CT shows a cross-section of the patient's chest at the point where the aorta arches over the dividing pulmonary artery. CT scans are usually shown as if the cross-section is being viewed from *below*, in other words, the left-hand side of the scan corresponds to the right-hand side of the body. X-ray contrast, which shows up white on the scan, has been injected into a cannula lying in the superior vena cava – the white dot in the otherwise dark vena cava is the contrast within the cannula. Blood which contains contrast is clearly visible in the ascending and descending aorta. There is blood in the right and left pulmonary arteries; however, dark areas are visible within these arteries which correspond to thrombus. This pulmonary embolus is a large one, and thrombus is visible in both pulmonary arteries.

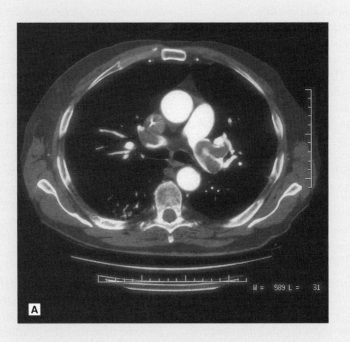

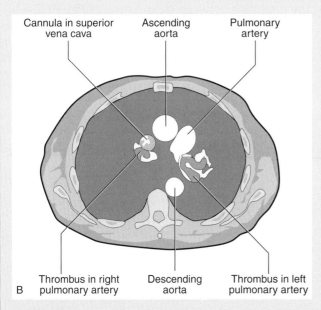

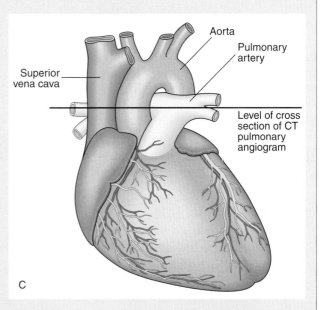

Fig. 7.5
CT pulmonary angiogram of a patient with a large pulmonary embolus (A). The CT represents a cross-section at about the level shown in (C). The clot is clearly visible in both pulmonary arteries as dark areas against the white of the X-ray contrast medium. (Courtesy Dr J. T. Murchison, Royal Infirmary, Edinburgh)

parts of the lungs tends to be directed towards maintaining as normal a $\dot{V}/\dot{Q}$ ratio as possible.

In the systemic circulation, blood flow through organs is almost entirely determined by high-resistance arterioles that regulate the blood flow through capillary beds. The arterioles in the pulmonary circulation do not have a high resistance and play only a small role in determining the blood flow to different parts of the lungs. The distribution of blood flow through the lungs is influenced instead by a number of different factors, including **gravity**, alveolar **gas pressure**, hypoxic pulmonary **vasoconstriction** and, to a lesser extent, the nervous control of blood vessel resistance.

Gravity

The diastolic blood pressure in the systemic circulation is about 80 mmHg, which is enough pressure to raise a column of water by a height of over a metre. In other words, there is more than enough pressure to carry blood from the heart up to the head. However, in the pulmonary circulation the diastolic blood pressure is about 12 mmHg, enough pressure to raise a column of water about 15 cm. In other words, there is only just enough pressure to pump blood from the right ventricle up to the lung apices. On the other hand, at the lung bases the blood pressure in the pulmonary circulation is equal to the pressure generated by the right ventricle *plus* the hydrostatic pressure of a column of blood extending up to the heart. Because the pressure generated by the right ventricle is not very high, this extra hydrostatic pressure makes a very significant difference. Thus there is a very considerable difference in arterial blood pressure between the bases and the apices of the lungs owing to gravity. In other words, gravity tends to direct blood towards the lung bases.

The regional flow of blood within the lungs can be demonstrated by dissolving a radioactive gas (usually Xenon-133 (^{133}Xe)) in saline and then injecting this into the right side of the heart via an intravenous catheter. During the injection the subject holds his breath, and some of the radioactive xenon leaves the blood and enters the alveoli. By measuring the level of radioactivity from outside the body it is possible to estimate the blood flow to different regions of the lungs (Fig. 7.6).

Although the difference in regional blood flow between the apices and bases of the lungs is thought to be due largely to the effect of gravity, it is nevertheless the case that the gradient remains in subjects who are in the supine position. Furthermore, the anatomy of the branching pulmonary vessels results in greater variation between different parts of the same level in the lung than between mean flow in adjacent levels.

Gravity is one factor influencing regional differences in blood flow within the lungs. However, other factors include the air pressure in the alveoli around the pulmonary capillaries, and hypoxic pulmonary vasoconstriction.

The pulmonary circulation: bringing blood and gas together Box 3

Treatment of pulmonary emboli

The mainstay of treatment is to prevent further emboli occurring. For this reason the patient is anticoagulated. Initially this is achieved with **heparin**, a drug which inhibits the coagulation cascade and is usually given as a continuous intravenous infusion, or the more modern **low molecular weight** heparins may be given subcutaneously. Later, the patient may be switched to **warfarin**, an oral drug which is also an anticoagulant and is often taken for several months following a pulmonary embolism. This combination of treatment is used for the type of pulmonary embolism suffered by Mrs Dodds.

Occasionally, following a very large pulmonary embolism an attempt may be made to break down the thrombus that is in the lungs. Drugs such as **streptokinase** may be used which activate the fibrinolytic pathway, resulting in breakdown of the clot. In extreme circumstances after a very major pulmonary embolus, a surgical operation may be carried out to remove the clot, particularly if it lies in the proximal pulmonary artery. If warfarin does not prevent further pulmonary emboli then it may be necessary to insert a **caval filter**, which is a small filter that fits into the inferior vena cava and is inserted folded through a puncture in the femoral vein before being opened up and wedged into the inferior vena cava under X-ray control. The filter 'catches' emboli from the lower limb veins and prevents them reaching the lungs.

Pulmonary emboli can sometimes have serious consequences and, as we have seen, are promoted by surgery and immobility. For this reason, patients undergoing surgery are often given small subcutaneous doses of heparin for a few days afterwards. This treatment has been shown to significantly reduce the risk of subsequent pulmonary emboli in these patients.

Pressure around the blood vessels

As we have seen, the pulmonary capillaries are influenced by the air pressure in the alveoli that surround them. If the blood pressure within a capillary is less than the pressure of the gas in the alveoli adjacent to it, there will be a tendency for the pressure in the alveoli to compress the capillary, limiting the blood flow through it. The pressure in the alveoli remains close to atmospheric during quiet breathing, but may become significantly positive during artificial ventilation or during heavy breathing. In these circumstances, alveolar gas pressure may have a significant effect on the distribution of pulmonary blood flow.

These two factors combine to influence the distribution of blood flow within the lungs. Three zones have been described related to the blood pressure at the beginning and end of a capillary and the gas pressure within the adjacent alveoli (Fig. 7.6):

- *Zone 1* In this zone, the pressure in the alveoli is always greater than the pressure in the capillaries. This means that in zone 1 there is no blood flow. It is unlikely that such a zone exists in healthy individuals, but if it does so it occupies a very small volume of the apices of the lungs, where the pulmonary blood pressure is lowest.
- *Zone 2* In this zone, the alveolar gas pressure is greater than the blood pressure at the venous end of the capillary but less than the blood pressure at the arterial end of the capillary. In zone 2, the flow through the capillaries is influenced by changes in blood pressure and changes in alveolar gas pressure. If alveolar gas pressure increases, then flow through the capillaries in zone 2 will be reduced.
- *Zone 3* In zone 3, the blood pressure throughout the capillaries, from the arterial end through to the venous end, is greater than the gas pressure in the surrounding alveoli. Therefore, in this zone, flow through the capillaries is influenced only by the difference in blood pressure along the capillary and is not influenced at all by changes in alveolar pressure. It is likely that in healthy humans, the *majority* of the volume of the lungs lies within zone 3, and blood flow is independent of alveolar gas pressure.

This 'three zone' model emphasizes the role of gravity in directing blood flow in the lungs although recent evidence suggests that gravity is not as important a factor in determining regional differences in blood flow in the lungs as was once thought. In particular, blood flow to the very lowest parts of the lung bases appears to be less than this model predicts and so the difference between the bases and the apices of the lungs in blood flow per unit lung volume is relatively modest.

Furthermore, at any given height from the base, there is a wide variation in blood flow to different lung regions. It is thought likely that this variation is due to the fact that when a blood vessel divides, the two vessels formed are not necessarily the same size. This effect leads to a random variation in blood flow

---

The pulmonary circulation: bringing blood and gas together Box 4

Massive pulmonary embolism – a rare medical emergency

Massive pulmonary embolism occurs when a large proportion (50% or more) of the pulmonary circulation is obstructed by an embolus. From your knowledge of respiratory physiology it is easy to predict what problems this will cause.

As we have seen, the entire cardiac output passes through the pulmonary circulation, therefore a major obstruction to the pulmonary circulation means a major obstruction to the circulation as a whole. Furthermore, the right ventricle as accustomed to pumping blood through a low-pressure, low-resistance vascular bed. A massive pulmonary embolus increases the pressure in the pulmonary circulation enormously. The right ventricle can produce only a modest increase in pulmonary artery blood pressure (say up to 60 mmHg systolic), which is insufficient to sustain an adequate blood flow. In doing so, the right ventricle is put under considerable strain and may start to fail, leading to crushing central chest pain similar to that of angina, as well as a raised central venous pressure.

The reduced blood flow to the lungs leads to a large mismatch in ventilation and perfusion, which leads to arterial hypoxia. The reduced blood flow through the lungs means that filling of the left ventricle starts to diminish, and the circulation as a whole therefore begins to fail. The patient may become pale and shocked and may lose consciousness. In severe cases, death follows quickly.

Treatment of massive pulmonary embolism is initially supportive, with the administration of oxygen and fluids. Anticoagulation, thrombolysis, acute surgery or heart bypass may be necessary. However, the result of a massive pulmonary embolus is often death.

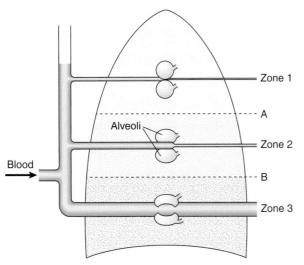

Fig. 7.6

The effect of blood pressure and alveolar pressure on regional blood flow through the lungs. In zone 1, the air pressure in the alveoli is greater than the pressure within the alveolar capillaries and therefore no blood flow takes place. If such a zone exists in healthy individuals, it is very small and situated at the apices of the lungs. In zone 2, the average alveolar gas pressure is lower than the pressure of blood entering the alveolar capillaries but higher than the pressure of blood leaving the capillaries. In zone 2, blood flow varies with changes in alveolar gas pressure. In zone 3, the blood pressure throughout the alveolar capillaries is higher than the alveolar gas pressure, and blood flow through the pulmonary capillaries is independent of alveolar gas pressure. In healthy individuals it is likely that most of the alveoli lie within zone 3.

between lung regions at the same height from the lung base. This effect is probably at least as important as gravity in producing variation in regional perfusion of the lungs.

Hypoxic pulmonary vasoconstriction

Arterioles in the lungs differ considerably from their systemic counterparts in their response to hypoxia. Systemic arterioles **vasodilate** in response to hypoxia. This tends to increase the blood flow to hypoxic tissues and therefore tends to increase oxygen delivery where it is required.

However, arterioles in the lungs **vasoconstrict** in response to hypoxia: this effect is called **hypoxic pulmonary vasocontriction**. Hypoxic pulmonary vasoconstriction is important in maintaining ventilation/perfusion matching and tends to direct blood *away* from underventilated parts of the lungs. Underventilated

regions of the lungs have a low oxygen concentration, and therefore blood leaving them tends to be relatively deoxygenated. Hypoxic pulmonary vasoconstriction in these areas directs blood towards better-ventilated parts of the lungs where there is a higher oxygen concentration. In other words, hypoxic pulmonary vasoconstriction tends to promote an optimum $\dot{V}/\dot{Q}$ ratio for the lungs as a whole by increasing the $\dot{V}/\dot{Q}$ ratio in areas of the lungs where it is lower than normal.

In its role in optimizing the $\dot{V}/\dot{Q}$ ratio, the vasoconstrictor response of the blood vessels to low oxygen concentrations is analogous to the bronchodilator response of bronchi to high levels of carbon dioxide (see Chapter 4). In addition, hypoxic pulmonary vasoconstriction plays an important role in limiting blood flow through the non-ventilated and therefore hypoxic lungs of the fetus. After the baby is delivered and takes its first breath, the oxygen concentration in its lungs increases, the hypoxic pulmonary vasoconstriction reduces and blood flow to the lungs is increased.

The mechanism behind hypoxic pulmonary vasoconstriction is not fully understood. What is known is that hypoxia causes membrane depolarization of the smooth muscle cells in the pulmonary blood vessels (Fig. 7.7). This is followed by contraction of the smooth muscles in the blood vessel wall. It is thought that the depolarization of the smooth muscle cells is mediated, at least in part, by a membrane potassium channel called the Kv channel. The conductance of Kv increases in response to hypoxia, resulting in membrane depolarization, although it is not certain whether the channel itself is sensitive to hypoxia or whether it responds to another detector of hypoxia.

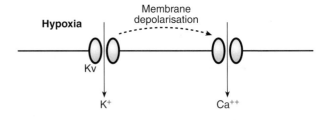

Fig. 7.7

Hypoxic pulmonary vasoconstriction. Pulmonary blood vessels constrict in response to hypoxia. The potassium channel K_v, which lies in the vascular smooth muscle membrane, opens in response to hypoxia, leading to membrane depolarization. This results in the opening of a calcium channel which allows extracellular calcium to enter the cell. This in turn triggers muscle contraction.

The membrane depolarization opens voltage-sensitive calcium channels that allow calcium to enter the cell. A rise in intracellular calcium concentration triggers smooth muscle contraction, resulting in vasoconstriction. Mediators such as endothelin (a vasoconstrictor) and nitric oxide (a vasodilator) released from the overlying endothelial cells also influence hypoxic pulmonary vasoconstriction, although they are not necessary for it to take place.

Although hypoxic pulmonary vasoconstriction is usually beneficial in maintaining ventilation/perfusion matching, it can cause problems in patients with lung conditions such as chronic obstructive pulmonary disease that result in long-term hypoxia. This chronic hypoxia affects all parts of the lungs and results in a widespread hypoxic pulmonary vasoconstriction. This means that the resistance of the pulmonary circulation as a whole is much higher than normal, and the pulmonary blood pressure increases. The right ventricle is not well suited to producing a high blood pressure and under these circumstances can start to fail. The patient may become increasingly breathless on exertion, as fluid tends to seep into the alveoli as cardiac output increases. Furthermore, the patient may notice oedema around their ankles. Failure of the right ventricle means that the pressure in the systemic veins increases. This sort of heart failure due to lung disease is called **cor pulmonale**.

Innervation of the pulmonary vessels

Fibres of the sympathetic and parasympathetic nervous system innervate the pulmonary vessels and may cause vasoconstriction or vasodilatation (Fig. 7.8). Sympathetic fibres release noradrenaline (norepinephrine), which acts predominantly on α_1 adrenoceptors on the smooth muscle of arteries and arterioles to produce vasoconstriction. Noradrenaline (norepinephrine) may also act on α_2 receptors to produce vasodilatation, but it is generally accepted that the overall effect of the sympathetic nervous system on the pulmonary vessels is vasoconstriction.

The parasympathetic nervous system produces most of its effects on the pulmonary blood vessels by the release of acetylcholine. The acetylcholine is thought to act on muscarinic M_3 receptors on the *endothelium* of the blood vessels, rather than on the smooth muscle cells themselves. It is thought that stimulation of the M_3 receptors by acetylcholine results in the release of nitric oxide (NO) from the vascular endothelial cells. Nitric oxide is a small gaseous molecule that is very rapidly broken down and is a very important mediator throughout many organ systems in the body. The NO released from the

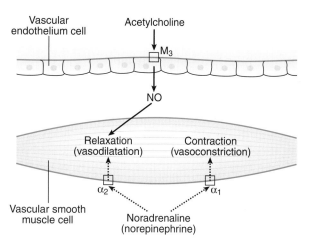

Fig. 7.8
Action of the sympathetic and parasympathetic nervous systems on pulmonary vessels.
Noradrenaline (norepinephrine) released from sympathetic nerve fibres acts on smooth muscle α_1 receptors to produce vasoconstriction and on α_2 receptors to cause vasodilatation. Overall, the effect of the sympathetic nervous system is to cause vasoconstriction. Acetylcholine acts on the vascular endothelium, causing the release of nitric oxide that causes vasodilatation of the underlying vascular smooth muscle.

endothelium in response to acetylcholine causes pulmonary vascular smooth muscle cells to relax, and therefore produces vasodilatation.

Like the bronchial smooth muscle, the pulmonary vascular smooth muscle also has a non-adrenergic, non-cholinergic parasympathetic innervation. There are many possible neurotransmitters in this system. It seems to produce vasodilatation, and may well act via NO. However, its importance in humans is not fully understood.

The sympathetic and parasympathetic innervation of the pulmonary blood vessels is probably not very important in maintaining ventilation/perfusion matching in humans. During a lung transplant the sympathetic and parasympathetic nerves cannot be reconnected, and the lack of sympathetic and parasympathetic innervation does not appear to be a serious problem to patients who have undergone this operation.

Regional differences in ventilation in the lungs

As we have seen, the blood flow to different regions of the lung is not uniform but tends to increase towards the bases of the lungs, as well as varying quite widely at a particular height from the lung base.

Fortunately, ventilation is also directed towards the bases. This happens essentially because the lungs 'sag'. The weight of the tissue making up the lungs tends to cause the alveoli and airways at the bases to collapse, while at the same time the airways and alveoli at the apices tend to be 'pulled' open by the lung tissue below them. This means that at the beginning of a breath, the alveoli at the apices of the lungs are nearer to being 'full' than the alveoli at the bases, and cannot take much 'fresh' air, and therefore ventilation tends to increase towards the bases. However, this difference in ventilation between the apices and the bases of the lungs becomes less pronounced (and may even reverse) with high airway gas flows. There is also variability in the distribution of gas flow to different lung regions at a given height from the lung base, similar to the variability that is seen in blood flow. This is probably due to random differences in the diameters of bronchi formed at the bifurcation of the airways, comparable to the same random variation that occurs in regional perfusion of the lungs.

We have seen that ventilation and perfusion, for a given volume of lung tissue, both increase towards the bases of the lungs. The rate of increase in perfusion is greater than the increase in ventilation, meaning that there is an increase in $\dot{V}/\dot{Q}$ ratio from the apices to the bases of the lungs.

We have also seen that at any given height above the base, there is a wide variation in regional ventilation and regional perfusion. Despite this, the range of $\dot{V}/\dot{Q}$ ratios found in the lung is relatively narrow. Figure 7.9 shows both ventilation and perfusion plotted against $\dot{V}/\dot{Q}$ ratio on a logarithmic scale. As you can see, most of the ventilation (open circles) and most of the perfusion (closed circles) take place in lung regions that encompass a relatively narrow range of $\dot{V}/\dot{Q}$ ratios. In other words, regions of the lung with relatively low ventilation tend to have relatively low perfusion.

How ventilation and perfusion are so closely matched is not fully understood. Matching is partly due to that fact that both ventilation and perfusion increase towards the lung bases and hypoxic pulmonary vasoconstriction plays a small part. Ignoring these effects, it nevertheless appears that compliant regions of the lung that are relatively well ventilated also seem to have lower vascular resistances and are therefore better perfused. It has been speculated that this relationship between lung compliance and vascular resistance in a given region is one that is formed in the developing lung.

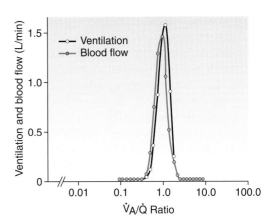

Fig. 7.9
Distribution of ventilation (O) and perfusion (•). Ventilation and perfusion are both plotted against $\dot{V}/\dot{Q}$ ratio on a logarithmic scale. Most ventilation and perfusion takes place in lung regions having a relatively narrow range of $\dot{V}/\dot{Q}$ ratio.

Although fairly well matched there is nevertheless a range of $\dot{V}/\dot{Q}$ ratios found in normal lungs. In diseased lungs, this variation is very much increased. What effect does variability in $\dot{V}/\dot{Q}$ ratios have on gas exchange?

Ventilation/perfusion matching and its effect on blood O_2 and CO_2 content

It is useful to think of ventilation and perfusion matching as representing the mixing together of air and mixed venous blood (although obviously blood and gas cannot be physically mixed). If the $\dot{V}/\dot{Q}$ ratio is high, the mixture contains more air than blood and therefore has a relatively high P_{O_2}, and a relatively low P_{CO_2}. If, however, the $\dot{V}/\dot{Q}$ ratio is low, the mixture contains a higher concentration of blood and therefore has a relatively low P_{O_2} and a relatively high P_{CO_2}. In fact, the $\dot{V}/\dot{Q}$ ratio can vary between zero and infinity. A $\dot{V}/\dot{Q}$ ratio of **zero** means that there is perfusion but **no ventilation**: in other words, an area of the lungs where shunting is taking place and there is perfusion but no ventilation and the gas concentrations are similar to mixed venous blood. A $\dot{V}/\dot{Q}$ ratio of **infinity** means that there is ventilation but **no perfusion**, in other words an area of the lungs that is dead space, where the gas concentrations are similar to those of air. Each value of the $\dot{V}/\dot{Q}$ ratio is therefore associated with a particular P_{O_2} and P_{CO_2}.

If the transfer of oxygen and carbon dioxide were based on a simple mixing effect then it would be straightforward to calculate the composition of gas in an alveolus in the same way we could calculate the composition of a beaker of saline (i.e. blood) to which various known amounts of water (i.e. alveolar gas) were added. Adding a small amount of water to the saline would result in a mixture with a composition close to that of the saline. Adding a large volume of water to the saline would result in a mixture with a composition similar to that of water. Figure 7.10 shows how the composition of the saline/water mixture varies with the proportions of each making up the mixture. If saline represents the composition of mixed venous blood ($\bar{v}$) and water represents the composition of air (I), then there would be a straight line joining point $\bar{v}$ (zero $\dot{V}/\dot{Q}$ ratio, dead space) and I (infinite $\dot{V}/\dot{Q}$ ratio, shunt). This straight line would represent the gas tensions at different parts of the lungs with ratios that lie between these two extremes.

However, gas exchange in the lungs is not a simple exchange of one molecule of carbon dioxide for one molecule of oxygen, and the line joining the two extremes of $\dot{V}/\dot{Q}$ ratio is, in fact, curved, mainly because the oxygen–haemoglobin dissociation curve is sigmoid in shape. In a region of lung with a high $\dot{V}/\dot{Q}$ ratio more CO_2 is removed from the blood but the blood does not take up much more oxygen. This is because at the higher Pa_{O_2}, that is found here the haemoglobin is already 97% saturated and can therefore carry very little extra oxygen. Similarly, in an area of lung with a low $\dot{V}/\dot{Q}$ ratio, relatively more oxygen is taken up by the blood because at the lower Pa_{O_2} here, haemoglobin is at the middle, steep part of the oxygen–haemoglobin dissociation curve. However, relatively little extra carbon

dioxide is released from the blood because the carbon dioxide dissociation curve is flatter than the oxygen–haemoglobin dissociation curve.

In other words, the ratio of carbon dioxide output to oxygen uptake (usually called the **respiratory exchange ratio, R**) varies throughout the lungs. The value of R for the lungs as a whole is about 0.8, varying according to what food is being metabolized. (The fact that this number is similar for the $\dot{V}/\dot{Q}$ ratio for the lungs is coincidental.) In regions near the lung apices with a high $\dot{V}/\dot{Q}$ ratio the value of R is high (up to 2.0), whereas in regions near the bases with a low $\dot{V}/\dot{Q}$ ratio the value of R is low (as low as 0.5).

The relationship between P_{O_2} and P_{CO_2} in regions of the lungs with different $\dot{V}/\dot{Q}$ ratios is usually expressed in a diagram such as Figure 7.11C. This is called the **oxygen–carbon dioxide diagram**, or **O_2–CO_2 diagram**. The values of P_{O_2} and P_{CO_2} at point '$\bar{v}$' are those of mixed venous blood (perfusion, no ventilation, $\dot{V}/\dot{Q}$ ratio of zero). The values of P_{O_2} and P_{CO_2} at I are those of moist air (ventilation, no perfusion, $\dot{V}/\dot{Q}$ ratio of infinity). The $\dot{V}/\dot{Q}$ ratio can take any value between these two extremes, and each value is associated with a particular respiratory exchange ratio as well as a particular P_{O_2} and P_{CO_2}.

It is possible also to draw separate hypothetical O_2–CO_2 diagrams for the composition of alveolar gas and for the gas tensions in the blood, although of course in reality neither arterial gas nor pulmonary capillary blood exists in isolation. Figure 11A shows the theoretical effect of different gas exchange ratios on the composition of alveolar gas. If R = 1.0, each molecule of O_2 removed from an alveolus is replaced by one molecule of CO_2. The P_{O_2} and P_{CO_2} change according to line 1.0. If R = 0.5, two molecules of O_2 are replaced by one of CO_2 and the gas tensions follow the 0.5 line; similarly, a line for R = 2.0 can be drawn. No line passes through the $\bar{v}$ point, as this would represent a value of R that lies outside the range of R in normal healthy lungs. Figure 7.11B represents the theoretical effects of different gas exchanges on the gas tensions in the blood. In this diagram, the relationships between P_{O_2} and P_{CO_2} are not straight lines, because the oxygen and carbon dioxide dissociation curves are not straight lines.

As we have said, the alveoli and the pulmonary capillaries do not act in isolation. Clearly, each molecule of CO_2 lost from the blood is gained by the alveolus, and each molecule of O_2 gained by the blood must have come from the alveolus. The alveolar gas and pulmonary capillary blood must have the same value for R. This means that for each value of R in a particular lung region, the values of P_{O_2} and P_{CO_2} must lie on both the alveolar gas R line and the blood R line, i.e. they must lie where the two lines intersect,

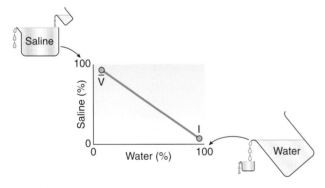

Fig. 7.10

An analogy of under- and overventilated regions of the lung. The exchange of gases is simplified as the displacement of saline by water. Saline represents mixed venous blood ($\bar{v}$) and pure water represents alveolar air. Point $\bar{v}$ represents the composition of blood in poorly ventilated regions of the lung, not enough water being added to wash the salt away. Point I represents regions with ventilation in excess. Nearly all the salt is washed away and the composition of I approaches that of pure water.

THE PULMONARY CIRCULATION: BRINGING BLOOD AND GAS TOGETHER

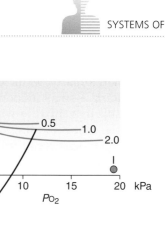

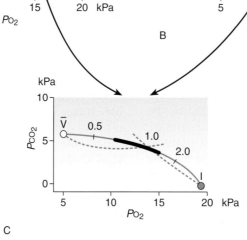

Fig. 7.11

The respiratory exchange ratio (R) for the gases in alveoli and the blood associated with them indicates how P_{CO_2} and P_{O_2} change in the alveolar gas and blood. Combination of the blood and gas lines enables us to determine the partial pressures of CO_2 and O_2 at any combination of ventilation and perfusion. Points $\bar{v}$ and I correspond to mixed venous blood and moist inspired air, respectively. The theoretical effects of different gas exchange ratios (R) are shown in (A), on the composition of the alveolar gas, and (B) on the blood gas tensions in the blood (in reality it is not possible for gas exchange to take place in either the alveoli or blood independently of each other). (C) shows the combined alveolar–blood gas tension relationships for different values of R. The gas R line for R = 1.0 and the blood R line for R = 1.0 have been drawn in interrupted lines. Because the gas tensions must be the same in the alveoli and the blood, the point where the gas and blood R lines intersect represents the blood gas tensions that are actually seen in the alveolar gas and the alveolar capillary blood. Plotting points for all values of R gives the O_2–CO_2 diagram for the lungs. The normal range of $\dot{V}/\dot{Q}$ ratios is shown by the heavy line.

as in Figure 7.11. Plotting points for every possible value of R leads to the O_2–CO_2 diagram for the lungs shown in Figure 7.11C. Notice how the line joining all the values of P_{O_2} and P_{CO_2} is curved. On the diagram, the heavy line represents the normal ranges of P_{O_2}, P_{CO_2}, $\dot{V}/\dot{Q}$ ratio and R that are found in healthy individuals.

As a result of regional differences in the $\dot{V}/\dot{Q}$ ratio and R, the alveoli at the apices of the lungs have a higher P_{AO_2} and a lower P_{ACO_2} than those at the bases of the lungs. Does this matter? After all, the blood from different regions of the lungs is mixed together in the left atrium. Surely the low P_{aO_2} and high P_{aCO_2} in blood leaving regions of the lung with a low $\dot{V}/\dot{Q}$ ratio will be 'balanced' by the high P_{aO_2} and low P_{aCO_2} in blood leaving regions of the lungs with a high $\dot{V}/\dot{Q}$ ratio?

In the case of carbon dioxide this is roughly true: blood leaving regions of the lungs with a high $\dot{V}/\dot{Q}$ ratio has a low P_{aCO_2} and low CO_2 content, and mixes with blood leaving regions of the lungs with a low $\dot{V}/\dot{Q}$ ratio, a high, P_{aCO_2} and high CO_2 content. The resulting mixture has a P_{aCO_2} and CO_2 content, which is 'normal'.

Unfortunately, this is not the case for oxygen, for two reasons:

1. The blood **flow** to the apices of the lungs is very much less than the blood flow to the bases, as we have already seen. The blood leaving the apices of the lungs has a higher P_{aO_2} than that leaving the bases; however, there is very much more blood leaving the bases of the lungs.

2. Although blood from the apices of the lungs has a higher Pa_{O_2} this does not translate into a higher blood oxygen **content**. The haemoglobin leaving regions of the lungs with a higher P_{O_2} is 97% saturated with oxygen and can therefore carry very little extra oxygen compared with regions of the lungs with a normal P_{O_2}. In other words, the content of oxygen in blood leaving regions of the lungs with a high P_{O_2} is very similar to that of blood leaving regions of the lungs with a 'normal' P_{O_2}. Clearly, then, it cannot 'compensate' for the low oxygen content of blood leaving regions of the lungs with a low P_{O_2}.

To summarize these two points: if there is a wide range of $\dot{V}/\dot{Q}$ ratios, blood in the left atrium will tend to have a *reduced* Pa_{O_2} (because the volume of blood with a low Pa_{O_2} from the bases of the lungs is greater than the volume of blood with a high Pa_{O_2} from the apices) and will also have a *reduced oxygen content* (the blood from the apices has a high Pa_{O_2}, but its oxygen content is only very slightly higher than normal because of the shape of the oxygen–haemoglobin dissociation curve). It is therefore very important that there is a relatively narrow range of $\dot{V}/\dot{Q}$ ratios within the lungs; in other words, ventilation and perfusion matching should be as good as possible. Poor ventilation/perfusion matching leads to deoxygenation. In healthy individuals, the degree of ventilation/perfusion matching is so good that arterial blood carries only 2% less oxygen than blood, leaving a theoretical 'ideal' set of lungs that have perfect ventilation/perfusion matching.

Although much of the difference in oxygen content between arterial blood and that of blood leaving an 'ideal' pair of lungs is due to ventilation/perfusion mismatching, there is a second source of relatively deoxygenated blood. This blood makes up part of the **anatomical shunt**. Anatomical shunt is deoxygenated blood that drains into the left (arterial) side of the circulation, and therefore is another reason why arterial blood does not contain as much oxygen as hypothetical blood from an 'ideal' pair of lungs.

Shunt

The content of oxygen in the systemic arteries is not as high as would be predicted from the alveolar gas equation. This is due partly to shunting (i.e. relatively deoxygenated blood being added to oxygenated blood leaving well ventilated alveoli) and partly to ventilation mismatching.

Shunted blood comes from two main sources. The blood draining the bronchial circulation via the deep bronchial veins has already been mentioned. The second source of shunted blood is the **thebesian veins**

in the myocardium. Most of the blood drains from the myocardium into the cardiac veins and then into the cardiac sinus. The cardiac sinus is essentially a large vein that drains into the right atrium. Deoxygenated blood draining through the cardiac vein system therefore does not form a shunt because it drains into the right-hand side of the circulation. The thebesian veins are small vessels that drain blood from the myocardium into the cavity of the underlying atrium or ventricle. Blood draining through the thebesian veins on the left-hand side of the heart therefore forms a shunt. Although the flow of blood through the left-sided thebesian veins is not great, the oxygen content of the blood is very low.

The amount of shunting and ventilation/perfusion mismatching may be expressed in a number of ways. One way is to calculate the difference in oxygen tension between the alveoli and the systemic arteries. The oxygen tension in the alveoli is calculated using the alveolar gas equation, and the oxygen tension in the systemic arteries is measured directly from a blood sample. In normal subjects the alveolar–arterial difference (A–a difference) is usually less than 5 kPa.

Another way of expressing the amount of shunting and ventilation/perfusion mismatching that is taking place is to calculate the **venous admixture**. This is defined as the amount of mixed venous blood that would need to be added to blood leaving a well-perfused and well-ventilated area of lung in order to produce the arterial oxygen concentration that is actually seen in the systemic arteries. The venous admixture is usually expressed as a proportion of the total cardiac output (**shunt fraction**). The venous admixture is a theoretical volume of blood, as the blood that actually flows through the physiological shunts has an oxygen content that may be higher (deep bronchial veins) or lower (thebesian veins) than that of mixed venous blood. The venous admixture may nevertheless be calculated using the **shunt equation**:

$$\frac{\dot{Q}s}{\dot{Q}t} = \frac{Cc'_{O_2} - Ca_{O_2}}{Cc'_{O_2} - C\bar{v}_{O_2}}$$

where $\dot{Q}s$ is the venous admixture flow, $\dot{Q}t$ is the total blood flow, Ca_{O_2} is the oxygen content of arterial blood, $C\bar{v}_{O_2}$ is the oxygen content of mixed venous blood and Cc'_{O_2} is the oxygen content of the capillary blood draining an alveolus with an ideal ventilation/perfusion ratio.

The oxygen content of blood can be calculated knowing the partial pressure of oxygen and the haemoglobin concentration, using the oxygen dissociation curve. Mixed venous blood needs to be obtained from a catheter placed in the pulmonary

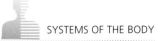

THE PULMONARY CIRCULATION: BRINGING BLOOD AND GAS TOGETHER

7

artery. How can the oxygen content of capillary blood draining an 'ideal' alveolus be measured? Of course it cannot, but it can be inferred by calculating the P_{AO_2} in an 'ideal' alveolus by solving the alveolar gas equation (see page 73) and then calculating the oxygen content of blood at equilibrium with such an alveolus, as above.

The shunt fraction in normal individuals is usually less than 5% of the total cardiac output. Most of the shunt is made due to ventilation/perfusion mismatching, rather than true shunting of blood from the deep bronchial and thebesian veins.

A salutary tale

A student illicitly eating peanuts in the library is surprised by the approach of the librarian. He inhales a nut, which completely blocks his *right* main bronchus. Leaping about in an attempt to expel the offending fruit our hero merely succeeds in dislodging a large clot which has formed in a leg vein due to the hours of immobility he has spent at his studies (this is a fairy story). If the clot obstructs his *right* pulmonary artery all will probably be well; although his right lung will be functionally nonexistent, his left lung will be normal and sufficient for him to survive. If the clot lodges in the *left* pulmonary artery the consequences of this extreme case of ventilation/per-

fusion mismatch will be grave. Despite the fact that his *total* lung ventilation and *total* lung perfusion may be sufficient for survival, both lungs will be functionally useless, but each for a different reason: one will have no ventilation and be a shunt and one will have no perfusion and be dead space. This story may help you understand the importance of matching ventilation and perfusion and a law-abiding lifestyle.

From Widdicombe JG, Davies A. 1991
Respiratory physiology

Further reading

Fishman AP. Normal pulmonary circulation. In: Pulmonary diseases and disorders, Vol 2. New York: McGraw-Hill, 1988

Glazier JB, Hughes JMB, Maloney JE, West JB. Measurements of capillary dimensions and blood volume in rapidly frozen lungs. Journal of Applied Physiology 1969;26:65–76

Hughes JMB. Distribution of pulmonary blood flow. In: Crystal RG, West JB, Barnes PJ, Weibel ER, eds. The lung: scientific foundations, 2nd edn. New York: Raven Press, 1997

Weir EK, Reeves JT (eds) Pulmonary vascular physiology and pathophysiology. New York: Marcel Dekker, 1989

West JB, Wagner PD. Ventilation–perfusion relationships. In: Crystal RG, West JB, Barnes PJ, Weibel ER, eds. The lung: scientific foundations, 2nd edn. New York: Raven Press, 1997

Self-assessment case study

A 69-year-old man has smoked heavily all his life. As a result, he suffers from quite severe chronic obstructive pulmonary disease and he is chronically hypoxic. He has started to develop swelling of his ankles.

① What effect do you think that chronic hypoxia will have on the blood vessels within his lungs?

② What effect will this have on the resistance of the blood vessels within his lungs?

③ How might his right ventricle be affected?

④ How might all this be related to the swelling of his ankles?

Answers see page 177

Self-assessment questions

① What is the normal arterial blood pressure in the systemic and pulmonary circulations?

② What is the normal blood flow through the systemic and pulmonary circulations?

③ What are the main anatomical differences between the systemic and pulmonary circulations?

④ What factors influence the distribution of blood within the lungs?

⑤ What are the consequences of a mismatch in ventilation and perfusion?

⑥ What are the important sources of shunt?

Answers see page 178

CARRIAGE OF GASES BY THE BLOOD AND ACID/BASE BALANCE

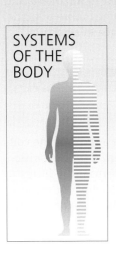

SYSTEMS OF THE BODY

Chapter objectives

After studying this chapter you should be able to:

① Define the O_2 capacity, saturation and content of the blood, and how they change in anaemia.

② Explain the advantages of having red cells and the problems of abnormal haemoglobin.

③ Describe the effect of changes in pH, $P\text{CO}_2$, temperature and 2,3-DPG on the oxyhaemoglobin dissociation curve.

④ Explain the differences between adult and fetal haemoglobin and myoglobin, and the problem of retention of fetal haemoglobin.

⑤ Explain carbon monoxide poisoning.

⑥ List the forms and proportions of CO_2 transported in blood.

⑦ Draw the relationship between CO_2 content and $P\text{CO}_2$ in oxygenated and deoxygenated blood.

⑧ Account for the chloride shift and carbonic anhydrase.

⑨ Define a buffer and the major buffers in the blood.

⑩ Explain how oxygenation of haemoglobin and its buffer power are linked.

⑪ Describe common acid–base defects found in disease and how these are compensated.

Introduction

The survival of the cells of our bodies requires the expenditure of energy. This energy is obtained by the oxidation of food, mainly in the form of glucose:

$$C_6H_{12}O_6 + 6O_2 = 6CO_2 + 6H_2O + \text{Energy}$$
(Equation 8.1)

This equation represents the reaction that takes place when we burn sugar (glucose), and when sugar is burned it releases its energy in a single burst, producing a high temperature. Of course this does not happen as a crude single step in our bodies: the reaction takes place in a series of small steps within the mitochondria of the cells, and most of the energy released is immediately stored as **adenosine triphosphate** (ATP), a high-energy molecule which is made by combining adenosine diphosphate (ADP) with inorganic phosphate:

$$ADP + \text{Phosphate} + \text{Energy} \Leftrightarrow ATP$$
(Equation 8.2)

Chemical oxidation can be by the addition of O_2 or by the removal of hydrogen (as H^+, a proton), and the latter is the mechanism used in the mitochondria. This removal of hydrogen cannot continue indefinitely, as a build-up of H^+ would stop the reaction, so the hydrogen is combined with O_2 to form water, as in Equation 8.1. This removal of hydrogen leaves behind the elements of CO_2 from the glucose. This simplistic description explains why the oxidative metabolism of our mitochondria, which keeps our cells alive, requires O_2 and produces CO_2 and water.

Oxygen moves into our cells and CO_2 moves out by the process of diffusion. In Chapter 6 we learned that there must be a difference in concentration of the diffusing substance for overall diffusion to take place. Outside the cell must have a higher concentration of O_2 and a lower concentration of CO_2 than inside the cell. High concentrations of O_2 and low concentrations of CO_2 are the conditions found in the air around us and, to a lesser extent, in the alveolar air. It is the business of the circulation to bring these conditions close to the individual cells.

Blood is a liquid tissue (plasma) containing formed elements (cells). The red blood cells (RBC, **erythrocytes**) play an important part in the transport of O_2 to and CO_2 away from the tissues. RBC should strictly be called corpuscles, because they contain no nucleus, but the term cell is in general use.

This exchange of gases between the cells and blood at our tissues is a repeat of the exchange between air and blood at the lungs, and results in the differences in composition between venous and arterial blood shown in Table 8.1. Although the RBCs play an important role in this carriage and exchange (carrying the majority of O_2 and processing CO_2 at both lungs and tissues), the gases must first enter into simple solution in the plasma before being carried or processed by the RBCs.

Oxygen in the blood is mainly carried in loose combination with haemoglobin (Hb) within the RBC. Carbon dioxide is carried partly in solution, partly in combination with proteins (particularly Hb), but mainly as bicarbonate in the plasma. The carrier mechanisms in blood have evolved so that the uptake or loss of O_2 promotes the loss or uptake of CO_2 and vice versa, a most useful arrangement.

The addition of CO_2 to the blood at the tissues would cause a dangerously large change in acidity if the blood did not contain efficient buffering systems, in particular protein, bicarbonate and phosphate, which take up hydrogen ions added to the blood and release them when the blood becomes more alkaline, thereby **buffering** (resisting) changes in acidity.

Oxygen transport

Haemoglobin (Hb)

Because we are complicated animals most of the cells of our bodies are far removed from the atmosphere. Oxygen has therefore to be carried from the lungs to these cells in the blood. All gases dissolve in water to a greater or lesser extent, but O_2 dissolves only to the extent of 3 mL L^{-1} in the watery plasma leaving the lungs.

Table 8.1
Some values for normal blood.

		Systemic arterial blood	Mixed venous blood
Oxygen			
Tension	(kPa)	13.3	5.3
Blood content	(ml litre^{-1})	200	150
Saturation	(%)	98	75
Carbon dioxide			
Tension	(kPa)	5.3	6.1
Blood content	(ml litre^{-1})	490	530
Plasma content	(ml litre^{-1})	600	640
Acidity			
Plasma [H^+]	(nM)	40	43
Plasma pH		7.40	7.37

Carriage of gases by the blood and acid/base balance Box 1

Carbon monoxide poisoning – a failure of oxygen transport

Mr Jones is a 31-year-old man who has recently lost his job and whose wife had left him a few months previously. He had been drinking increasingly heavily and had been slipping further and further into debt. Such was his despair that, one afternoon, following a heavy drinking session, he decided to try to commit suicide.

He went into the garage, connected a length of hosepipe to the exhaust of his rather old car, and fed the other end of the pipe through one of the car windows. He sat in the driver's seat with a bottle of whisky and started the engine. The interior of the car began to fill with exhaust fumes.

The combination of the alcohol that he had consumed and the carbon monoxide in the exhaust fumes meant that Mr Jones soon started to lose consciousness. Fortunately, a neighbour found Mr Jones in the car. He turned off the ignition and tried to wake him. Mr Jones was just rousable but his speech was slurred and he remained drowsy. The neighbour called an ambulance and attempted to remove Mr Jones from the car. When they arrived, the paramedics from the ambulance administered oxygen to Mr Jones from a face-mask and transferred him to hospital.

On his arrival at the Accident and Emergency department an arterial blood sample was taken from Mr Jones for analysis of blood gas tensions. The sample revealed that his arterial blood gases were close to normal. However, his carboxyhaemoglobin level was measured at 52%, confirming the diagnosis of carbon monoxide (CO) poisoning.

He was treated with high concentrations of oxygen and was closely monitored on the high-dependency ward. Gradually, he regained consciousness as the CO was displaced from his blood by oxygen and the effects of the alcohol he had consumed began to wear off. The carboxyhaemoglobin levels in his blood were measured later than day and were found to be 12%.

In this chapter, we will consider:

① Why carbon monoxide is poisonous.
② Symptoms of carbon monoxide poisoning.
③ The treatment of carbon monoxide poisoning.

While exercising vigorously we may need up to 3 L of O_2 per minute. This implies that if O_2 was only carried to the tissues in simple solution we would need a blood flow of 1000 L min^{-1} to supply our bodies with O_2. Olympic athletes can increase the output of their hearts to about 30 L min^{-1} which you can see is still several hundred times too little to supply their tissues with O_2. The answer to this problem is that, like all other vertebrates, we have evolved a carrier molecule in the blood which picks up and then releases a great deal of O_2. In us this molecules is **haemoglobin** (Hb).

Haemoglobin has remarkable O_2-carrying properties which are related to its molecular structure (Fig. 8.1.)

Each haemoglobin molecule consists of a protein (globin) and haem (protoporphyrin and ferrous iron). The globin is made up of four polypeptide chains, each carrying a haem group. This structure is repeated four times in each molecule, which means there are *four sites, each capable of carrying one O_2* on each Hb molecule. This explains many of the properties of Hb, as we will see in a moment. Each of the four chains can vary, which will vary the O_2-carrying properties of the blood. The chains are described chemically as α or β, depending on their structure. The types of polypeptides that make them up give rise to the various forms of normal and abnormal Hb.

Adult Hb consists of two α and two β chains, with 141 and 146 amino acid residues per chain, respectively. Each Hb molecule thus has 574 amino acids and four haems, which gives the molecule a weight of about 64 500. Fetal Hb is slightly, but importantly, different. Men have about 150 g L^{-1} Hb in their blood, women about 130 g L$^{-1.}$

Oxygen combination with haemoglobin

This reversible reaction can be summarized as follows:

$$Hb + O_2 \Leftrightarrow HbO_2 \qquad \text{(Equation 8.3)}$$

which will be driven to the right (HbO_2) by increased P_{O_2} and to the left by low P_{O_2}. The Hb of this equation is deoxyhaemoglobin – often, and incorrectly, referred to as 'reduced haemoglobin', despite the fact that the Hb is not chemically reduced. The HbO_2 in this equation is oxyhaemoglobin, and by the same token that Hb is not chemically oxidized, the combination between Hb and O_2 is **oxygenation**, a much looser combination than oxidation.

Each of the four haem groups of the Hb molecule represents a site for combination with O_2. It might be more correct to consider each haemoglobin molecule as Hb_4, with which association or dissociation with O_2

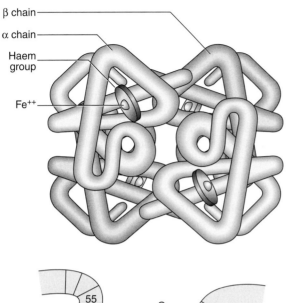

β chain
α chain
Haem group
Fe^{++}

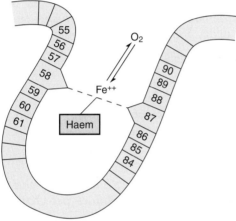

Fig. 8.1

The structure of haemoglobin. Each of the four globin chains (the wormlike structures in the figure) is made up of a spiral of just over 100 amino acids. Each chain is attached at one point to an iron-containing haem group. Each haem group can carry a molecule of O_2, so each haemoglobin molecule has four 'hooks', each of which can carry one O_2.

takes place in four steps, in which case Equation 8.3 should be written:

$$Hb_4 + O_2 \Leftrightarrow Hb_4O_2$$
$$Hb_4O_2 + O_2 \Leftrightarrow Hb_4O_4$$
$$Hb_4O_4 + O_2 \Leftrightarrow Hb_4O_6$$
and finally $Hb_4O_6 + O_2 \Leftrightarrow Hb_4O_8$ (Equation 8.4)

It is conceptually useful to consider each Hb molecule as having only four 'hooks'. On each hook can hang one O_2.

Carriage of gases by the blood and acid/base balance Box 8

Why carbon monoxide is poisonous

Carbon monoxide (CO) is a colourless, odourless, tasteless gas formed from the incomplete combustion of organic substances. Poisoning with CO may be the result of inhalation of fumes from a faulty heating system, inhalation of smoke from house fires, or deliberate self-injury by the inhalation of car exhaust fumes (although modern cars with catalytic converters do not emit much CO).

CO produces its toxic effect by causing hypoxia in peripheral tissues. It does this by interfering with the transport of oxygen by haemoglobin, and also by interfering with cellular respiration.

CO binds to haemoglobin with an affinity about 250 times that of oxygen, to form carboxyhaemoglobin. Carboxyhaemoglobin cannot carry oxygen, and so the amount of haemoglobin available for the carriage of oxygen is reduced. This means that even if the *partial pressure* of oxygen in arterial blood is normal and therefore the *oxygen saturation* of the available haemoglobin is maintained, the *oxygen content* of the blood is reduced because the amount of haemoglobin available to carry oxygen is reduced. Furthermore, in the presence of carboxyhaemoglobin the oxygen–haemoglobin dissociation curve is distorted and shifted to the left. As a result of this, oxygen tends to remain bound to haemoglobin in the peripheral circulation rather than being released into the tissues. In other words, less oxygen is carried in the circulation, and of the oxygen that is carried, much remains bound to haemoglobin and is not available for tissue respiration.

In addition to these effects on oxygen carriage by the blood, CO also interferes with electron transport in mitochondria and with other cellular processes. Overall, then, its effect is to reduce oxygen delivery to peripheral tissues, and also to reduce the ability of these tissues to use what oxygen they obtain. Cellular ATP levels fall and vital cellular functions begin to fail. In severe cases of poisoning this may lead to impairment of the respiratory and cardiovascular systems, which exacerbates oxygen transport even more.

The haem and the globin of each molecule are held in a fixed relationship to each other by links (salt bridges) between the polypeptide chains. In each of the steps in Equation 8.4, when a molecule of O_2 binds to the iron atom in each haem the molecular shape is distorted, making the attachment of the next O_2 molecule easier. This distortion is called an allosteric effect and, together with the fact that there are only four 'hooks' for O_2 per molecule, explains the sigmoid shape of the graph obtained when we plot percentage saturation of Hb by O_2 against PO_2 (Fig. 8.2). This S-shaped curve is called the **oxyhaemoglobin dissociation curve**, and it is so important to our understanding of the transport of O_2 that a description of how it is obtained is well worthwhile.

Obtaining a dissociation curve

If you take, say, five test tubes of blood and expose each of them to a different partial pressure of O_2 (say 0, 2, 4, 8, 16 kPa O_2, as in Fig. 8.2), in each tube a different percentage of haemoglobin will be converted to oxyhaemoglobin, depending on the partial pressure it has been exposed to, and have a different colour because oxyhaemoglobin is brighter red than haemoglobin (arterial blood is red; venous blood is purple). An instrument called a spectrophotometer can use this colour to measure what percentage of the Hb has been converted to HbO_2, and so we can plot a graph of percentage saturation (percentage of the O_2-carrying 'hooks' occupied) against the PO_2 to which that particular sample of blood was exposed (Fig. 8.2A). We have talked about each Hb molecule having four hooks, each of which can carry one O_2 molecule. This might suggest that blood can only be 25% (one hook), 50% (two hooks) 75% (three hooks occupied) or 100% (four hooks). This is true for each individual molecule, but would ignore the fact that even a drop of blood contains millions of Hb molecules, any one of which can be carrying from zero to four O_2 molecules.

Properties of the oxyhaemoglobin dissociation curve

When 100% saturated (all 'hooks' occupied), 1 g of Hb carries about 2 mg – 1.36 ml – of O_2 at normal body temperature. Therefore, 1 L of your blood, containing 150 g of Hb, can transport 200 ml of O_2 as HbO_2. Comparing this with the 3 ml carried in simple solution gives some idea of the advantage having Hb in our blood bestows.

The carriage of O_2 in our blood is not quite as simple as hanging O_2 molecules on hooks, like coats on a stand: evolution has refined this already efficient process even further. To understand these refinements requires the definition of four terms:

A Saturation curve

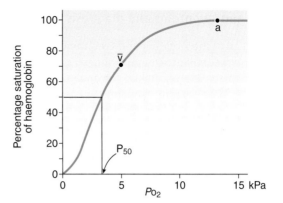

B Content curve

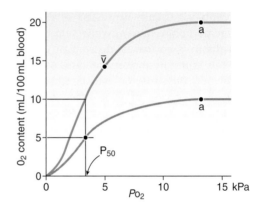

Fig. 8.2
The oxyhaemoglobin dissociation curve. This curve is obtained by exposing blood to a number of partial pressures of O_2 and measuring how much of its total O_2 carrying capacity is occupied. This can be expressed in two ways. The saturation curve (A) represents the percentage of the total number of 'hooks' for O_2 that are occupied (the 50% occupancy, P_{50}, is shown). This curve gives us no idea of the amount of O_2 being carried, which depends on the amount of Hb present and is shown by the content curve (B). That content depends on the amount of Hb is shown by the lower curve, which represents anaemic blood. Both this and the normal curve are equally saturated at different PO_2, as shown by their identical P_{50}, but the amount they are carrying is very different. Because temperature and pH affect the properties of Hb we must state that these curves were obtained at pH 7.4 and 37°C. The important loading and unloading conditions for blood are from arterial blood at (a) and into mixed venous blood at ($\bar{v}$). Note that the slope of the curve is very different at these two points.

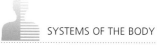
Carriage of gases by the blood and acid/base balance Box 3

Signs and symptoms and diagnosis of carbon monoxide poisoning

On arrival at the Accident and Emergency department, Mr Jones was still drowsy, with slurred speech. An arterial blood sample was taken for analysis of blood gas pressures. The sample revealed that the partial pressure of carbon dioxide in Mr Jones' arterial blood was high, suggesting that he was hypoventilating. The partial pressure of oxygen in his blood was slightly higher than normal because he was breathing oxygen. However, his carboxyhaemoglobin level was measured at 52%, confirming the diagnosis of carbon monoxide poisoning.

Measurement of carboxyhaemoglobin levels is the key to diagnosing CO poisoning. The carboxyhaemoglobin is usually expressed as a percentage of total haemoglobin. In city dwellers up to 5% carboxyhaemoglobin is normal, and levels of up to 10% are very often found in smokers. In cases of CO poisoning levels of over 20% may be associated with symptoms, and levels in excess of 60% often result in coma. However, although measuring carboxyhaemoglobin levels is useful in diagnosing CO poisoning, it is often difficult to relate these measurements to the patient's clinical condition. This is because once the patient is removed from the source of CO blood levels fall very quickly, and the clinical picture is thought to be more closely related to peak carboxyhaemoglobin levels.

The signs and symptoms of CO poisoning are all related to the tissue hypoxia that it causes. Many organs, but particularly the brain, the heart and the lungs, can be affected.

In mild cases of CO poisoning patients develop a frontal headache that may be associated with drowsiness or agitation and confusion, particularly in the elderly. Often these symptoms are associated with nausea or vomiting. In more severe cases of poisoning, patients may lose consciousness or start to fit.

CO may also affect the heart and cause ECG abnormalities, and is recognized as a cause of cardiac failure and myocardial infarction. Its effects on the lungs include hyperventilation and pulmonary oedema.

It may affect the nervous system, producing hemiplegia or peripheral nerve damage, and recovery from poisoning may be complicated by long-term psychiatric problems such as personality changes and memory loss, which are thought to be a consequence of hypoxic brain damage.

Classically, patients with CO poisoning are said to have pink skin and mucosae owing to the presence of carboxyhaemoglobin, which has a bright red colour. This is not a reliable sign, and in severe cases of CO poisoning associated with a failing circulation it may not be apparent.

- *Oxygen tension (Po_2; kPa)* We have met this term before, but revision of its meaning might be useful. Oxygen **tension** is sometimes called the **partial pressure** of O_2 in solution. The difference in Po_2 between two sites determines the rate and direction of diffusion of O_2. This is because the partial pressures correspond to the concentrations *in solution* (Henry's Law). Thus dissolved O_2 will diffuse down its concentration gradient. The Po_2 of active skeletal muscle may be as low as 1 kPa. Arterial blood supplying that muscle has a Po_2 of about 13 kPa, and this large pressure difference 'pushes' O_2 strongly into the tissues.

- *Haemoglobin content (Hb, g L^{-1})* It is Hb that has the 'hooks' that carry the O_2. The number of 'hooks' determines the maximum O_2-carrying capacity per mL of blood. If blood has only 50% (say) of the normal amount of Hb (it is anaemic), it will only have 50% of the normal number of 'hooks', and even when fully saturated with O_2 it will only be able to carry 100 mL rather than 200 mL of O_2.

- *Haemoglobin saturation (%)* This is the percentage of the total number of 'hooks' available for O_2 that are in fact occupied. It is nothing to do with the *number* of 'hooks' present. The number present may be increased (polycythaemia), normal or reduced (anaemia). Measurement of Hb saturation is technically simple using the spectrophotometer as described (Obtaining a dissociation curve, p. 113) and gives useful information for clinical assessment as 100% saturation of arterial blood implies the lungs are doing a good job of gas exchange. However, other measurements, particularly Po_2 and Hb content, are necessary to provide a complete picture.

  Students sometimes find it helpful to think of saturation as the 'appetite' haemoglobin has for O_2. If haemoglobin finds itself in a Po_2 where its saturation should be high (say 10 kPa in Fig. 8.2) it is 'hungry' and will readily accept O_2 until it is appropriately saturated, 'full'. At low Po_2 (say 2 kPa in Fig. 8.2) it is not so hungry; in fact, it is overstuffed for these conditions and vomits off its excess oxygen.

Carriage of gases by the blood and acid/base balance Box 4

Treatment of carbon monoxide poisoning

After the diagnosis of carbon monoxide poisoning had been made Mr Jones was treated with high concentrations of oxygen (60% inspired oxygen) and was closely monitored on the high-dependency ward. Gradually, he regained consciousness as the carbon monoxide was displaced from his blood by oxygen and the effects of the alcohol he had consumed began to wear off. The carboxyhaemoglobin levels in his blood were measured later that day and were found to be 12%.

Oxygen is the treatment of CO poisoning. By administering high concentrations of oxygen, carbon monoxide is dissociated from carboxyhaemoglobin, producing haemoglobin, which is then free to combine with oxygen. In some centres CO poisoning is treated with hyperbaric oxygen: in other words, the patient is placed in a pressurized chamber and breathes 100% oxygen. Under these circumstances, the partial pressure of oxygen is very high because the ambient pressure is high. The high partial pressure of oxygen leads to an even more rapid removal of CO. It is also possible that an improvement in oxygenation occurs because the administration of a high partial pressure of oxygen results in an increase in the amount of dissolved oxygen in the blood, possibly to a clinically significant level. The use of hyperbaric oxygen remains controversial, however, and it is only useful if it is quickly available, which is not the case in most centres.

- *Oxygen content* (mL L^{-1}) We have seen ('Haemoglobin content', above) that the amount of oxygen in a litre of arterial blood is limited by the amount of Hb it contains. It also depends on the P_{O_2} of the air in the lungs driving O_2 into the blood. This underlies the difference between 'saturation' and 'content', which is very important to understand. An analogy that might help is to consider the RBC as a cloakroom used to store coats. The number of coats (O_2 molecules) that can be stored depends on the number of hooks (Hb molecules) present. The number that are actually stored (O_2 *content*), up to the theoretical maximum when all hooks are occupied (100% *saturation*), depends on the size of the cloakroom (amount of Hb) and the pressure from customers wishing to leave their coats (P_{O_2}).

  So, if everything else is normal:

- O_2 content in blood depends on the amount of Hb present *and* P_{O_2}.
- O_2 saturation depends only on oxygen partial pressure (P_{O_2}).

The shape of the curve (Fig. 8.2)

The oxyhaemoglobin dissociation curve (Fig. 8.2) can express the relationship between P_{O_2} and saturation, which is independent of blood Hb content, or P_{O_2} and O_2 content which is not. In terms of content the curve is displaced downwards in anaemia (where Hb content is low).

Whether expressing the relationship between P_{O_2} and saturation or content, the curves in Figure 8.2 have the same characteristic shape, which has an important influence on function. The major function of Hb is to *load* with O_2 at the lungs and *unload* at the tissues. This function is carried out at the flat **loading region** at the top of the curve and at the steep **unloading region**. The difference in slope of the curve at these two points has the following consequences:

- *Loading region (the lungs)* Above about 10 kPa Hb cannot take up much more O_2: it is saturated, because most of the molecules of Hb are carrying their full complement of four O_2 molecules and this number cannot be exceeded however high the P_{O_2}. Alveolar ventilation can decrease by up to 25% or increase indefinitely without affecting O_2 *content* significantly. O_2 *tension* varies, however. The evolutionary advantage of this is that normal activities such as talking, sighing, coughing etc. do not greatly alter the amount of O_2 per litre of blood leaving the lungs for the tissues.

- *Unloading region (the tissues)* Blood in the capillaries of active tissues finds itself in an environment of low P_{O_2}. Oxygen diffuses from blood to tissues, and even a small fall in blood P_{O_2} causes a large unloading of O_2, i.e. the blood is working on the steep part of the HbO$_2$ dissociation curve. If it stays in the tissue long enough blood P_{O_2} will equilibrate with tissue P_{O_2}. If the blood is anaemic (low Hb content), however, removal of even a small amount of O_2 causes a large fall in P_{O_2} because there is little O_2 in the blood to begin with. A situation is quickly reached where there is little possibility of further supply to the tissues and a reduced P_{O_2} to drive it in. Thus anaemia can cause tissue hypoxia even though arterial blood has normal P_{O_2} and Hb saturation.

To identify the position of the steep part of the oxyhaemoglobin dissociation curve (usually to see if it is being oxygenated properly) the P_{O_2} at which 50% of the Hb is saturated is measured: this is called the P_{50} and is about 3.2 kPa for normal adult human arterial blood.

Displacement of the oxyhaemoglobin dissociation curve (Fig. 8.3)

The evolution of Hb with a dissociation curve of the shape described has been a wonderful advantage to the species that possess it. Even more wonderful is the displacement of this curve along the P_{O_2} axis of the graph that takes place with each circuit of the blood between lungs and tissue and between tissue and lungs. This displacement of the dissociation curve represent cyclic changes in the properties of Hb which make it an even more efficient carrier of O_2.

We have seen (Fig. 8.2) that abnormal amounts of Hb in the blood will displace the O_2 *content* curve vertically but will not affect the *saturation* curve. We will now look at factors that displace the curve horizontally and the way in which this improves the supply of O_2 to the tissues.

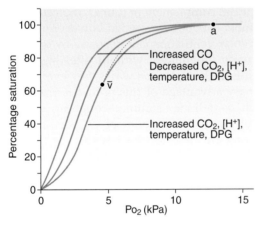

Fig. 8.3
Shifts of the dissociation curve. Conditions in terms of [H⁺], CO_2, temperature and 2,3-diphosphoglycerate are very different at the sites of loading (the lungs) and unloading (the tissues) of Hb with O_2. These differences shift the dissociation curve and improve its carrying properties. For example, the effects of increased H⁺ and CO_2 at the tissues is to shift the curve to the right (this is called the Bohr shift), and this steepens the functional dissociation curve to that shown as a dotted line.

- *Hydrogen ion concentration* Increased [H⁺] (decreased pH, increased acidity) displaces the curve to the *right* (Fig. 8.3). This **Bohr shift** is due to H⁺ acting on the Hb molecule to decrease its affinity for O_2. This does not affect the loading region of the curve because it is horizontal, and so movement to left or right does not produce a change in saturation.

  The steep unloading region of the curve is a different matter. In metabolizing tissues the release of acids or of CO_2 (which increases [H⁺]) shifts the curve to the right. This has two major consequences, the first fairly obvious, the second less so:

  1. Take a vertical line at some P_{O_2} on the steep part of the curve, say 4 kPa in Figure 8.3. If the curve moves to the right the saturation appropriate for that P_{O_2} will fall. The Hb has less 'appetite' for O_2 and it 'vomits off' the excess (see Haemoglobin saturation, p. 114, above). This is clearly an advantage, liberating O_2 to diffuse down the concentration gradient to the tissues.
  2. What is not so immediately obvious but equally important is revealed if you take a *horizontal* line, at, say 50% saturation. When the curve moves to the right the P_{O_2} appropriate for that saturation *increases*!! This increases the partial pressure gradient driving O_2 into the tissues.

  These effects of acidity are so powerful that a decrease of 0.2 pH units can increase O_2 release by 25% at low P_{O_2}.
- *Carbon dioxide* In addition to its acid properties, which are dealt with above, CO_2 reacts with Hb to form **carbamino Hb**. This also moves the curve to the right. If hypercapnia (increased P_{CO_2}) persists for several hours, with chronic acidosis, red cell **2,3,diphosphoglycerate** (DPG, see below) is decreased, shifting the curve back to the left.
- *Temperature* A decrease in temperature shifts the curve to the left. Blood therefore gives up its O_2 less readily in cold tissues, and blood leaving them may be well oxygenated because of this effect. Also, cold will reduce the metabolic demand for O_2. For this reason, children playing in the snow have pink ears and noses when their vasoconstricted skin might have been expected to turn blue. This effect is not very important in the lungs because the air in them is so well warmed. It is important, however, in patients made hypothermic during open heart surgery. In these patients, even if arterial P_{O_2} is low the Hb is relatively well saturated and the patient does not look hypoxic.
- *2,3-Diphosphoglycerate (DPG)* In most cells under anaerobic conditions 1,3-diphosphoglycerate (1,3-DPG) is converted to 3-phosphoglycerate, with the release of energy which is stored in the form of adenosine triphosphate (ATP).

In red cells, however, 1,3-DPG is converted to 2,3-DPG without the release of energy (Fig. 8.4), an apparently pointless metabolic reaction.

It was discovered that this DPG reacts with HbO_2, causing a release of O_2 by shifting the dissociation curve to the right, and this suggested that DPG was important:

1. in chronic hypoxia of disease, or residence at high altitude, when DPG is increased, releasing O_2 in hypoxic tissues
2. during prolonged exercise, when again DPG increases
3. when blood is stored, as in blood banks, and DPG decreases. This blood will not give up its oxygen so easily, a disadvantage to patients receiving transfusions
4. red cells containing abnormal haemoglobins, as in sickle cell anaemia, or patients with enzyme abnormalities, may have abnormal levels of DPG.

Unfortunately, despite the excitement caused by the discovery of the action of DPG, it has yet to be demonstrated as having any significant effect under normal and pathological conditions. Even under the conditions cited above other physiological effects are much more important, and DPG remains an evolutionary oddity.

Other types of haemoglobin

There are a number of respiratory pigments that occur naturally and carry oxygen under normal physiological conditions. There are also a number of abnormal carriers, and situations when the carrying capacity of Hb is compromised. It is clinically important for clinicians to recognize when the O_2 content of blood is reduced for whatever reason, and this is frequently first detected as cyanosis.

Cyanosis

Clinicians are often alerted to reduced blood O_2 content by **cyanosis**, a bluish tinge to the skin. This arises because the colour of blood depends on the Hb content, and the proportions of this that are in the oxygenated (red) or deoxygenated (purple) state. In normal blood the appearance of cyanosis corresponds to about 70% saturation and a Po_2 of 5 kPa: this means the blood contains 50 g L^{-1} deoxygenated haemoglobin, which gives cyanosed skin its blue colour. If the patient is anaemic there is not sufficient Hb to produce this effect, and anaemic patients can be severely hypoxic without cyanosis. On the other hand, polycythaemic patients, with excess Hb, may be cyanosed with little hypoxia.

Myoglobin

Myoglobin is found in muscle and, in part, gives muscle its red colour. Unlike haemoglobin, with its four chains carrying oxygen, myoglobin consists of one molecule of haem and one polypeptide chain. Its dissociation curve is to the left of Hb (Fig. 8.5), so it readily takes up O_2 from Hb in capillary blood. Myoglobin may act as a small store of O_2 available during anaerobic conditions. This would be useful

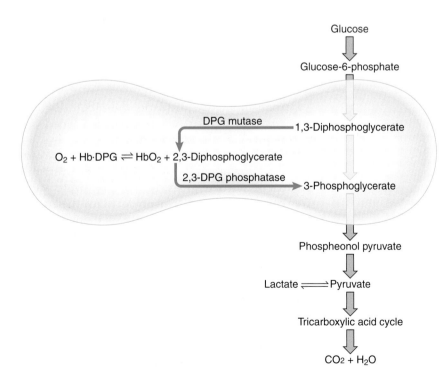

Fig. 8.4
The 2,3-diphosphoglycerate (2,3-DPG) shunt. The metabolic glycolytic pathway of red corpuscles has an extra 'shunt' which produces 2,3-DPG. This substance shifts the oxyhaemoglobin curve to the right, but this effect is of little functional importance and this metabolic pathway remains a biochemical oddity.

during the contraction of muscle, particularly heart muscle, because contraction cuts off blood flow. This effect is very limited in the case of sustained contraction of skeletal muscle because the oxygen stored in myoglobin is depleted in a few seconds.

Fetal haemoglobin

The human fetus, dependent on its mother for O_2, is always threatened with hypoxia. To alleviate this threat, fetal haemoglobin has a high affinity for O_2 and this facilitates transfer from mother to fetus. Fetal Hb has two γ-polypeptide chains in place of the β chains of adult Hb, and inside red cells fetal Hb has a greater affinity for O_2 than does adult Hb (Fig. 8.5). Fetal blood in the uterine/placental circulation takes up O_2 mainly because its P_{O_2} is lower than that of the maternal uterine arterial blood. In addition, inspection of Figure 8.5 will show that, because its dissociation curve is to the left of the maternal one, at most P_{O_2} fetal blood is more saturated – 'hungry' for O_2. The transfer of O_2 from mother to fetus is aided by a further mechanism produced by the unloading of CO_2 in the other direction, from fetus to mother. We have seen above (Displacement of the oxyhaemoglobin curve, p. 116) that the acidic effects of CO_2 cause the release of O_2 from oxyhaemoglobin. The effect of the transfer of CO_2 from fetus to mother first moves the fetal dissociation curve to the left (CO_2 is leaving this blood), and

then the same CO_2 moves the mother's dissociation curve to the right (CO_2 is being added to this blood). The overall effect of this **double Bohr shift** is to widen the gap between the two dissociation curves, shifting the balance of transfer to the fetus. The mechanisms that make fetal haemoglobin so efficient at obtaining O_2 from the mother also make it less efficient at releasing it at the fetal tissues. This results in a degree of hypoxia, which the fetal tissues are better able to withstand than those of the adult. Furthermore, because fetal Hb is more acid than adult Hb it is less able to carry CO_2, and so the fetus tends toward acidosis.

There is a mixture of fetal and adult haemoglobin in fetal blood. The fetal form is gradually replaced in the first few months after birth, except in the hereditary disorder **thalassaemia**, which as the name suggests (Greek, *thalassa*, sea) is particularly prevalent in Mediterranean peoples. In this disease the persistence of fetal haemoglobin means the blood releases its O_2 less readily. Thalassaemia is treated by blood transfusion at 4–6-week intervals throughout life.

Abnormal haemoglobins

- *Carboxyhaemoglobin (HbCO)* Carbon monoxide (CO) binds to Hb 250 times more strongly than does O_2 and competes with it for sites on Hb to form HbCO. This means that as there is 21% O_2 in air it only takes 0.1% CO to 'compete' on equal terms for the O_2-carrying sites on Hb and results in arterial blood having 50% HbO_2 and 50% HbCO, which is useless to the tissues. This is equivalent to being 50% anaemic. For this low concentration of CO to come into equilibrium with the blood takes over an hour, but once there the CO takes equally long to be cleared from the blood. Ventilation with 100% O_2 will speed the elimination of CO because the high P_{O_2} displaces the CO more efficiently than atmospheric P_{O_2}.

  Carbon monoxide displaces the HbO_2 dissociation curve to the left, so the poisoned blood less readily gives up the little O_2 it has.

  When domestic gas was made from coal it contained a large amount of CO as does the untreated exhaust of petrol engines. These fumes were at one time popular methods of suicide. Since the advent of natural gas, which does not contain CO, and catalytic converters for cars which change CO to CO_2, these methods have ceased to be available. The cherry-red colour of HbCO gives patients poisoned by CO a deceptively pink and healthy appearance.

- *Methaemoglobin (Met-Hb)* Methaemoglobin is formed by the oxidation of the ferrous atom of Hb into the ferric form. This can occur because of a congenital defect or as a result of oxidizing poisons, such as

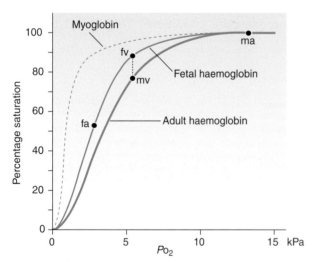

Fig. 8.5
The dissociation curves for fetal haemoglobin and adult myoglobin.
These curves are to the left of the normal adult curve, indicating that these respiratory pigments are more 'avid' for O_2 than the adult form, and promote a flow of O_2 in the required direction – to the muscles or to the fetus. Maternal and fetal arterial and venous saturations are shown.

nitrites. The Met-Hb cannot combine with O_2. The **methaemoglobin reductase** found in red blood cells slowly converts Met-Hb back into Hb.

- *Genetically abnormal haemoglobins* More than 100 different types of human Hb have been discovered, with variants of the peptide patterns in the four polypeptide chains. Some of these Hbs have abnormal dissociation curves because the Hb itself is changed, or because the changes lead to changes in the red cell, such as abnormal DPG content. Abnormalities of Hb may change the shape of the red cell and make it more fragile, as in sickle cell disease.

Sickle cell disease

Most variations in the structure of haemoglobin consist of the substitution of a single amino acid in the globin chain, the haem group being normal. These differences are usually identified electrophoretically and only a few result in clinical manifestations. In the genetically determined **sickle cell disease** deoxygenation of the abnormal haemoglobin (HbS) causes it to polymerize and distort the red blood corpuscle.

Heterozygotes for this disease are said to carry the trait for sickle cell: about 40–50% of their total Hb is HbS and they are asymptomatic except under hypoxic conditions. Homozygotes always manifest the disease, which may be fatal in childhood. The disease is found in regions where falciparum malaria is endemic, and people who carry the sickle cell gene are protected against malaria.

Clinical symptoms develop at about 6 months old. They include bone pain and painful vaso-occlusive crises caused by sickled erythrocytes blocking small blood vessels. Leg ulceration is common, and splenic infarction results in splenic atrophy.

Fetal haemoglobin reduces the risk of sickling, which explains why symptoms do not develop before the age of 6 months, by which time HbF has been almost completely replaced by adult Hb.

No specific therapy has been found to prevent sickling. The steady state of anaemia in this condition frequently requires no treatment. Acute attacks require intravenous fluids, oxygen, and antibiotics if necessary. Transfusions are only given if there is severe anaemia. Genetic counselling should be given to prospective parents who carry the trait.

Dissolved oxygen: do we really need Hb and why keep it in red cells?

Having Hb isolated from the plasma by packaging it in red cells has the following advantages:

1. The presence of DPG displaces the dissociation curve to the right and so aids the unloading of O_2 at active tissues.
2. If the 150 g L^{-1} Hb were free in plasma it would raise the viscosity to intolerable values, and colloid osmotic pressure would also increase considerably. The viscosity effect would be particularly important in capillaries, where containing the Hb in red cells gives blood an anomalously low viscosity (the Fahraeus–Lindqvist effect).
3. Hb molecules are just small enough to escape from the blood through the glomeruli of the kidneys and thus be lost in the urine.
4. There are enzyme systems in the red cells which help prevent Hb breakdown. For example, methaemoglobin reductase converts ferric methaemoglobin back to ferrous haemoglobin.
5. Carbonic andhydrase is restricted to the red cells and is crucial in the role of red cells in CO_2 transport.

Although red blood cells are clearly of great importance in the transport of O_2 the only way O_2 can get to the red cells in the lungs, or leave them in the tissues, is by going into solution in plasma and tissue fluid. These fluids are essentially water, and O_2 is not very soluble in water. Henry's Law tells us that the amount dissolved is proportional to the pressure of O_2 (its partial pressure in a mixture such as air). Normal arterial blood contains only 3 mL of O_2 per litre in solution, compared to 200 mL attached to haemoglobin (about 180 mL in women, because they have less Hb). So, about 60 times as much O_2 is carried by Hb as in solution.

However, by Henry's Law the amount dissolved can be increased by increasing the pressure (unlike the amount attached to Hb, which reaches a maximum at atmospheric pressure). If a subject breathes pure oxygen the alveolar and arterial P_{O_2} increases over sixfold, and the amount of O_2 in solution rises to 20 mL per litre of blood. Table 8.1 illustrates the important point that we do not extract all the oxygen present in arterial blood. Mixed venous blood is still 75% saturated with O_2, and there is an arteriovenous content difference of 50 mL O_2 per litre of blood. If a subject breathes pure O_2 at 3 atmospheres pressure he can theoretically obtain sufficient O_2 from that dissolved in plasma, and Hb is not necessary as an O_2 transporter.

Readers interested in even wilder speculation on the importance of Hb might consider an alternative system of supplying our tissues with O_2 simply by increasing the flow of Hb free plasma carrying O_2 in solution – and speculate what we would look like having cardiovascular systems 60 times larger than they are.

Carbon dioxide transport

Carbon dioxide is a major product of our metabolism. It is a most potent acid substance and has to be removed from our bodies.

Almost all the CO_2 in the blood comes from tissue metabolism. Just like O_2 moving in the opposite direction, CO_2 diffuses down its concentration gradient from the cell interior to extracellular fluid, to plasma and into the red cell. Here its chemical conversion into bicarbonate (HCO_3^-) is accelerated, and the bicarbonate so formed is stored largely in the plasma. At the lungs the whole process is reversed, releasing CO_2 to the alveolar air. Carbon dioxide in the blood is found in simple **solution**, in the form of HCO_3^- and combined with the amino groups of **proteins**. Very small amounts of carbonic acid (H_2CO_3) and carbonate ion (CO_3^{2-}) are also present.

Carbon dioxide in plasma

Plasma water reacts with CO_2 to form HCO_3^- and H^+:

$$CO_2 + H_2O \Leftrightarrow H_2CO_3 \Leftrightarrow HCO_3^- + H^+$$
(Equation 8.5)

Like any chain reaction the overall speed of this reaction is determined by its slowest step.

In plasma the first stage of this reaction is slow, taking 100 s to reach 90% equilibrium at body temperature (this impediment is relieved within the RBC, as we will see below). One of the products of reaction 8.5 is H^+ (a **proton**), and to prevent unacceptable increases in acidity [H^+] this has to be **buffered**. A chemical buffer is a substance that accepts or releases H^+ and so minimizes changes in [H^+].

The H^+ formed in Equation 8.5 is buffered by plasma proteins which take up or release H^+.

The amino groups of plasma proteins themselves carry CO_2 in the form of carbamino compounds:

$$Protein\text{-}NH_2 + CO_2 \Leftrightarrow Protein\text{-}NHCOO^- + H^+$$
(Equation 8.6)

and this H^+ has to be buffered.

Carbon dioxide in whole blood

The first part of the reaction described by Equation 8.5 ($CO_2 + H_2O \Leftrightarrow H_2CO_3$) is normally slow, and the second part of the equation ($H_2CO_3 \Leftrightarrow HCO_3^- + H^+$) rather limited in plasma. Adding even small quantities of CO_2 to whole blood will therefore increase plasma P_{CO_2} appreciably, and as this occurs at the tissues CO_2 will diffuse into the red blood cells (Fig. 8.6).

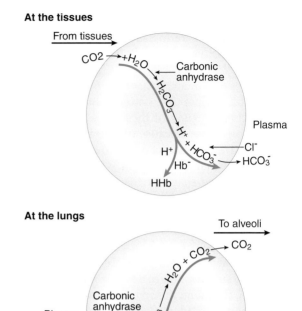

Fig. 8.6
Bicarbonate formation. The erythrocytes, because of the Hb and carbonic anhydrase they contain, are essential for the rapid loading and unloading of the plasma with CO_2 in the form of HCO_3^-.

Reaction 8.5 also occurs inside the red cells, but with important differences. The presence of the enzyme **carbonic anhydrase**, not found in plasma, accelerates the normally slow formation of H_2CO_3 from CO_2 and H_2O. Thus in the red cell reaction 8.5 goes quickly to the right, increasing [H^+] and [HCO_3^-]. These ions are quickly removed, allowing the reaction to continue moving to the right. [H^+] is mopped up by Hb and HCO_3^- diffuses out of the cell into the plasma down its concentration gradient. The HCO_3^- ions carry a negative charge out of the cell and, to maintain electrical neutrality in the cell, chloride ions. (Cl^-) move in. This exchange of ions is called the **chloride shift** (Fig. 8.6). If this did not occur HCO_3^- would be held in the red cell by its negative charge, reaction 8.5 would be blocked by the build-up of HCO_3^- and less CO_2 could be converted to HCO_3^-. The proteins involved in reaction 8.6 include, most importantly, haemoglobin, which has a three times greater affinity for CO_2 and is present at four times a greater concentration than plasma proteins in blood. **Carbaminohaemoglobin** is formed by the combination of CO_2 and Hb at the tissues

(Equation 8.7). This is a special case of the reaction represented by Equation 8.6:

$$Hb\text{-}NH_2 + CO_2 \Leftrightarrow Hb\text{-}NHCOO^- + H^+$$

(Equation 8.7)

It releases CO_2 very readily at the lungs, and the first 30% of the total CO_2 released at the lungs is from this source (Fig. 8.7).

The H^+ formed in the red cells is buffered by Hb, and because deoxygenated Hb is a weaker acid than HbO_2 it has more sites available to accept H^+ (protons). It therefore absorbs more H^+ and reaction 8.7 shifts to the right. In other words, the release of O_2 from HbO_2 into active tissues allows the Hb to take up and carry more CO_2 for the same P_{CO_2}. This effect of deoxygenation increasing the ability of blood to carry CO_2 is called the **Haldane effect**, and should be considered along with the Bohr effect (p. 116), when the beauty of the interaction of these two effects in augmenting the

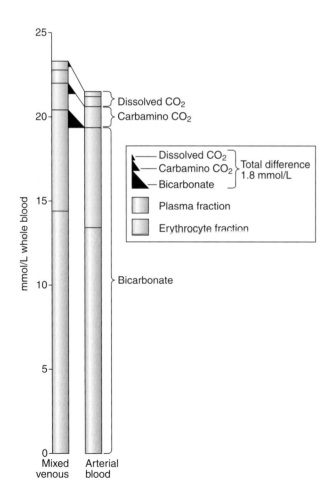

Fig. 8.7
The quantities of CO_2 carried in the blood. The amounts lost at the lungs are shown; note that different proportions are lost from different sources.

transport of the two most important respiratory gases will be appreciated.

Gas exchange at the lungs

At the lungs the processes taking place at the tissues are reversed (Fig. 8.6). As CO_2 is blown off, reactions 8.5, 8.6 and 8.7 move to the left and the chloride shift is reversed. The oxygenation of Hb aids the release of CO_2 from the red cells into the plasma and alveoli. It should be remembered that, as with O_2 moving in the opposite direction, although the amount in simple solution in plasma water is small, before CO_2 can move from red cell to air it must enter into solution in plasma.

The quantities of transported carbon dioxide

The quantities of the forms of CO_2 carried in venous blood are shown in Figure 8.7 and Table 8.1. Although the total *amount* of CO_2 carried in the red cells is much less than that carried in the plasma, the chemical reactions of CO_2 in the red cells and the buffering of H^+ produced are much greater than in the plasma. The red cells act like factories, processing CO_2 and producing HCO_3^- to be stored in the plasma. Thus the *exchange* of CO_2 at lungs and tissues depends more on the processing power of the red blood cells than the plasma content. This is clearly demonstrated by inhibiting carbonic anhydrase in the red cells with a suitable drug. Carbon dioxide entering the blood is then only slowly converted to HCO_3^- and the amounts of CO_2 in solution and as plasma carbamino compounds build up, causing acidosis.

The dissociation curve for carbon dioxide

The relationship between P_{CO_2} and the concentration of CO_2 in whole blood is shown in Figure 8.8. This plot is similar to that for oxygen (Fig. 8.2), except that for CO_2 we cannot plot *saturation* against *partial pressure* because in the case of CO_2 there is no carrier molecule (Hb in the case of O_2) to be saturated.

The relationship between P_{CO_2} and total CO_2 in blood is approximately linear over the physiological range of P_{CO_2}s: from mixed venous (6.1 kPa) to arterial blood (5.3 kPa). Oxyhaemoglobin has a weaker affinity for CO_2 than has deoxygenated haemoglobin. This means that oxygenation of blood causes the curve to be displaced to the right (the Haldane shift). Also HbO_2 is a stronger acid than deoxygenated Hb and releases H^+, which drives reactions 8.5, 8.6 and 8.7 to the left with the formation of free CO_2. The Haldane

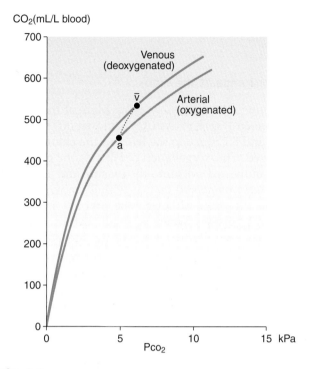

CO$_2$(mL/L blood)

Venous (deoxygenated)

Arterial (oxygenated)

Pco_2

kPa

Fig. 8.8

The CO$_2$ dissociation curve. Oxygenated blood carries less CO$_2$ at the same Pco_2 than does deoxygenated blood. This means that the 'true' dissociation curve as occurs in the body is steeper than might be expected (the broken line), because this Haldane effect results in Pco_2 being about 0.5 kPa lower than if the blood were oxygenated, which helps unloading of CO$_2$ from the tissues.

shift results in the 'functional' CO$_2$ dissociation curve (the normal range of blood Pco_2 over which we function) being steeper than would be expected, because it joins points a and $\bar{v}$ on Figure 8.8. We have seen for oxygen that a steep curve improves unloading, and as a result of this shift at any Pco_2 blood loads and unloads extra CO$_2$ when it is unloading or loading with O$_2$. Because the quantity of Hb in a sample of blood is fixed, the O$_2$ capacity of that blood is also fixed. Because the CO$_2$ dissociation curve cannot be saturated, the CO$_2$ content of our blood is much more variable, even in health, than its O$_2$ content.

Acid-base balance

A little chemistry

Our metabolism is largely aerobic – i.e. it uses oxygen. The word oxygen means 'acid producer' in Greek, and acids are continually being produced in our bodies. Oxidation of proteins and nucleic acids produces sulphuric and phosphoric acids, CO$_2$ is hydrated to

carbonic acid and, in the absence of oxygen, lactic and other acids are released in anaerobic metabolism of fats and carbohydrates, for example in heavy exercise. These acids dissociate (ionize) to increase the [H$^+$] (H$^+$ concentration) of the blood. H$^+$ is a proton and acids, by definition, are proton donors. When an acid releases a proton it forms a **base** which, as an anion, is a proton acceptor.

$$HB \Leftrightarrow H^+ + B^-$$
(acid) (proton) (base, anion)

(Equation 8.8)

In aqueous solution acids increase [H$^+$] and the H$^+$ combines with H$_2$O to form H$_3$O$^+$, but it is conventional, and more convenient, to speak of hydrogen ions, H$^+$.

Because the concentration of [H$^+$] in a solution involves very small numbers, chemists sometimes express it in terms of pH, which makes the numbers manageable and understandable:

pH is the negative log to the base 10 of [H$^+$]
$$= - \log_{10} [H^+]$$

(Logs because that compresses the scale, thus log 10 = 1, log 1 000 000 = 6, etc., and negative because the raw numbers are less than 1, which would result in negative logs, which is awkward, so we use the mathematical trick of

$$- \times - = +$$

In this system pH 7.0 represents neutrality, higher pH represents alkalinity, and lower pH represents acidity.)

The problem with pH is that when hydrogen ion concentration rises (i.e. the solution gets more acid) the pH gets less. This does not lead to an intuitive grasp of what is happening when changes take place.

Also, because there is not a linear relationship between pH and [H$^+$], increases or decreases of equal amounts of pH are brought about by different changes in [H$^+$]. Thus a solution containing 40 nmol/L [H$^+$] has a pH of 7.4. To raise the pH 4 points (to 7.8) we must remove 24 nmol/L of [H$^+$], but to lower the pH 4 points (to 7.0) we need to add 60 nmol/L of [H$^+$].

Life is only possible within a range of blood pH from 7.0 to 7.8, which represents only a sixfold range of [H$^+$], from 10.0×10^{-8} to 1.6×10^{-8}. It is therefore becoming more usual to express acidity directly as hydrogen ion concentration [H$^+$], although we frequently resort to pH when describing the bigger chemical picture of the chemists.

The most immediate and serious effect of a build-up of [H$^+$] in the body is to interfere with enzyme activity, which is obviously 'a bad thing'. Changes in [H$^+$] in the body are resisted by chemicals known as **buffers**. Buffers are chemicals, or combinations of chemicals, which 'mop up' or release H$^+$ when acids or

Carriage of gases by the blood and acid/base balance Box 5

Interpretation of arterial blood gases

The analysis of blood gas tensions, usually in arterial blood, provides key information about a patient's respiratory system. Generally a blood gas analyzer measures the partial pressures of oxygen and carbon dioxide in the blood as well as its pH. From these measurements the machine then calculates other values such as actual and standard bicarbonate concentrations and the base excess. An example of blood gas results from a patient without respiratory disease is given below, with normal ranges for the measured variables:

		Normal range
pH	7.1	(7.35–7.45)
$[H^+]$	40 nmol.l^{-1}	(36–44)
P_{CO_2}	5.3 kPa	(4.4–6.0)
P_{O_2}	12.4 kPa	(12.0–14.0)
$HCO_{3\ act}$	24 mmol.l^{-1}	
$HCO_{3\ std}$	24 mmol.l^{-1}	
Base excess	0.1 mmol.l^{-1}	

In this example, pH has been given alongside hydrogen ion concentration $[H^+]$. pH is related to $[H^+]$ by the equation:

$$pH = -\log_{10}[H^+]$$

In other words, a change in pH of one unit is equivalent to a 10-fold change in hydrogen ion concentration. This makes the pH scale very versatile in fields of chemistry where hydrogen ion concentrations may vary widely. In medicine, blood hydrogen ion concentrations vary comparatively little and for this reason a logarithmic scale is not necessary. However, pH and $[H^+]$ are both still used in medical practice and both are quoted in the following examples. Remember that a $[H^+]$ of 10 nmol.l^{-1} is equivalent to a pH of 8.0 and a $[H^+]$ of 100 nmol.l^{-1} is equivalent to a pH of 7.0.

Plasma bicarbonate is calculated from pH and P_{CO_2} using the Henderson–Hasselbalch equation. Two values of bicarbonate are often quoted: the actual bicarbonate ($HCO_{3\ act}$ in this example) and the standard bicarbonate ($HCO_{3\ std}$). The actual bicarbonate is calculated at the P_{CO_2} measured in the blood sample and standard bicarbonate is calculated using a 'normal' value for P_{CO_2} (often 5.3 kPa). In other words, the actual bicarbonate is an estimate of the bicarbonate concentration in the sample and the standard bicarbonate is what the concentration of bicarbonate would be, *if the P_{CO_2} were normal*. The purpose of calculating these two values is to differentiate between respiratory and metabolic acidaemia and alkalaemia. If a patient has a purely respiratory acidosis, then his *actual* bicarbonate will be *abnormal* but his *standard* bicarbonate will be *normal* since all the abnormalities in the bicarbonate are due to the abnormal P_{CO_2}. On the other hand, a metabolic acidosis or alkalosis will tend to cause a change to the standard bicarbonate.

Another way to differentiate between respiratory and metabolic acidaemia and alkalaemia is to calculate the base excess. This is defined as the amount of hydrogen ions that need to be added to a litre of blood to bring the pH back to normal *at a normal P_{CO_2}*. The key part of this definition is 'at a normal P_{CO_2}': in other words the base excess is a measure only of metabolic abnormalities in acid base status. If a patient has an *acidosis*, then the base excess will be *negative*, since hydrogen ions will have to be *removed* to return the pH to normal.

Armed with all this information, you should be able to answer the following questions about a patient by studying their blood gases:

① Is the patient's oxygenation adequate?
② Does the patient have an acidaemia or an alkalaemia?
③ Does the patient have a respiratory acidosis or alkalosis?
④ Does the patient have a metabolic acidosis or alkalosis?

Is the patient's oxygenation adequate?
This question can be answered knowing the patient's P_{O_2} and inspired oxygen concentration. Knowing the P_{O_2} alone is not enough: a patient with a P_{O_2} of 11 kPa breathing room air clearly has better gas exchange than a patient with a P_{O_2} of 12 kPa breathing 60% of oxygen.

Does the patient's blood have a normal pH/$[H^+]$?
If the answer to this question is 'yes' it does not mean that the patient's acid base balance is normal. Remember, a patient may have a respiratory acidosis that is partially compensated by a metabolic alkalosis leading to a near normal pH. A high $[H^+]$ (or low pH) is an acidaemia and a low $[H^+]$ (or a high pH) is an alkalaemia.

Does the patient have a respiratory acidosis or alkalosis?
This question is answered by looking at the P_{CO_2}. A raised P_{CO_2} results in a respiratory acidosis whereas a low P_{CO_2} results in a respiratory alkalosis.

Does the patient have a metabolic acidosis or alkalosis?
This question is answered by looking at either the standard bicarbonate or the base excess. A low standard bicarbonate indicates a metabolic acidosis whereas a raised standard bicarbonate indicates a

CARRIAGE OF GASES BY THE BLOOD AND ACID/BASE BALANCE

metabolic alkalosis. Similarly, a large negative base excess indicates a metabolic acidosis and a large positive base excess indicates a metabolic alkalosis.

These principles are best illustrated by a few examples:

		Normal range
pH	7.26	(7.35–7.45)
$[H^+]$	55.6 nmol.l^{-1}	(36–44)
P_{CO_2}	8.84 kPa	(4.4–6.0)
P_{O_2}	7.66 kPa	(12.0–14.0)
HCO$_{3\ act}$	28.7 mmol.l^{-1}	
HCO$_{3\ std}$	24.1 mmol.l^{-1}	
Base excess	–0.3 mmol.l^{-1}	(+2.0–−2.0)

This patient suffered from severe chronic obstructive pulmonary disease. She had sustained a fractured leg and had been given rather a lot of morphine to control her pain. At the time this sample was taken, she was receiving oxygen with an inspired concentration of 35%. These results show:

① There is impaired oxygenation – this patient's P_{O_2} is low, particularly given the fact that she is breathing 35% oxygen.
② The pH of the patient's plasma is low and the $[H^+]$ is high – she is acidaemic.
③ There is a respiratory acidosis – the P_{CO_2} is high.
④ There is neither a metabolic acidosis or alkalosis – standard bicarbonate and base excess are both normal.

The combination of this patient's respiratory disease and opioid administration had resulted in hypoxia and carbon dioxide retention. The carbon dioxide retention had led to a respiratory acidosis.

These are the results for the same patient 36 hours later. The patient is still breathing 35% oxygen. However, the patient is no longer receiving opioid drugs and analgesia is now being provided by an epidural local anaesthetic, which does not cause respiratory depression:

		Normal range
pH	7.40	(7.35–7.45)
$[H^+]$	40.0 nmol.l^{-1}	(36–44)
P_{CO_2}	6.43 kPa	(4.4–6.0)
P_{O_2}	9.5 kPa	(12.0–14.0)
HCO$_{3\ act}$	29.1 mmol.l^{-1}	
HCO$_{3\ std}$	27.6 mmol.l^{-1}	
Base excess	+3.5 mmol.l^{-1}	(+2.0–−2.0)

① The patient's oxygenation has improved, although it is still abnormal.
② The patient's blood is at a normal pH and $[H^+]$.
③ The patient still has a respiratory acidosis (high P_{CO_2}) although this has improved.
④ The patient has a metabolic alkalosis (high standard bicarbonate, positive base excess).

The patient is clearly improving: her oxygenation is better since her opioids were stopped and her P_{CO_2} is coming back towards normal. She has developed a metabolic alkalosis which in this case has compensated fully for her respiratory acidosis. Note that this has taken many hours – a metabolic alkalosis develops in response to increased acid excretion by the kidneys and this takes time. It is unusual for a metabolic alkalosis to compensate completely for a respiratory acidosis: in this lady's case it is likely that her respiratory acidosis was improving anyway.

bases are added to them, and so resist changes in $[H^+]$. Buffers within the cells and buffers in the blood neutralize H^+, but their ability is limited and only give respite against the constant stream of acid produced by metabolism. Over the long term the body must get rid of as much acid as it produces. Buffers are a kind of 'overdraft' that enables the body to keep going, but eventually the acid 'debt' has to be got rid of.

Metabolic acids can be categorized as **volatile acids** (which are removed in gaseous form, and of which the only one of interest to us is carbonic acid, removed as CO_2 by the lungs) and **fixed** or **non-volatile acids**, which are removed by the kidneys, in particular as sulphate and phosphoric acid. As the normal pH of urine is about 6.0 (acidic) the body is producing an excess of acid over that removed by respiration,

although the acid load removed by the lungs is about four times greater than that removed by the kidneys. The lungs do not, of course, 'excrete' acid: they excrete CO_2, which as you can see from Equation 8.5 is in equilibrium with H^+ in the plasma. The $[H^+]$ determines pH, and it doesn't matter where the H^+ comes from or in what form it is removed: every H^+ is equivalent to every other. When acids such as lactic acid are added to the blood they add H^+, which displaces Equation 8.5 to the left, forming CO_2 and water. Water is harmless and diffuses away; removal of CO_2 by the lungs allows reaction 8.5 to continue moving to the left, removing H^+ and limiting the acidosis.

More than 50 mmol of non-volatile acids are produced each day by a normal healthy man. It is essential that this be disposed of, but in quantitative

Carriage of gases by the blood and acid/base balance Box 6

Analysis of results example 1

These results were obtained from a gentleman who had recently returned to the ward following major emergency surgery for an obstructed bowel:

		Normal range
pH	7.29	(7.35–7.45)
[H⁺]	51.8 nmol.l⁻¹	(36–44)
P_{CO_2}	6.27 kPa	(4.4–6.0)
P_{O_2}	21.08 kPa	(12.0–14.0)
HCO_3 act	21.9 mmol.l⁻¹	
HCO_3 std	20.6 mmol.l⁻¹	
Base excess	−4.7 mmol.l⁻¹	(⁺2.0–⁻2.0)

Patient breathing 40% oxygen.
  These results show:

① Good oxygenation. The patient's P_{O_2} is well above normal.
② A raised [H⁺] and low pH – the patient is acidotic.

③ The patient has a respiratory acidosis: his P_{CO_2} abnormally high.
④ The patient has a metabolic acidosis: his standard bicarbonate is abnormally low and his base excess is abnormally negative.

This patient has both a respiratory and metabolic acidosis. The respiratory depression causing his respiratory acidosis may be due to the administration of postoperative opioids or as a result of drowsiness due to the hangover effects of the general anaesthetic. Notice that this degree of respiratory impairment in a man with healthy lungs does not cause a problem with oxygenation if he is breathing supplemental oxygen.

A metabolic acidosis is not unusual following major, emergency surgery. It is likely that the patient was relatively dehydrated prior to his surgery and this may have led to poor organ perfusion and oxygenation. This in turn often leads to the production of lactic acid.

terms this is very small compared to the 12 mol of CO_2 (250 times as much 'acid') that is produced each day. If acids formed by metabolism did not ionize in solution and could be excreted in their non-ionized form by the kidneys they would not present a problem; however, the only metabolic acids that do not ionize strongly are monobasic phosphoric acid, β-hydroxybutyric acid and creatinine. All others are almost completely ionized, producing the problem of excess H⁺. We cannot produce urine with a pH below about 4.5: at this pH no more H⁺ can be added, although some additional H⁺ can be buffered by ammonia secreted by the kidney. Under these conditions the power of the kidney to eliminate further acid is curtailed.

When you consider the relative amounts of acid disposed of by the lungs and by the kidneys you will understand why some respiratory physiologists dismiss the kidneys as mere minor extensions of the lungs.

Buffer compartments of the body

As this is a textbook of respiration we only consider acid–base control in relation to the effects of respiration on the blood. This is only one of the three fluid compartments of the body involved in buffering (blood, interstitial fluid and intracellular fluid), and in terms of *total* CO_2, H⁺ and HCO_3^- the least impor-

tant. In terms of purely chemical buffering, the cells of our bodies, with their high protein content, are by far the most important chemical buffer, but as we will see shortly this system is finite, whereas the mechanisms that have evolved for the respiratory system have an almost infinite capacity. We will see that the cell system is like a non-rechargeable battery: once used it is finished, but the system involving respiration is rechargeable and is used over and over again. To explain how this system works we can consider it in isolation, but in clinical situations the interactions between the three buffer compartments (blood, interstitial fluid, intracellular fluid) are of great importance.

Normal plasma hydrogen ion concentration

Normal plasma [H⁺] = 40 nmol (pH 7.40). Increases or decreases cause, respectively, **acidaemia** or **alkalaemia**. Because the pH scale is logarithmic, a shift of one pH unit represents a tenfold change in [H⁺], and one should be careful not to be *too* impressed by the precision with which acidity is controlled. The addition or removal of H⁺ to the blood activates compensatory changes in respiratory excretion of CO_2 and changes in excretion of H⁺ and HCO_3^- by the kidneys.

Carriage of gases by the blood and acid/base balance Box 7

Analysis of results example 2

These blood gases were taken from a lady in intensive care, on a mechanical ventilator with an inspired oxygen concentration of 40%:

		Normal range
pH	7.04	(7.35–7.45)
[H+]	91.2 nmol.1^{-1}	(36–44)
P_{CO_2}	5.9 kPa	(4.4–6.0)
P_{O_2}	18.8 kPa	(12.0–14.0)
HCO$_3$ act	10.8 mmol.1^{-1}	
HCO$_3$ std		
Base excess	–18.9 mmol.1^{-1}	(+2.0–-2.0)

These results show:

① Adequate oxygenation P_{O_2} is18.8.
② The patient is very severely acidaemic: a very high [H+]/low pH.
③ The patient does not have a respiratory acidosis/ alkalosis.
④ The patient has a severe metabolic acidosis (base excess –18.9).

This patient is very ill and has a very severe metabolic acidosis which was thought to be due to renal and liver disease. If this patient were able to breathe spontaneously, her tidal volume would probably be very large and she would produce a respiratory alkalosis in an attempt to compensate for her metabolic acidosis. As she is on a mechanical ventilator, this did not happen.

Blood buffering

A **strong acid** is one that dissociates vigorously and almost completely in solution. Strong in this chemical sense should not be confused with concentrated. Hydrochloric acid, for example, is a strong acid and dissociates vigorously into H+ and Cl−, whether it is in concentrated or dilute solution.

We have already noted that buffers are solutions that resist changes in [H+] when acids or bases are added to them. Buffers consist of a weak acid (H+B−) which only weakly dissociates into H+ and anion B− and its salt, in this case a sodium salt NaB, which dissociates more strongly into its ions Na+ and B−. In an aqueous solution of the two the following reaction takes place with the equilibrium well to the left:

$$H^+B^- + B^- + Na^+ \Leftrightarrow B^- + H^+ + Na^+B^-$$
(weak   (ions of   (ions of   (salt)
acid)   salt)   acid)

(Equation 8.9)

The addition of a strong acid such as H+Cl− will shift the equilibrium further to the left because of the strong affinity of B− for the added H+. Thus the potential increase in H+ is minimized. The added Cl− associates with Na+ to form neutral Na+Cl−.

pK of a buffer

The pK of a buffer system is the pH at which the buffer works best to resist changes in *either* direction.

From Equation 8.9 you can see that the source of the ions on the left side is the acid, and on the right side the salt. For this buffer to work most efficiently at reducing changes of pH in *either* direction there should be equal amounts of acid or salt. If there is already a lot of acid in the buffer system it can resist the effects of added base very well, but cannot deal with the addition of more acid. If there is a lot of salt then the buffer system can deal with acid but not base. So, in the ideal state for resisting changes of pH in either direction, the system is 'in the middle', with the buffer salt and the acid both half dissociated; the pH at which a buffer system is in this ideal state is called its **pK**. Normal plasma has a pH of 7.40, and a buffer system with a pK of this value will be at its most powerful in the blood. Figure 8.9 illustrates the performance of the buffer systems for phosphate and HCO$_3^-$. It would seem that the HCO$_3^-$ system, with its pK far from plasma pH, would be a poor buffer in the body, but it has other attributes that make it perhaps the most important buffer we have, and we will consider these a little later. The main buffers in the blood are bicarbonate, proteins – in particular haemoglobin – and phosphate.

Proteins as buffers

Plasma proteins and haemoglobin constitute the major **chemical** blood buffers of added acid (we will see shortly that another system which does not rely solely on chemical means is at least as important). Haemoglobin is more important than plasma protein, because molecule for molecule it is a more efficient buffer, and also because there is more of it (150 g L^{-1} for Hb, compared to 40 g L^{-1} plasma protein).

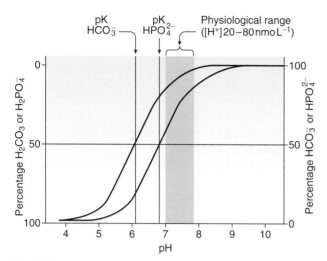

Fig. 8.9

pK. The pK of a buffer is where there are equal amounts of its two components. At this point the curve is at its steepest, so changes in the proportions of the components produces the minimum effect on pH, i.e. the buffer is at its most efficient at stabilizing pH. For reasons explained in this chapter, the bicarbonate buffer system is probably the most important in the blood even though its pK is not the pH of plasma. The phosphate buffer system has a pK close to intracellular pH.

Buffering action is based on Equation 8.6, where the protein can be haemoglobin or plasma protein.

Phosphates as buffers

The phosphate system illustrated in Figure 8.9 is made up of the acidic (H_2PO_4) and basic ($NaHPO_4$) forms of **phosphoric acid** and its salts, respectively. In plasma, phosphate buffers are not very important because the concentrations of the radicals involved are small. In the kidney, however, the system is particularly important in regulating the excretion of H^+. At pH 7.4 urine contains four part of basic to one part of acidic phosphate. If more acid is excreted and the pH of the urine is reduced to 5.8, say, then the ratio of acidic to basic phosphate becomes 10:1. Phosphates may form a more important buffer system inside the cells than in plasma or interstitial fluid.

Bicarbonate as a buffer

At the beginning of this section on CO_2 transport we saw that:

Carbonic acid is formed when CO_2 dissolves in water:

$$CO_2 + H_2O \Leftrightarrow H_2CO_3$$

(Equation 8.10)

Carbonic acid is a weak acid which dissociates:

$$H_2CO_3 \Leftrightarrow H^+ + HCO_3^-$$

(Equation 8.11)

This is a buffer system: the addition of H^+ will shift the reaction to the left, and the H^+ will be taken up with little change in pH. Removal of H^+ will shift the reaction to the right, producing more H^+ and again minimizing the change in pH.

The Law of Mass Action describes the equilibrium of reversible reactions, such as Equation 8.7, as follows:

$$\frac{[H^+]\,[HCO_3^-]}{[H_2CO_3]} = K_A$$

(Equation 8.12)

where K_A is the dissociation constant for H_2CO_3.

Equation 8.12 can be converted to a special equation relating CO_2, HCO_3^- and pH in the blood: **The Henderson–Hasselbalch Equation**, as follows:

pH is the negative logarithm of $[H^+]$ so, taking logs of both sides of Equation 8.12 and transposing, we get:

$$\log \frac{[H^+]\,[HCO_3^-]}{[H_2CO_3]} = \log K_A$$

(Equation 8.13)

$$\log[H^+] + \log \frac{[HCO_3^-]}{[H_2CO_3]} = \log K_A$$

(Equation 8.14)

$$\log[H^+] = \log K_A - \log \frac{[HCO_3^-]}{[H_2CO_3]}$$

(Equation 8.15)

pH and pK_A are the negative logarithms of $[H^+]$ and K_A, respectively.

Therefore

$$pH = pK_A + \log \frac{[HCO_3^-]}{[H_2CO_3]}$$

(Equation 8.16)

The problem with using this equation to calculate blood pH, or if we know pH blood $[HCO_3^-]$, is that there is so little $[H_2CO_3]$ in blood that it is very difficult to measure. However, this very small quantity means that the addition of H^+ to whole blood shifts the reaction rapidly and almost completely to the left. Like water added to a container in Figure 8.10, H^+ added on the right is soon mostly shared with container CO_2 on the left, with very little being retained in the small container H_2CO_3 in the middle.

CARRIAGE OF GASES BY THE BLOOD AND ACID/BASE BALANCE

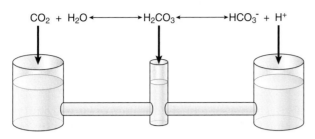

$$CO_2 + H_2O \longleftrightarrow H_2CO_3 \longleftrightarrow HCO_3^- + H^+$$

Fig. 8.10
'Water finds its own level', just like CO_2, H_2CO_3 and H^+ in this reaction.

At equilibrium, which is reached very rapidly because of carbonic anhydrase in the red cells, $[CO_2] = 809[H_2CO_3]$. Thus Equation 8.16 can be written:

$$pH = pK' + \log \frac{[HCO_3^-]}{[CO_2]}$$

(Equation 8.17)

(pK_A has changed to pK' because we have changed from $[H_2CO_3]$ to $[CO_2]$).

The amount of CO_2 dissolved $[CO_2]$ is proportional P_{CO_2} (Henry's Law), and the Henderson–Hasselbalch equation is usually written:

$$pH = pK' + \log \frac{[HCO_3^-]}{\alpha\, P_{CO_2}}$$

(Equation 8.18)

where α is the solubility of CO_2 in plasma per kPa P_{CO_2} at body temperature (0.23 mmol kPa^{-1} L^{-1}). Expressing the equation this way has the advantage that P_{CO_2} is easy to measure in blood with a 'CO_2 electrode'.

Although this system buffers H^+ added to the blood by other acids it is not a buffer system for CO_2 for the following reasons. Remember the reaction:

$$CO_2 + H_2O \Leftrightarrow H_2CO_3 \Leftrightarrow HCO_3^- + H^+$$

The reaction reaches equilibrium to the right, bicarbonate concentration $[HCO_3^-]$ being 20 times greater than $[CO_2]$. You can see from the equation that every molecule of CO_2 involved forms not only a HCO_3^- but also an H^+, and so this is not buffering of CO_2.

It may seem illogical that CO_2 and therefore H_2CO_3 can cause acidosis because each H^+ (acid) produced is accompanied by the production of an HCO_3^- (base), but the effect of adding one H^+ to a concentration of 40 nmol/L hydrogen ion is much greater than adding one HCO_3^- to 26 mmol/L bicarbonate ion.

Although the system is not a good buffer in the chemical sense it is an excellent **transport** of CO_2, and so by carrying CO_2 for excretion by the lungs it performs the same function as a buffer very well. It minimizes the acidaemia that results from the addition of CO_2 to the blood.

The ability of the blood to *transport* CO_2 makes up for its weakness as a purely chemical buffer. By transporting CO_2 to the lungs and HCO_3^- to the kidneys it 'enlists their aid' in controlling the levels of these substances and hence pH.

The lungs excrete or retain CO_2 and the kidneys eliminate or reabsorb HCO_3^-: both work to maintain the HCO_3^-/CO_2 ratio at 20:1. Although not a buffer system in the chemical sense of the word, the kidney – HCO_3^-/CO_2 – lung combination is a more powerful controller of blood pH than excellent chemical buffers such as Hb. The ability of Hb to deal with excess acid or base is limited by the amount of Hb present. When that is 'used up' that is the end of its buffering. The kidneys and lungs, on the other hand, can deal with an almost infinite excess of acid or base because they simply pass them to the outside.

An analogy that students find helpful is that of a man in a leaky rowing boat. The water leaking in is the constant metabolic production of acid which, if allowed to accumulate, will lead to disaster (drowning). He is far worse off with a large supply of best-quality sponges (Hb), with which he can mop up the water but is not allowed to wring over the side, than he would be with two pumps (kidneys and lungs), with which he can eject the encroaching water simply by putting a little energy into them.

We must therefore modify the dismissive remarks about the kidneys as 'mere minor extensions of the lungs' (A little chemistry, p. 122) and admit them as full partners in the regulation of the HCO_3^-/CO_2 ratio and therefore of pH. Indeed, the Henderson–Hasselbalch equation has been qualitatively rewritten (Gilman and Brazeau, 1953) as follows:

$$pH = a\ constant + \frac{kidneys}{lungs}$$

Calculation and illustration of acid–base status

The Henderson–Hasselbalch equation is important because if any two of the variables (pH, $[HCO_3^-]$ or P_{CO_2} is known the third can be calculated. Furthermore, theoretically it allows calculation of what would happen if one of the three variables were changed. For example, if CO_2 were added to the blood, pH and/or $[HCO_3^-]$ must change in a clearly defined way. Knowing the values of the three variables allows an accurate assessment of the acid–base status of the blood to be made. For example, normal arterial blood has a pH of 7.40 and pK = 6.10, and because

$$pH = pK + \log \frac{[HCO_3^-]}{[CO_2]}$$

$$7.4 - 6.1 = \log \frac{[HCO_3^-]}{[CO_2]} = \log \frac{20}{1}$$

So, knowing pK and measuring pH, the $[HCO_3^-]/CO_2$ ratio can be calculated. In patients with acid–base abnormalities the Henderson–Hasselbalch equation can be applied to discover the source of the abnormality. Many automated systems for analyzing arterial blood now carry out these calculations to provide this information.

The figures provided by these systems are of little use if their relevance is not understood, and one of the most useful systems of displaying the relationship between pH, CO_2 and $[HCO_3^-]$ is known as the **Davenport diagram**.

The problem with displaying the Henderson–Hasselbalch relationship graphically on a page is that you have to display three variables on a two-dimensional surface. The Davenport diagram gets round this by displaying P_{CO_2} as a series of **isobars** (lines consisting of points of equal partial pressure)

plotted against plasma $[HCO_3^-]$ and pH, laid out along axes as in a conventional graph (Fig. 8.11).

Disturbances in the normal acid–base situation may be **acidosis** or **alkalosis** and result from:

- *Respiratory* malfunction, where ventilation is too great (respiratory alkalosis) or too little (respiratory acidosis)
- *Metabolic* malfunction, where excess acid is ingested or generated (metabolic acidosis) or acid is lost from the body, perhaps by vomiting gastric contents (metabolic alkalosis). The acute changes (1) and the chronic compensatory changes (2) that take place primarily to restore pH to normal are shown in Figure 8.11.

Clinical measurements

In the clinical situation $[H^+]$ and P_{CO_2} are measured in arterial blood samples in an instrument known reasonably enough as a blood gas analyzer which consists of a series of ion-sensitive electrodes. The blood samples are usually taken from the brachial or radial artery into a syringe containing an anticoagulant (heparin). It is important to exclude air from the sample, as the partial pressures between blood and air will equilibrate. If the sample is to be kept for any length of time before analysis it should be stored in ice to arrest metabolism of white cells.

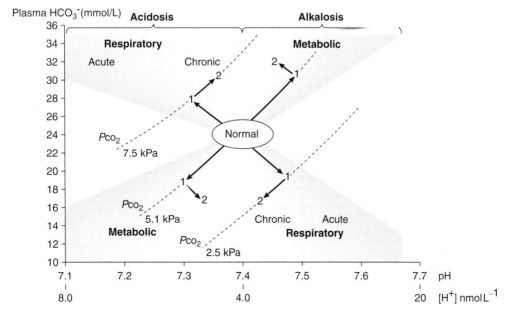

Fig. 8.11

The Davenport Diagram. This illustrates the relationship between CO_2, pH and $[HCO_3^-]$ under normal conditions, and during acidosis and alkalosis.

Modern blood gas analyzers measure [H⁺] and P_{CO_2} directly and calculate a multitude of other values of varying importance. These include:

- *Standard bicarbonate*, which is the [HCO₃] expected if the arterial blood sample were equilibrated to a normal P_{CO_2} of 5.3 kPa, and
- *Base excess*, which is the amount of acid (or base, in the case of a *base deficit*) which has to be added to the blood (which is first restored to a physiological P_{CO_2} to remove any respiratory component), to restore the pH to normal. Base excess is therefore zero in normal situations, and is represented in the pathological situation by the broken line in Figure 8.11.

When interpreting acid–base results these biochemical measurements are only a means of quantifying the severity of the disorder. The patient's clinical history is the most important factor in deciding the nature of the disorder, or whether more than one disorder is present.

Further reading

Baumann R. Blood oxygen transport. In: Farhi L, Tenney SM, eds. Handbook of physiology. The respiratory system, Vol 4 Section 3, 147–172. Bethesda, MD: American Physiology Society, 1987

Davenport HW. The ABC of acid–base chemistry, 6th edn. Chicago: University of Chicago Press, 1974

Klocke RA. Carbon dioxide transport. In: Crystal RG, West JB, Barnes PJ, Weibel ER, eds. The lung: scientific foundations, 2nd edn. New York: Raven Press, 1997

West JB. Gas transport to the periphery. In: Respiratory physiology: the essentials, 4th edn. Baltimore: Williams & Wilkins, 1990

Self-assessment case study

A 65-year-old lady is being investigated for anaemia. She had been to see her GP as a result of feeling tired and listless most of the time, with a few episodes of feeling faint. Her doctor measured her blood haemoglobin concentration and found it to be 91 grammes per litre. A normal haemoglobin concentration in females is 122–152 g/L.

Further investigation of the lady revealed that her anaemia was due to a chronically bleeding duodenal ulcer. After treatment, the lady's symptoms resolved.

From your knowledge of the carriage of oxygen by the blood, you should be able to attempt the following questions.

① What effect will anaemia have on the carriage of oxygen by the blood?

② How might the cardiovascular system respond to anaemia?

③ What adaptive changes to anaemia might be seen in the red cell?

Answers see page 178

Self-assessment questions

① List four factors that would displace the oxyhaemoglobin dissociation curve to the right.

② In carbon monoxide poisoning what values would you expect for
a) arterial P_{O_2},   b) arterial O_2 content,   c) arterial O_2 saturation?

③ In which direction does chloride ions (Cl⁻) move across the red cell membrane, a) at the tissues,   b) at the lungs?

④ Write the Henderson–Hasselbalch equation and define the terms used.

⑤ Which enzyme catalyses the reaction $CO_2 + H_2O \Leftrightarrow H_2CO_3$, and where is it found in the blood?

⑥ At the same P_{O_2}, which is more saturated, fetal or adult haemoglobin?

Answers see page 178

CHEMICAL CONTROL OF BREATHING

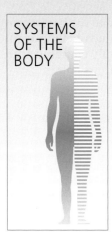

SYSTEMS
OF THE
BODY

Chapter objectives

After studying this chapter you should be able to:

① Explain the different roles of chemical and neural control of breathing.

② Describe the location and adequate stimulus of chemoreceptors.

③ State the effects of changes in Pa_{CO_2}; Pa_{O_2} and $[H^+]$ on breathing.

④ State the relative potency of the above stimuli.

⑤ Discuss the interaction of chemical stimuli on breathing.

⑥ Explain how the adaptation of chemoreceptors affects breathing in obstructive pulmonary disease.

Introduction

This chapter is only separated from the following one on neural control of breathing for your ease of understanding. All control of breathing is fundamentally neural. The sensory cells that detect changes in the external environment and the composition of the blood and cerebrospinal fluid, the central processors in the brain and the outputs that activate the muscles of breathing are all nerves.

A major difference between 'neural control', dealt with in the next chapter, and chemical control of breathing is the difference in timescale of their responses. Neural control responds in fractions of a second and changes the size and duration of individual breaths. Chemical control is normally much slower in its response, changing breathing minute by minute. In essence, chemical control determines minute ventilation, whereas neural control determines the most efficient pattern to achieve that ventilation with the minimum expenditure of work.

The 'objective' of respiration is homeostasis of arterial blood in terms of O_2 and CO_2 (which is closely related to arterial $[H^+]$). This is achieved by matching ventilation to the metabolic activity of the body. This matching requires monitoring of the chemical composition of arterial blood, and the sensors which act as monitors are known as **chemoreceptors**.

Just as we have divided the subject of control of breathing into neural and chemical, so we can divide chemical control of breathing into sections in terms of the anatomical location of the sensors or, alternatively, what they are sensitive to. Those within the central nervous system are called **central chemoreceptors** and those outside **peripheral chemoreceptors**. Central chemoreceptors are most sensitive to excess CO_2; peripheral chemoreceptors are most sensitive to lack of O_2.

It is rare for excess CO_2 or lack of O_2 to occur alone: they usually occur together, and the whole chemoreceptor system is shown schematically in Figure 9.1.

Oxygen lack

The term for a lack of oxygen in any gas mixture or solution is **hypoxia**. Lack of O_2 in arterial blood is termed **hypoxaemia**. Total absence of O_2 is **anoxia**. It is very easy to change the amount of a gas in the arterial blood by utilizing the powerful gas transporting properties of the lungs. Simply giving a subject a gas mixture to breathe will result in his or her arterial blood taking on the composition of that gas mixture within remarkably few breaths. The rate at which equilibrium is reached depends on the solubility of the

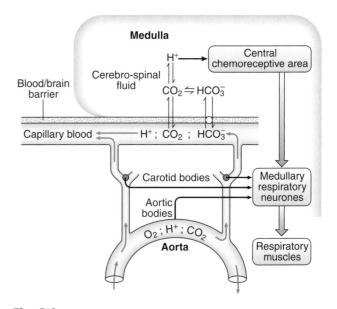

Fig. 9.1
A schematic of the chemoreceptors, and structures associated with the chemical control of breathing.

gas in body fluids, and this has important consequences in anaesthesia. However, for the gases we are concerned with here equilibrium is approached within a few dozen breaths. The chemoreceptors that sense lack of arterial O_2 are the **carotid bodies** and the **aortic bodies**. In humans it is the carotid bodies that are mainly responsible for the respiratory response. They are small (5.0 mm diameter) nodules of glomus tissue (Latins *glomerus*, a skein or ball of thread) situated near the bifurcation of each common carotid artery. Unlike the carotid bodies, which mainly respond to Pa_{O_2}, the aortic bodies are stimulated by reductions in arterial O_2 content, e.g. carbon monoxide poisoning and anaemia affect them more. So it seems that the aortic bodies are sensitive to the total amount of O_2 delivered to them, and the carotid bodies are sensitive to Pa_{O_2}. The carotid bodies are situated close to the **baroreceptor** region of the carotid arteries, which help to regulate blood pressure, and are frequently confused with them. The carotid bodies are *not* baroreceptors.

Histology, embryology and anatomy of the carotid bodies

The function of the carotid bodies is related to their unusual structure. They have an extremely high metabolic rate (about three times that of the brain) but their rate of perfusion by blood from the carotid arteries is even higher: 10 times that which would be

Chronic obstructive pulmonary disease

Mrs Andrews is a 69-year-old lady who suffers from chronic obstructive pulmonary disease (COPD). This has been brought about by many years of heavy smoking – Mrs Andrews smokes 30 cigarettes per day and has done since she was a teenager. Mrs Andrews has a cough that is usually productive of white sputum. She often feels breathless and 'wheezy', and takes two bronchodilator drugs via an inhaler. She frequently suffers from chest infections that are usually treated with antibiotics by her doctor.

One winter, Mrs Andrews contracted a particularly severe chest infection. She had a cough productive of large volumes of green sputum and became very breathless indeed. Her own doctor decided to admit her to hospital for treatment.

In hospital, Mrs Andrews was found to be cyanosed and arterial blood gases indicated that she was hypoxic with a Pa_{O_2} of 6.2 kPa breathing. Her blood gases also indicated that her Pa_{CO_2} was raised at 7.3 kPa. Initially, she was given oxygen to breathe. Although this resulted in the Pa_{O_2} increasing to 10.8 kPa, it also resulted in an increase in Pa_{CO_2} to 8.4 kPa. At this stage, she was becoming very breathless and the effort of breathing was starting to exhaust her. The decision was taken to ventilate her lungs artificially while she received treatment for her infection and she was taken to the intensive care unit.

In this chapter we will consider:

① What causes chronic obstructive pulmonary disease.
② The clinical features of chronic obstructive pulmonary disease.
③ Oxygen therapy and chronic obstructive pulmonary disease.

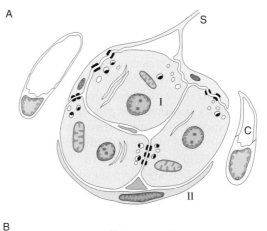

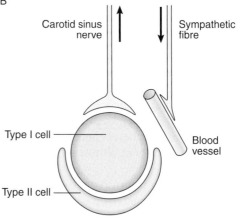

Fig. 9.2
(A) Sketch of cells of the carotid body. I, type I cell; II, type II sustenticular cell; C, capillary; S, sensory nerve. **(B)** Schematic of cell types and nerve fibres of the carotid body.

expected. This blood flows through capillaries (Fig. 9.2A and B) which surround the sensory elements (the glomus or type I cells) that monitor blood P_{O_2}. The type I cells seem to be supported by type II (sustentacular) cells, whose function is still not clear. The type I cells send their information to the brain via the carotid sinus nerve, a branch of the glossopharyngeal nerve (Fig. 9.2A and B), which also provides them with sympathetic and parasympathetic innervation. A separate supply of sympathetic fibres from the nearby superior cervical ganglion innervates the carotid bodies' blood vessels.

The overall effect of this extensive sympathetic and parasympathetic supply *to* the carotid bodies is that their sensitivity can be altered by:

1. neural influences on the glomus cells themselves
2. neural influences on the blood vessels supplying the glomus cells.

As far as these influences on neurotransmission *from* the chemoreceptor cells to the afferent sensory nerve endings is concerned it has become frustratingly obvious that, like many CNS synapses, there is a complex interplay of neuromodulators. However, the general consensus is that whereas sympathetic activity may mildly modulate carotid body function it does *not* have powerful effects on hypoxic ventilation. Dopamine, on the other hand, appears to be an important neuromodulator in the carotid body, inhibiting ventilatory responses to hypoxia.

The embryological origin of the carotid bodies provokes an interesting speculation. As a mammalian embryo develops its structure changes, resembling successive adult forms of more primitive species, starting with the most primitive and finally reaching mammalian form. This is the (now questionable) concept that 'ontogony recapitulates phylogeny'. During our fish-like phase those structures that are going to become our O_2-sensitive carotid bodies are represented by the gill arches of the fish-like embryo. It is the gills of fish that are their sensors of O_2 lack. It is therefore postulated that our carotid bodies are a residue of the mechanism by which our fishy ancestors detected O_2 lack in their watery environment.

Hypoxic stimulation

Activity in the carotid bodies is measured experimentally as the frequency of discharge of action potentials in the carotid sinus nerve: increased activity expresses itself in the whole animal as an increase in ventilation. Hypoxia stimulates peripheral chemoreceptors, which is unusual, as the activity of almost all other organs is depressed by it.

During eupnea under normoxic conditions most of the **drive to breathe** comes from central chemoreceptors, and also neural mechanisms associated with wakefulness. Evidence that the peripheral chemoreceptors provide some drive to breathe comes from the observation that in patients who have been subjected to carotid body denervation arterial P_{CO_2} is elevated by up to 6 torr.

The effect of decreasing a subject's arterial P_{O_2} by giving them increasingly hypoxic gas to breathe is shown in Figure 9.3.

It can be seen that Pa_{O_2} must be reduced considerably (to about half normal) before breathing is stimulated, and that very low partial pressures of O_2 depress breathing.

Hypercapnic stimulation

Increased levels of arterial CO_2 (**hypercapnia**) also stimulate peripheral chemoreceptor activity, probably by increasing [H^+] within the glomus cells, in the same way as increased extracellular acidity increases chemoreceptor activity and breathing.

What is the actual physiological stimulus to the carotid bodies? It is difficult to see how the *absence* of something, in this case O_2, can be a stimulus. A number of different observations combine to give us a clue:

1. Chemoreceptors have a very high metabolic rate and so rapidly use up O_2 supplied to them.

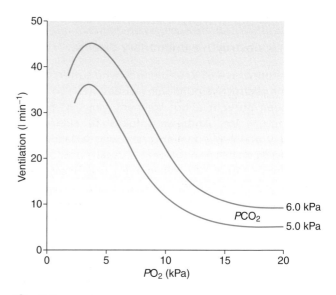

Fig. 9.3
The relationship between minute ventilation and inhaled oxygen tension. The relationship at two levels of CO_2 is shown.

2. They have a very high blood flow, gram for gram 40 times that of the brain.
3. Pa_{O_2} must be reduced considerably before there is stimulation of breathing, but then the increase is profound.
4. Increasing Pa_{O_2} above normal (13 kPa) by inhaling O_2-rich mixtures only produces a small reduction in breathing by depressing chemoreceptor activity.
5. Increasing arterial [H^+] does not have a great effect on central chemoreceptors but stimulates peripheral chemoreceptors.
6. Peripheral chemoreceptors are much less sensitive to increases in Pa_{CO_2} than are the central chemoreceptors.
7. Sympathetic activity has only a small effect on chemoreceptor blood flow and sensitivity during hypoxic stimulation.

These observations explain the two clinical conditions that result in vigorous activation of peripheral chemoreceptors: **hypoventilation** and **hypotension** due to haemorrhage. Under these conditions there is a build-up of metabolites resulting from the supply of O_2 to the chemoreceptors being insufficient for their high metabolic needs, owing to the inadequate oxygen content of the blood or inadequate blood flow to carry O_2 to the chemoreceptors and wash metabolites away.

In summary, peripheral chemoreceptors are stimulated by lack of O_2, excess of CO_2 and excess of [H^+]. These factors cause a build-up of metabolites, which are the specific stimulus to these receptors. Lack of O_2 is a stimulus unique to peripheral chemoreceptors, but

O_2 lack must be pretty severe to produce an effect on breathing. Why is there such a modest response to the lack of such an important requirement of the body?

Hypoxia and breathing

The answer to the above question is that it would be a waste of time having a more sensitive detector of O_2 lack because the shape of the oxyhaemoglobin dissociation curve would defeat its sensitivity. You can see from the oxyhaemoglobin dissociation curve shown in Figure 8.2 (p. 113) that even if P_{O_2} is reduced to 8 kPa, haemoglobin is still 90% saturated. Also, P_{O_2} can rise to infinity and haemoglobin can only be 100% saturated. This useful situation means that ventilation of the lungs can halve or double without the amount of O_2 being carried changing very much. But by the same token, a mechanism that relied on O_2 saturation to control breathing under normal circumstances would lack sensitivity, because saturation does not change much over a large range of partial pressure.

The importance of the peripheral chemoreceptors lies in the fact that they are the only mechanism in the body by which low O_2 tension can stimulate breathing, and when tension falls sufficiently this stimulation is very vigorous.

Hypoxic stimulation of breathing is also opposed by changes in CO_2 and $[H^+]$, because as breathing begins to be stimulated CO_2 is washed out of the blood, arterial $[H^+]$ falls and the drive to breathe from these two sources is reduced, producing what is sometimes called the **hypocapnic brake** (Fig. 9.4). Just how powerful a drive to breathe hypoxia can be is demonstrated if this braking effect is prevented by adding CO_2 to the inspired air to keep its levels constant in the blood. Under these circumstances hypoxia produces 10 times the effect produced if CO_2 is allowed to be washed out.

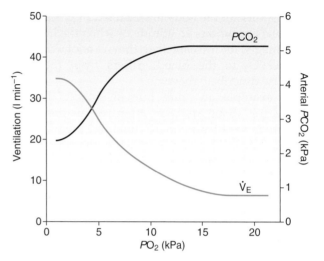

Fig. 9.4

The hypocapnic brake. Increased ventilation caused by hypoxia washes out CO_2, the reduced Pa_{CO_2} reduces drive to breathe and so the overall response is less than if Pa_{CO_2} was maintained.

Chemical control of breathing Box 2

What causes chronic obstructive pulmonary disease?

Chronic obstructive pulmonary disease (COPD) is nearly always the result of long-term smoking. It results in changes throughout the respiratory system, from the large airways to the alveoli, as a result of prolonged irritation by smoke.

In the larger airways, there is inflammation of the airway mucosa accompanied by an increase in thickness of the airway wall and an increase in the mucus secreting glands. Smaller airways are also inflamed and may be significantly narrowed or obstructed by secretions. This narrowing and obstruction of the smaller airways results in the characteristic increase in airways resistance that is a feature of COPD.

Outwith the airways there is a generalized loss of lung tissue with the destruction of alveoli and pulmonary capillaries, as well as the loss of supporting connective tissue. The loss of alveoli and capillaries results in a very significant impairment of gas exchange as a result of a severe mismatch of ventilation and perfusion. Loss of connective tissue means that there is a generalized increase in the lung volume as a whole but very little of this additional volume is ventilated. Loss of connective tissue also tends to worsen the narrowing of the smaller airways. This is because these airways rely on tension in the surrounding connective tissue to keep their lumens patent as, unlike larger airways, they do not have cartilage or other supportive tissue in their walls.

COPD used to be termed 'chronic bronchitis and emphysema', a name which related to the airway inflammation (chronic bronchitis) and the loss of alveolar tissue (emphysema). However, the newer term emphasizes the usually single aetiology behind the condition as well as emphasizing airways obstruction, which is a cardinal feature of the condition.

Peripheral chemoreceptor activity primarily increases breathing; however, it has minor effects in constricting peripheral blood vessels (except those of the skin), reflexly increasing heart rate and stimulating secretion of the adrenal glands. These three effects combine to increase arterial blood pressure.

Long-term hypoxic stimulation and anaesthesia

The response of the body to sustained hypoxia, of the kind one encounters at altitude or when the lungs are so damaged by disease that they cannot efficiently transfer O_2 to the blood, differs from the acute response described above.

For example, in adult human subjects hypoxia lasting for about an hour produces an immediate increase in ventilation (in 3–5 minutes) followed by a decrease to a steady state level higher than the control, normoxic level. This occurs even when P_ACO_2 is kept constant and this phenomenon is called **hypoxic ventilatory decline**. This may be due to hypoxic CNS depression. On a longer time scale, in animals at least, there is a ventilatory acclimatization characterized by a time dependent increase in ventilation which stabilizes at a value greater than the response to acute hypoxia (Fig. 9.5). This response is somewhat confusingly called acclimatization to short-term hypoxia (ASTH) if only to distinguish it from acclimatization to long-term hypoxia (ALTH) which involves the situation found in natives or very long-term residents at altitude. The major mechanism of ASTH appears to be an increased sensitivity of the carotid body to hypoxia (Fig. 9.5) and not, as was once thought, changes in the CSF surrounding the central chemoreceptors.

However, in the longer lasting clinical condition, or at altitude, arterial P_O2 is reduced, causing stimulation of the peripheral chemoreceptors, which in turn increases ventilation. In the high-altitude situation this hyperventilation washes out CO_2 from the blood and cerebrospinal fluid and they become more alkaline, reducing the drive to breathe (mainly at the central chemoreceptors) below the increased level that is appropriate for the reduced atmospheric P_O2. After a day or two the active transport system of the blood–brain barrier returns the $[H^+]$ of the CFS to normal. This restored drive from CO_2 and the extra drive from O_2 lack goes part-way to achieving the required ventilation. Within a few weeks at altitude the kidneys excrete extra HCO_3^- and restores blood $[H^+]$ which, together with the hypoxic drive to the peripheral chemoreceptors, stimulates breathing to an appropriate level.

Some unfortunate patients with respiratory disease do not make this compensation, particularly if they are

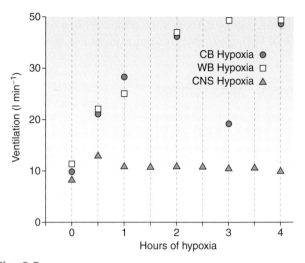

Fig. 9.5
Ventilatory acclimatization to hypoxia. This type of acclimatization is called acclimatization to short term hypoxia (ASTH), although it takes place over hours, to distinguish it from long term acclimatization – over years or a lifetime. The graph shows that hypoxia of the carotid body (CB) has the same effect as whole body hypoxia (WB) while hypoxia of the CNS has little effect. (Adapted from Bisgard et al 1993)

of the type picturesquely described as a 'blue bloater'. This piscine description relates to patients with chronic obstructive pulmonary disease who have marked arterial hypoxaemia and CO_2 retention but do not seem to be breathless. They are blue because they are cyanosed and bloated by congestive heart failure. These patients have adapted to high arterial P_CO2, and so the majority of their drive to breathe comes from O_2 lack detected by the peripheral chemoreceptors. These individuals are particularly at risk if they require a general anaesthetic (see below).

Chemical control of breathing Box 3

Clinical features of chronic obstructive pulmonary disease

The term chronic obstructive pulmonary disease (COPD) describes the airway condition that is largely caused by many years of smoking. Clinically, the disease is characterized by a chronic, productive cough. The sputum is generally white, but during periods of airway infection it may become thick and green coloured. As the disease progresses, patients become increasingly breathless on exertion and in severe cases may become breathless at rest. On examination, patients with COPD may often have a hyperinflated chest and may have an audible wheeze. They may be centrally cyanosed and may exhale through pursed lips in an attempt to increase their airway pressure and therefore keep their smaller airways open. On auscultation, there may be widespread wheeze throughout the chest and coarse crackles may also be heard. In the early stages of the disease, spirometry may reveal an obstructive pattern with a reduction in FEV_1, but in more severe cases, a restrictive pattern with a reduction in FVC is seen. Chest X-rays reveal a hyperinflated chest and may show changes of lung infection, if this is present.

The impaired gas exchange that occurs as a result of COPD means that there is a reduction in Pao_2. Initially, the $Paco_2$ is normal, as an increase in minute ventilation can compensate to some extent for the failing lung function, but in severe cases and during acute exacerbations of the disease the $Paco_2$ starts to rise.

Treatment of COPD is largely symptomatic. Patients are encouraged to give up smoking, often with only limited success. Acute infections are treated with antibiotics when required. Patients often derive some benefit from inhaled bronchodilators, such as the beta-adrenergic agonists salbutamol, and anticholinergic drugs, such as ipratropium. Whereas in asthmatic patients beta adrenaergic agents are generally thought to be more effective bronchodilators than anticholinergics, in patients with COPD these two types of agents are often equally effective. Patients may administer bronchodilators via an inhaler device, but in the later stages of the disease they may require a nebulizer to obtain an adequate dose of bronchodilator drug. In some patients, inhaled steroids may also bring about an improvement. In very severe cases of COPD, gas exchange is so impaired that the patient need to breathe oxygen on a long-term basis and require oxygen therapy at home.

Anaesthetists measure anaesthetic effect in terms of MAC (minimal alveolar concentration for anaesthesia). The peripheral chemoreceptors are extremely sensitive to inhalation anaesthetics (Fig. 9.6). The consequences of this for patients with lung disease receiving anaesthesia are important. They cannot respond when challenged by hypoxia and, if of the 'blue bloater' type, who has already lost his drive to breathe from CO_2, will stop breathing when anaesthe-

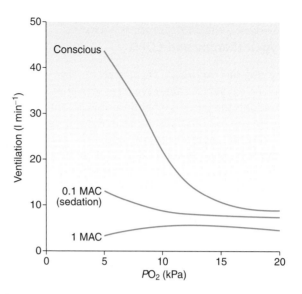

Fig. 9.6
Effect of anaesthesia on hypoxic response. General anaesthesia can almost abolish sensitivity to hypoxia. Response to CO_2 is maintained.

sia abolishes his drive from hypoxia. You can see from Figure 9.6 that quite low levels of anaesthesia, of the order of those found in the postoperative period, when the patient appears able to look after himself, can seriously blunt the response to hypoxia.

Carbon dioxide excess

High levels of CO_2 are known as **hypercapnia** and low levels as **hypocapnia**. The $Paco_2$ of the blood reaching the brain is the major chemical factor normally regulating ventilation. Those sites in the brain stimulated by CO_2 to increase breathing are *not* the components of the **central pattern generator**, which is discussed in the next chapter, but a separate region which comprises the **central chemoreceptors**.

Ambient air normally contains very little CO_2 (0.03%) and, unlike reductions in Pao_2, any increase in inhaled CO_2 stimulates breathing in a linear manner (Fig. 9.7) until levels are reached which act as an effective anaesthetic. (CO_2 has been used in this way in clinical practice.)

Central chemoreceptor response

Unlike the peripheral chemoreceptors the central chemoreceptors are not stimulated by hypoxia. In fact, severe hypoxia depresses breathing in adults by a direct action on the respiratory complex in the brainstem.

Chemical control of breathing Box 4

Oxygen therapy and COPD

Why did Mrs Andrew's Pa_{CO_2} start to rise when she received oxygen therapy? We have seen that in normal individuals the Pa_{CO_2} is what determines ventilation on a minute to minute basis. A rise in Pa_{CO_2} is detected by the central chemoreceptors and this provokes an increase in minute ventilation that in turn tends to bring the Pa_{CO_2} back towards normal. In a small sub-group of patients with severe COPD this mechanism for controlling ventilation fails. In these patients, the Pa_{CO_2} is higher than normal, and their ventilatory response to carbon dioxide is very much reduced or even absent. For these individuals, the ventilatory response to hypoxia is more important. The chronic hypoxia resulting from COPD is their 'stimulus' to breathe. If these patients are given supplementary oxygen to breathe, their Pa_{CO_2} rises and the magnitude of this stimulus is reduced and their minute ventilation may start to reduce. This may in turn result in an increase in Pa_{CO_2}. In very severe cases, the increase is Pa_{CO_2} may be so large that it actually results in a further decrease in ventilation (remember that although carbon dioxide usually *stimulates* ventilation, in very high concentrations it can act on the respiratory centres to *inhibit* ventilation).

In a *small number* of patients with COPD, oxygen therapy may therefore result in an increase in Pa_{CO_2}, and occasionally this increase can be dangerous. It is important to stress, however, that this occurs only in a small minority of COPD patients. It does mean, though, that oxygen therapy in these patients has to be administered with care (using masks that administer a known concentration of oxygen and with regular monitoring of blood gases). However, hypoxia is usually more dangerous that a rise in carbon dioxide, which, in any case, usually takes a while to happen. For this reason it is very important that oxygen therapy is not withheld from patients with COPD. Where an increase in Pa_{CO_2} is provoked by oxygen therapy, often the patient will require artificial ventilation, as happened in Mrs Andrew's case.

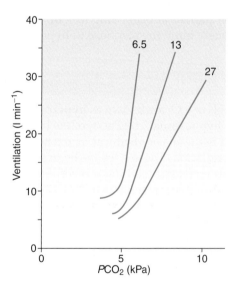

Fig. 9.7
The ventilatory response to asphyxia. The response to varying levels of CO_2 at fixed levels of O_2 is shown. This relationship might equally well be demonstrated with fixed levels of CO_2 and varying levels of O_2 (Fig 9.3).

Furthermore, the peripheral chemoreceptors respond to changes in P_{CO_2} within seconds, whereas the response of central chemoreceptors takes about 5 minutes to reach equilibrium. This delay is thought to contribute to the instability of breathing in patients with Cheyne–Stokes respiration, where breathing waxes and wanes for no apparent reason.

Although slower to respond than the peripheral receptors, central chemoreceptors are responsible for about 80% of our sensitivity to CO_2. The difference in speed of response can be understood as the central receptors are situated in the brain, behind what is known as the 'blood–brain barrier'.

The site of central chemoreceptors

Although no discrete structures such as the carotid bodies have been identified as central chemoreceptors, perfusing the ventrolateral surfaces of the medulla with acidic solutions or solutions with a high P_{CO_2} stimulates breathing. Intracellular recordings in the neurons 500 μm or so below the surface of the brain in the regions shown in Figure 9.8 reveal that the frequency of discharge of these cells increases as the acidity or P_{CO_2} of the interstitial fluid surrounding them increases. This leads to the question, is it CO_2 or H^+ produced by the acidifying effects of CO_2 that is the stimulus? A great deal of careful research indicates that the specific stimulus to the central chemoreceptor neurons is intracellular $[H^+]$, which is determined primarily by the P_{CO_2} of the cerebrospinal fluid.

A

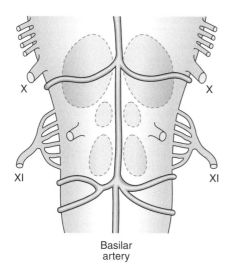

Basilar
artery

B

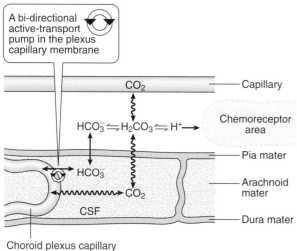

Choroid plexus capillary

Fig. 9.8
Central chemoreceptive areas of the brain. (A) These
are not the traditional 'respiratory centres' dealt with
in Chapter 11. (B) Their environment is closely
controlled by the blood–brain barrier which is
permeable to passive diffusion of CO_2 and actively
transports HCO_3^-.

Blood/CSF relationships

As well as being acidic, CO_2 is a highly diffusible gas
which is important in the relationship between arterial
blood and cerebrospinal fluid (CSF) which is established across the **blood–brain barrier**. The activity of
the blood–brain barrier makes the CSF bathing the
brain and spinal cord the most closely controlled environment in the body. Lipid-soluble molecules such
as O_2 and CO_2 diffuse freely between blood plasma
and brain. Ions such as H^+ and HCO_3^- move under

strict control, and are often pumped against their concentration gradients by active transport when it is necessary to control the environment of the brain. The
capillaries whose walls form the blood–brain barrier
are specialized to produce the CSF from plasma in a
region known as the choroid plexus (Fig. 9.8B).

Carbon dioxide acidifies the intracellular environment of the central chemoreceptors by displacing the
reaction

$$CO_2 + H_2O \Leftrightarrow H_2CO_3 \Leftrightarrow H^+ + HCO_3^-$$

to the right, producing H^+, which is probably the
specific stimulus of the central chemoreceptors. It is
difficult to see at first glance why the above reaction,
which produces both acid (H^+) and base (HCO_3^-),
acidifies a solution (remember, it is the *ratio* of
H^+/HCO_3^- that determines acidity, and there is a lower
concentration of H^+ than HCO_3^- in plasma; therefore,
the addition of one of each of the ions has a bigger
effect on H^+ (see p. 128). Because H^+ passes through the
blood-brain barrier with difficulty, increases in arterial
$[H^+]$ do not affect the central chemoreceptors if arterial
P_{CO_2} is kept constant.

The ion-pumping activity of the blood–brain barrier
is particularly important in compensating for chronic
disturbances of the composition of the CSF, such as
occur during long stays at altitude or in chronic lung
disease. Small and acute decreases in blood CO_2,
caused by singing, for example, do not depress breathing because of the horizontal part of the $P_{CO_2}/\dot{V}_E$ curve
(Fig. 9.7). On average, increasing people's P_{CO_2} by
0.3 kPa doubles their minute ventilation.

Asphyxia

It is very rare for either arterial P_{O_2}, P_{CO_2} or $[H^+]$ of a
healthy individual to change without changes in the
other two (unless you fall into the hands of a respiratory
physiologist). The stimulus to breathe that builds up
when you hold your breath or rebreathe from a plastic
bag involves changes in all three of these variables.

The overall effect of changes in all three was
described by a formula devised by Gray in 1945:

$$VR = 0.22[H^+] + 0.26\, P_{CO_2} - 18 + 105/10^{0.038}\, P_{O_2}$$

where VR is the ratio of ventilation during asphyxia to
unstimulated ventilation. This formula is more important as an illustration that no single factor controls
ventilation than as a quantitative estimate.

The way in which hypoxia and hypercapnia
combine to stimulate breathing is shown in Figure 9.7,
where each curve represents a $P_{CO_2}/\dot{V}_E$ relationship at
a different P_{O_2}. With progressive hypoxia the curves

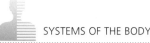
are seen to steepen, producing a greater ventilatory response than would be produced by the simple sum of the two stimuli. On the other hand, it is not unusual for the arterial P_{O_2}, P_{CO_2} or $[H^+]$ of patients to be changed independently by their disease. Most usually this change consists of a fall in P_{O_2} while P_{CO_2} is maintained close to normal.

Chemical control of breathing determines minute ventilation, with changes taking place over a matter of one or more minutes. The pattern of breathing that makes up this minute ventilation is determined by the neural control of ventilation, which can bring about changes in pattern in fractions of a second. This process is dealt with in Chapter 10.

Further reading

Bisgard et al 1993 Respiratory control, central and peripheral mechanisms. Lexington: Univerity of Kentucky; 191–194

Farhi LE. Ventilation–perfusion relationships. In: Farhi LE, Tenney SM, eds. Handbook of physiology. Section 3, The respiratory system. Vol IV Gas exchange, p. 199. Bethesda, MD: American Physiological Society, 1987

Rahn H, Fenn WO. A graphical analysis of the respiratory gas exchange. The O_2–CO_2 diagram. Washington, DC: American Physiological Society, 1955

West JB. Ventilation/blood flow and gas exchange, 5th edn. Oxford: Blackwell Science, 1990

West JB, Wagner PD. Ventilation–perfusion relationships. In: Crystal RG, West JB, Barnes PJ, Weibel ER, eds. The lung: scientific foundations, 2nd edn. New York: Raven Press, 1997

Self-assessment case study

A party of fairly novice mountaineers are climbing a mountain in South America. They are making good progress and are pleased with the speed with which they are ascending. However, on the second evening one of the members of the expedition starts to become unwell. He feels tired and lethargic and starts to develop a severe headache. He goes on to develop dizziness and nausea and starts to vomit. A colleague suggests that he might be suffering from acute mountain sickness and advises that he should descend to a lower altitude.

Mountain sickness is a common disease that occurs when unacclimatized individuals ascend quickly to a high altitude. At altitude, the concentration of oxygen in the air is about 21%, just as at sea level. However, the total atmospheric pressure is decreased. This means that the *partial pressure* of oxygen is decreased, although the *concentration* does not differ. Remember that partial pressure is concentration multiplied by total pressure. Remember also that the oxygen–haemoglobin dissociation curve has the partial pressure of oxygen along the ordinate, not concentration. This means that at altitude, the haemoglobin starts to desaturate.

Initially, affected individuals develop a hyperventilation in response to the hypoxia, but not to a degree that would be expected given the severity of the hypoxia. Later, the hyperventilation increases. Mountain sickness may be treated by drugs such as acetazolamide that cause the plasma to become more acidic.

From your knowledge of the chemical control of ventilation, you should be able to attempt the following questions.

① Why is there an initial hyperventilation on ascent to altitude?

② Why is this hyperventilation less than would be expected, given the severity of the hypoxia that occurs?

③ Why are drugs such as acetazolamide effective in treating acute mountain sickness?

④ Do you know what other symptoms may develop in acute mountain sickness?

Answers see page 179

Self-assessment questions

① What are the roles and time scales of operation of chemical and neural control of breathing?

② What are the names and anatomical sites of the sensors involved in the chemical control of breathing?

③ Define three types of stimulus to breath that can be produced by changing the composition of inspired air.

④ What is meant by 'the hypocapnic brake'?

⑤ How do the respiratory responses to hypoxia and hypercapnia differ when applied singly and combined?

Answers see page 179

NERVOUS CONTROL OF BREATHING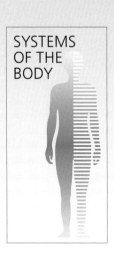

10

SYSTEMS
OF THE
BODY

Chapter objectives

After studying this chapter you should be able to:

① Identify the major sites in the brainstem which contribute to the control of pattern of breathing.

② Describe the changes in pattern of breathing seen in COPD.

③ Explain why 'respiratory centre' is not a precise term.

④ Outline the major afferent neural influences on pattern of breathing.

⑤ Describe three classes of vagal mechanoreceptor in the lungs, together with their effect on breathing.

⑥ Discuss termination of inspiration.

⑦ Discuss dyspnoea.

⑧ Compare the afferent and efferent innervation of the respiratory muscles.

⑨ Discuss neuromuscular disorders of breathing.

⑩ Compare voluntary and automatic control of breathing.

⑪ Explain how expiration may be active or passive.

Introduction

This chapter is closely related to Chapter 9, which described chemical control of breathing. This division of the subject of control is a semantic one, designed to make learning easier. All chemical control involves neural sensory mechanisms, and it is neural mechanisms that determine and bring about breathing, which in turn plays such an important part in the homeostatic control of the chemical composition of the body. The difference between chemical and neural control is really a matter of time: chemical control, which we have dealt with, takes place over seconds or minutes; neural control reacts in fractions of a second to influence breathing breath by breath.

The coordinated act of 'breathing' is ancient in origin. Sea anemones open their mouths and contract their bodies to expel and replace their coelenteric fluid every half-hour or so to ensure O_2 supply to their cells. This opening of the mouth and body contraction obviously involves a coordinating system, which is most probably neural, but next to nothing is known of this. Even more wonderful, the humble sea-cucumber achieves the majority of its respiratory exchange by 'breathing' water into and out of its cloaca, and, in a way that inevitably invites comparison with the gasp and breath-hold we make when startled, the sea-cucumber 'holds its breath' when poked.

We are not normally conscious of the automatic systems of our bodies. The kidneys, gut, cardiovascular and respiratory systems, for example, carry on their tasks of homeostasis largely beyond our control and without affecting our consciousness. That is, with the exception of the respiratory system which, when required, can be subjugated to assist in conscious tasks such as speaking, and even to take part in non-respiratory acts, such as when we fix our ribcage to act as a framework against which the arms can work when lifting a weight. When not being used in this conscious way the respiratory system carries on automatically, producing a minute ventilation which is appropriate for metabolism at that time and controlling levels of O_2, CO_2 and $[H^+]$ in the blood. It is the neural control of breathing that determines the *pattern* of that minute ventilation.

Minute ventilation ($\dot{V}_E$) is described by the equation:

$$\dot{V}_E = V_T \times f$$

where V_T and f are the tidal volume of each individual breath and the frequency of breathing, respectively. The equation tells us that a particular minute ventilation can be made up of an infinite variety of volumes and frequencies, from high frequencies and small volumes to low frequencies and large volumes. How

and why we unconsciously 'choose' a particular pattern is the province of neural control of breathing.

Economy of energy is an evolutionary advantage, and the pattern of breathing chosen by our bodies is aimed at minimizing the amount of work we have to do to produce a particular minute ventilation. This work is directly related to the force exerted by the respiratory muscles, and it may be that we aim to minimize the tension in our respiratory muscles and/or minimize work. It seems that we get our respiratory systems to 'resonate'. The resonant frequency for any particular minute ventilation depends on the value of that minute ventilation and the mechanical properties of the lungs (which have been dealt with in Chapters 3 and 4).

The process of matching pattern of breathing to the physical properties of the lungs can be likened to pushing someone on a swing. If you get the timing right it requires very little effort to keep the swing going, and the timing of the push depends on the physical properties of the swing (the length of the ropes).

Breathing originates in the brainstem (Fig. 10.1) which is made up of the **medulla** (which means marrow, as in bone marrow) and the **pons** (which means bridge), which connects the medulla to the rest of the brain. The neural basis of breathing within the brainstem is the **central pattern generator**, whose output to the respiratory muscles is modulated by numerous afferent inputs. Nerve impulses leave the central nervous system via the **phrenic** and intercostal nerves to bring about breathing by contraction of the respiratory muscles, mainly the diaphragm and intercostals. Other nerves to accessory muscles (e.g. of the larynx) synchronize their contractions with the phases of breathing.

The rhythm generator

Breathing is a rhythmic process, and this rhythm starts in a generator in the central nervous system appropriately called the central pattern generator. This produces a 'rough and ready' pattern of breathing. This pattern is modified and improved on in terms of efficiency by other regions of the brain, and by afferent inputs from receptors in the lungs and chest in particular, to produce a pattern which is efficient and can respond to changed conditions.

The basic pattern of breathing originates in that part of the brainstem which joins the spinal cord to the midbrain and cerebellum, shown in Figure 10.1 and in more detail in Figure 10.5. This region consists of the medulla and pons. If the brain above the medulla is removed (as by Transection II in Figure 10.5) the breathing pattern is remarkably normal. Breathing only ceases when connections between the medulla and spinal cord are cut. (There is some evidence that

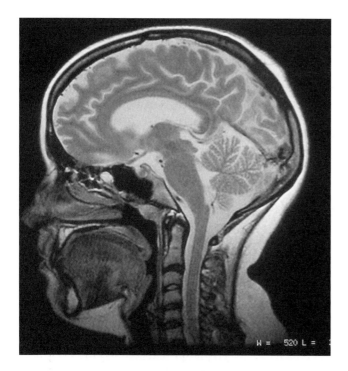

The importance and site of the central pattern generator is clearly seen when people are executed by the process of hanging. The cause of death is not asphyxiation by the noose, as many people think, but rather a snapping of the spinal cord. This arrests breathing by cutting off the output from the medulla to the phrenic nerve and diaphragm.

The neural mechanisms that bring about the rhythm of breathing, consisting of an oscillation of inspiration followed by expiration, followed by inspiration and so on, are still not completely clear.

The idea that oscillating activity in the phrenic nerve could originate in a group of neurons that simply increase and decrease their activity is untenable because there is no reason why such a system should not simply 'stick' in the on or off position, which would result in the subject being 'stuck' in inspiration or expiration. This argument also applies to the old but persistent idea of two groups of neurons that produce either inspiration or expiration and reciprocally inhibit each other (Fig. 10.2).

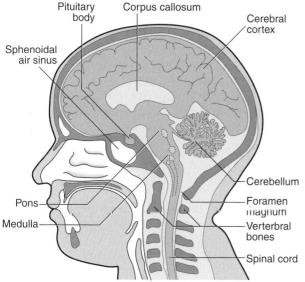

Fig. 10.1
The anatomical origin of breathing rhythm. This scan shows the areas of the central nervous system from which our pattern of breathing originates. These areas are influenced by many afferent inputs.

there are rhythm generators capable of producing breathing movements in the spinal cord itself, but this is a very minor effect occurring under very limited conditions.) The major generator of basic respiratory rhythm is situated in the medulla and is influenced by higher regions of the brain and by activity from **receptors** in other parts of the body.

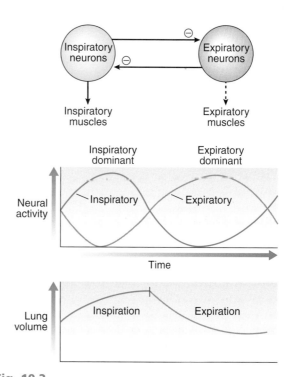

Fig. 10.2
A simple oscillator model of the generation of breathing. Groups of inspiratory and expiratory neurons alternately become dominant by inhibiting the other group. This model implies there is a 'self-inhibition' within each group that causes it to switch itself off. If that were not so breathing would 'stick' in inspiration or expiration.

All plausible models of the central pattern generator start with inspiratory neurons, because to generate a pattern of quiet breathing that is all that is required, expiration in quiet breathing being passive. Most of these models involve some sort of self-limiting negative feedback in the medulla, which operates an **'off switch'** that limits inspiration (Fig. 10.3).

The durations of the two phases of breathing (inspiratory duration, **t_I**, and expiratory duration, **t_E**) are under independent control and so can change independent of each other, or both can change at the same time. Both are influenced by the volume of the lungs. Thus when breathing is accelerated t_E is the first to be shortened as V_T increases, with t_I remaining fairly constant until a threshold is reached, after which it begins to shorten significantly (Fig. 10.4).

These relationships are partly the result of the influence of **peripheral mechanoreceptor** activity on the rhythm generator (p. 142). These influences are still not completely understood, but some simple statements about the generation of the basic pattern of breathing can be made:

- All brainstem neurons involved in inspiration are linked and all brainstem neurons involved in expiration are linked by *self-exciting* connections which synchronize their activity.
- On the other hand, there are *self-inhibiting* connections between all the neurons of the inspiratory group and all the neurons of the expiratory group, which limit the duration of action of each group.
- If any activity in the expiratory neuron group during eupnoea (quiet breathing) does not reach a level that activates the expiratory muscles of the abdominal wall, expiration is passive in normal quiet breathing.

Pattern of breathing in COPD

The relationship between V_T, t_I and t_E shown in Figure 10.4 is disrupted in disease. In chronic obstructive pulmonary disease, for example, overall minute ventilation ($\dot{V}_E$), which can be thought of as the physical expression of the neural drive to breathe, increases as the disease progresses. This offsets to some extent the decrease in efficiency caused by in $\dot{V}/\dot{Q}$ mismatching and changes in lung mechanics.

Within this increase in V_E the pattern of breathing also changes. There is initially an increase in V_T, but as airways resistance increases as the disease progresses V_T decreases below normal. Frequency of breathing increases throughout the progress of the disease. The relationship of inspiratory duration to tidal volume (t_I to V_T) reflects the drive to breathe. The relationship between inspiratory duration and the total breath

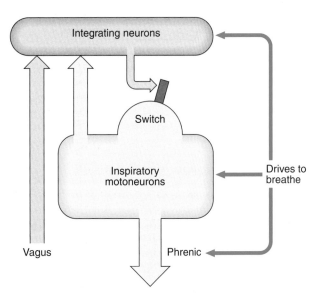

Fig. 10.3

An off-switch model of breathing. This model proposes that inspiratory drive (which is related to lung volume) builds up and puts pressure on an 'off-switch'. When this pressure is sufficient the switch flicks off, expiration commences and the whole system is reset. This idea has been refined to include activity of vagal afferents, which signal lung volume and rate of change of volume and drives to breath whose activity is integrated with feedback from inspiratory neurones themselves before acting on the off-switch.

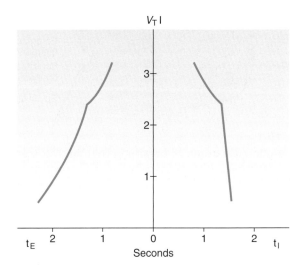

Fig. 10.4

Breathing pattern in man. Tidal volume (V_T) increases while inspiratory duration (t_I) and expiratory duration (t_E) decrease as breathing is stimulated to increase minute ventilation. The actual pattern is highly variable between individuals.

duration (t_I to t_{Tot}) reflects the way a single breath is divided up into the time to fill the lungs (t_I) and the time to empty back to the start position (t_E). These two phases are of course governed by the mechanical properties of the lungs and airways. Central drive to breathe must increase as airflow limitation progresses, reaching a maximum with respiratory failure. This increased drive effectively increases V_T until the increased work of breathing resulting from airflow limitation overpowers it and actually causes a fall in V_T. The only way the patient can now increase his minute ventilation is to increase his frequency of breathing. The problem with this strategy is that the expiratory airflow limitation produced by the disease demands that a greater proportion of each breath be devoted to expiration, and the fraction of each breath devoted to inspiration has to be reduced. Air trapping and a subjective sensation of relief when breathing at high volume (which holds the airways open in what has been termed 'auto-PEEP') causes the patient with severe COPD to breathe with a rapid shallow pattern at increased lung volumes. This is an inefficient pattern because, in addition to the airflow obstruction, it places the respiratory muscles at a mechanical disadvantage to such an extent that the increased work of breathing can exhaust the patient.

The respiratory 'centres'

The different effects of damage at different levels of the brainstem, and the profound effects of cutting off afferent information in the **vagus nerves** by cutting or blocking activity in them, led early investigators to the erroneous idea that there were a variety of anatomical 'centres' in the pons. These centres, together with afferent activity from the peripheral nervous system (mainly in the vagus nerve), modified the activity of the medullary rhythm generator into an efficient pattern of breathing. The term 'respiratory centre' is incorrect if it is taken as implying that there are discrete anatomical bodies or regions of the brain that can be identified macroscopically or microscopically. Respiratory 'centres' are more correctly thought of as diffuse networks of neurons which are active together to bring about the same respiratory effect. Higher densities of neurons with a common purpose are, however, found in specific regions of the brain, and these regions can, if you wish, be considered as centres for ease of description.

Disconnecting the upper pons from the brainstem (Transection I in Figure 10.5) removes the effect of the pontine respiratory group (PRG). The neurons that make up this centre are found in and around the nucleus parabranchialis medialis (NPBM).

When Transection II (Fig. 10.5) is made, with the vagi cut, breathing becomes slower and deeper. This rate-controlling, volume-limiting effect of the PRG is probably a result of the inspiratory neuron group of the medulla stimulating the PRG during inspiration. When stimulated in this way the PRG, after a short delay, sends inhibitory impulses back to the inspiratory neurons, cutting short their activity (and hence phrenic nerve discharge to the diaphragm) in a classic negative-feedback arrangement. Shortening one breath in this way means that the next breath can start earlier, that is, the frequency of breathing is increased and the volume of breaths reduced. It has been suggested that the PRG evolved as a means of mediating rapid shallow breathing (panting), initiated for thermal or emotional reasons by higher parts of the brain.

Nervous control of breathing Box 1

Coning

Coning is when raised intracranial pressure squashes the respiratory regions of the brain.

John Thompson is a 21-year-old man who was riding his bicycle to work early one dark and wet morning. Although he has bought a cycle helmet, he very rarely wore it and today was no exception.

Unfortunately, John was involved in an accident. He turned out of a side-street without looking properly and a car driving at speed hit him from the side, throwing him from his bicycle. John's right leg was broken in two places in the collision and he struck his head hard on the nearby kerb. John lay unconscious on the road in a pool of blood.

An ambulance arrived quickly and John was rushed to the nearby hospital. On arrival, John was found to be quite deeply unconscious with a low blood pressure. Because of this, an endotracheal tube was passed into his trachea and his lungs were ventilated artificially. His leg fractures were stabilized and he was given blood and other fluids intravenously to increase his blood pressure to normal values. Following this he as taken to the CT scanner and a brain scan was performed.

In this chapter we will consider:

① How a severe head injury can be recognized and why raised intracranial pressure is a problem.
② How raised intracranial pressure can be treated.
③ How raised intracranial pressure can lead to death by compression of the brainstem.

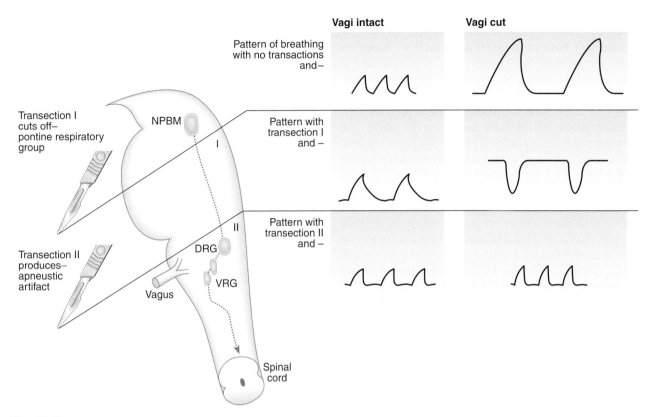

Fig. 10.5
Breathing patterns after brainstem and vagal transections. Experiments such as transecting nerve pathways in the brain have been used to isolate different effects of parts of the brain on pattern of breathing. Such experiments are very disruptive and the results should be interpreted with caution.

The effects of removing the PRG are only seen when the vagi are cut, because *either* the PRG *or* the vagi can produce the same effect of cutting short inspiration and limiting inspiratory volume.

Removing the PRG *and* cutting the vagi results in **apneusis** – long powerful inspiratory efforts interspersed with brief expirations (Greek, *apneusis, without breath*). This led to the suggestion that there was an **apneustic centre** in the lower pons. This idea is no longer popular, and the effects produced by this transection are thought to be the result of general damage rather than the disconnecting of a specific centre.

The medullary groups

The pons connects the medulla to the higher regions of the brain. From direct electrical recording and observations of the clock-like unmodulated rhythms (slow deep patterns of breathing and apneusis) seen when these regions are damaged two functionally dis-tinct groups of neurons in the medulla have been identified (Fig. 10.6).

The dorsal respiratory group (DRG)

This is made up of exclusively inspiratory neurons in the region of the nucleus of the tractus solitarius (solitary tract). These neurons integrate information from chemoreceptors and mechanoreceptors related to breathing. The nerve cells of the DRG have a spontaneous rhythm of discharge, similar to that of breathing and synchronized with inspiration, which can be altered by environmental changes that alter breathing rate. This suggests that the neurons of the DRG may be the origin of the most basic respiratory rhythm.

The ventral respiratory group (VRG)

This consists of both inspiratory and expiratory motor neurons (unlike the exclusively inspiratory DRG). Inspiratory activity in the DRG excites inspiratory and inhibits expiratory activity in the VRG. The

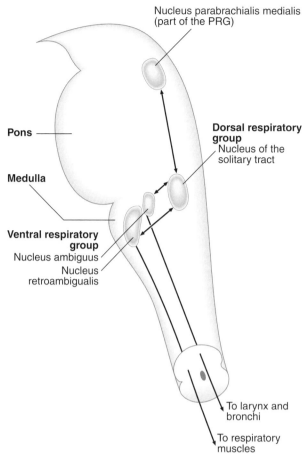

Fig. 10.6
Brainstem respiratory 'centres'. The areas of the brainstem shown in this diagram have a large percentage of neurons whose activity is locked to a specific phase of breathing. The idea that there are specific anatomical 'centres' is not a helpful one but the term 'centre' has been hallowed by usage. PRG, pontine respiratory group.

VRG cells are found rostrally in the nucleus ambiguus and caudally in the nucleus retroambigualis. The rostral part of the nucleus retroambigualis innervates the **accessory muscles** of respiration on the same side of the body – those of the larynx for example. The caudal part of the nucleus innervates the contralateral diaphragm, contralateral expiratory intercostal and abdominal muscles, and the ipsilateral and contralateral inspiratory intercostal muscles. The VGR is probably also a switching station for the PRG and (if it exists) the apneustic centre of the pons.

Conscious control of breathing

The control of breathing described so far is automatic and independent of the brain above the pons. In unanaesthetized humans, however, the higher parts of the brain affect breathing both involuntarily, during emotion, hyperthermia, and probably during exercise, but also during conditions that require **voluntary control** of our respiratory muscles. These conditions may be primarily respiratory, speaking, blowing, whistling; or be for other purposes, such as when we lock the ribcage to provide a framework against which the arms can act, or when we increase intra-abdominal pressure during defecation. In all cases voluntary control is always bilateral: we cannot contract one half of our diaphragm or one half of our larynx. The origin of this control is probably the **motor cortex**, and the voluntary pathways bypass the PRG and rhythm generator in the brainstem to descend in the pyramidal tracts (Fig. 10.7).

These voluntary pathways can be destroyed independently of the involuntary pathways, for example by a stroke. Patients with such a stroke breathe normally, respond to reflex and chemical stimuli, but cannot voluntarily change their pattern of breathing; they will cough if their larynx is stimulated, but cannot cough on command. Very rarely, the opposite situation is seen, where the automatic

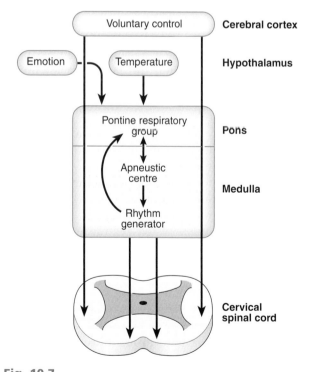

Fig. 10.7
An outline schematic of central neural structures involved in breathing. The centres and generator are collections of neurons that function together rather than specific anatomical structures.

Nervous control of breathing Box 2

How a severe head injury can be recognized and why raised intracranial pressure is a problem

The scan showed that John had suffered a severe head injury. His skull was fractured and there had been a good deal of brain damage. There was quite severe bruising to his brain and there had been bleeding into the intracerebral ventricles. The scan also suggested that because of his brain injuries the pressure inside his skull was high. John was taken to the intensive care unit and was kept on a ventilator and given fluids and sedative drugs.

A tiny pressure monitor was inserted through a small hole drilled in his skull. This showed that the pressure within John's skull (intracranial pressure) was very high.

There are many causes of raised intracranial pressure, including brain injury and brain tumours. Raised intracranial pressure is a very serious condition and in many patients can lead to death.

Anything that increases the volume of the brain, such as bruising, bleeding or a tumour, increases the pressure because the brain in encased within a solid box,

the skull. Raised pressure in the brain can result in a reduction in its blood supply. This in turn can lead to ischaemia, which can cause swelling of the brain tissue, which itself leads to a further increase in intracranial pressure. A 'vicious circle' of increasing intracranial pressure can therefore be set up.

The largest 'hole' in the skull is the foramen magnum, through which the spinal cord passes. Just above the foramen magnum lies the medulla, in which are contained the respiratory regions. If there is a sudden large rise in intracranial pressure or a prolonged increase in intracranial pressure, the brainstem is squashed against the foramen magnum. The rim of the foramen magnum compresses the brainstem, reducing the blood supply to the structures it contains (see Fig. 10.1). Damage to these important structures, which include not only the respiratory centre but other areas important in maintaining life, can eventually lead to death.

pathways have been destroyed but the pyramidal tracts are left intact. The patient can breathe deliberately but not automatically, as in sleep. This condition is called 'Ondin's curse' after the folk-tale of the mortal man who formed a liaison with an ondin or water-nymph. Her father, the king of the ondins, objected to this relationship (the way fathers do) and put a curse on the man that if he did not remember to keep his vital functions, such as heartbeat and breathing, going, they would stop. Of course, when he fell asleep he died. Fortunately, this condition, and ondins, are very rare.

The pathways for automatic and voluntary breathing are also separate in the spinal cord. The automatic pathways from the brainstem run in the anterior region near the outlets of the ventral roots, whereas the voluntary pathways pass down in more lateral areas.

Respiratory muscle innervation

Motor innervation of the diaphragm is very unusual. Unlike most other skeletal muscle the diaphragm is controlled almost entirely **directly** by α motor neurons from the cervical region ('C 3, 4 and 5 keep the diaphragm alive'). These α motor neurons are also unusual in lacking feedback to Renshaw cells which, in other motor neurons, controlling other muscles of

the body, cut short the afterdischarge of activity. Furthermore, as if to prevent fatigue of the diaphragm, the motor neurons 'take turns' to be active, and so stimulate different populations of muscle fibres in the diaphragm, which themselves 'take turns' to bring about successive inspirations.

The inspiratory motor neurons of the spinal cord are inhibited during expiration and the expiratory motor neurons are inhibited during inspiration. This reciprocal inhibition prevents the opposing inspiratory and expiratory muscles contracting simultaneously. Unlike opposing skeletal muscle groups this inhibition is *not* brought about by **muscle-spindle** reflexes but is the direct result of the dorsal and ventral respiratory groups activating specific motor neurons sequentially. This type of direct control of opposing inspiratory and expiratory muscle groups is necessary because the diaphragm is very poorly supplied with muscle spindles, which carry out this reciprocal inhibition in other opposing muscle groups. This absence of spindles probably explains why we do not feel fatigue of the diaphragm in the same way as we feel fatigue in other muscles. Some activity in the diaphragm continues into expiration, causing a 'brake' on the rate of expiration and extending its duration.

The **larynx** exhibits movements synchronized with breathing. These movements are brought about by the muscles of the larynx, which are innervated by the superior laryngeal and recurrent laryngeal nerves.

Nervous control of breathing Box 3

Treatment of raised intracranial pressure

John's raised intracranial pressure was treated with mannitol and frusemide. The way in which these drugs work to reduce intracranial pressure is not fully understood, but they may improve oxygenation by decreasing blood viscosity and they may act by reducing intracerebral oedema.

Despite the best efforts of everyone in the intensive care unit, John's condition continued to deteriorate over the next days and it became increasingly difficult to control his intracranial pressure.

After several days the intensive care doctors decided that John's brain was probably no longer functioning. To confirm this, they performed a series of brainstem death tests. One of these involved disconnecting John from the ventilator, having oxygenated his lungs with 100% oxygen and while introducing oxygen into his lungs with a catheter.

John did not make any respiratory effort even after his blood carbon dioxide had been allowed to rise to a level that would be sufficient to stimulate ventilation. After the brainstem death tests had been performed and then repeated by a different doctor, John was pronounced dead.

Damage to the respiratory and other vital regions in the brainstem can lead to brainstem death. Because the heart can function independently of nervous control from the brainstem, and because John's lungs were being ventilated artificially, it was not immediately evident that his brain was no longer functioning and that his organs would not again be able to function without life support. The brainstem death tests confirm that vital areas in the brainstem have been irreparably damaged, and under these circumstances continuing with intensive care was futile.

These are branches of the vagus nerve. During inspiration the vocal folds are pulled apart and this reduces the resistance to airflow into the lungs. During expiration the vocal folds come together, slowing down expiratory flow. These movements are automatic – we are not conscious of them, and the nerve impulses that cause them arise from the rostral part of the ventral respiratory group in the nucleus ambiguus. We can, of course, consciously control our larynx, as in vocalization. The larynx is therefore almost a model of the control of respiration, with an automatic rhythm that can be consciously overridden.

The major **expiratory muscles** are those of the abdomen and the internal intercostal muscles. Unlike the diaphragm, these muscles are well supplied with spindles and behave more like other voluntary muscles, in that their contraction is caused by a combination of direct activation of extrafusal muscle fibres plus indirect activation via stimulation of the intrafusal fibres of muscle spindles which produces reflex contraction. Both internal and external intercostal muscles are active, but to only an insignificant degree in quiet breathing.

The abdominal muscles only become involved when forced expiration is required during exercise or coughing. As exercise becomes more intense, or breathing becomes more laboured, as in disease, more accessory muscles, for example those of the shoulder girdle, are recruited. The muscles of the abdomen and chest are also involved in posture, locomotion, and in the movement of the arms in lifting heavy weights. During almost all of these activities, if not too extreme, it is possible to breathe and vocalize, which involves well controlled modification of airflow. This ability reaches its peak in opera singers, who seem to be able to sing in the most unusual positions.

Neuromuscular disorders

Breathing is initiated by several steps, from the respiratory neurones in the brain via the spinal cord through peripheral nerves to the respiratory muscles. At each of these steps and the junctions between them the process is susceptible to disorder.

With respiratory muscle weakness comes a reduction in lung volume, particularly vital capacity and its components. This leads to a reduction in ventilation consequent on the weakness of inspiratory muscles. Equally, if not more important, is the weakness of expiratory muscles which reduces the efficiency of cough. This can result in inefficient clearance of mucus and frequent pulmonary infections.

- *Central nervous system* Trauma to the brain and spinal cord can result in partial or total loss of respiratory function, depending on the degree and site of the lesion. Frequently, as a result of trauma, vasoconstriction, hypertension, mucus secretion and oedema result from increased uncontrolled activity of airways innervation.

149

Nervous control of breathing Box 4

Compression of the brainstem

Raised intracranial pressure is a very serious condition and in many patients can lead to death. There are many causes of raised intracranial pressure, including brain injury and brain tumours.

Anything that increases the volume of the brain, such as bruising, bleeding or a tumour increases the pressure in the brain because the brain is encased within a solid box, the skull.

As explained in Box 10.2 (p. 148), raised intracranial pressure can cause damage to important structures, which include not only the respiratory neurones but other areas important in maintaining life, which can eventually lead to death.

In the case of John, who was on life support, this only became evident when the machines supporting his ventilation were temporarily removed. The brainstem death tests that are carried out test for the function of other regions in the medulla, such as the vestibular centre.

Hemispheric strokes interfere with the voluntary pathways of breathing. Brainstem strokes that affect the dorsal medullary centres (see Fig. 10.6) cause fatal apnoea.

Patients with Parkinson's disease frequently complain of dyspnoea (see below), respiratory muscle weakness and impaired ability to clear respiratory secretions. This leads to pneumonia, which is a common cause of death in these patients.

- *Poliomyelitis* This disease is now rare owing to the advent of vaccines. About 25% of those infected require mechanical ventilation during the acute stage. Many recover respiratory muscle strength thanks to the reinnervation of denervated fibres.
- *Diphtherial Corynebacterium diphtheriae* produces an exotoxin that provokes a demyelinating neuropathy, which results in respiratory failure if the respiratory muscles are involved. Antitoxin is the only specific therapy.
- *Botulism* The anaerobe *Clostridium botulinum*, which can be foodborne, colonizes the gut of infants or infects wounds and produces a toxin which blocks the release of acetylcholine at the neuromuscular junction. When innervation of the respiratory muscles becomes involved artificial ventilation is required. Even then 10% of patients may die. The innervation of the respiratory muscles seems particularly vulnerable, and ventilation may be

required for several months. Treatment includes debridement of infected wounds, penicillin, and antitoxin in the early stages.

- *Duchenne's muscular dystrophy* This X-linked recessive genetic disorder affects the gene for the production of protein dystrophin. From the age of 10 vital capacity declines inexorably in these patients. They first develop nocturnal hypoxaemia and commonly die from respiratory failure secondary to pulmonary infection at about 20 years of age. Mechanical ventilation is the only option to relieve respiratory failure.

Vagal reflexes

Perhaps because of our unique power of speech, reflex control of breathing seems to be very different in human beings from that in other animals, and is not yet satisfactorily explained (at least not to the satisfaction of your author).

The control of breathing pattern in most mammals is profoundly influenced by inputs travelling in the **tenth cranial nerves** (the vagus nerves). These are two very large nerves which run in the neck, one either side and parallel to the trachea. These nerves carry information from other parts of the body, but the information coming from the lungs is of particular importance in the control of breathing. It originates in three types of receptor:

- Slowly adapting pulmonary stretch receptors (PSR)
- Rapidly adapting (sometimes called irritant) receptors (RAR)
- C-fibre receptors (J receptors).

The stretch and rapidly adapting receptors send their information to the brain in large- and small-diameter myelinated fibres, receptively.

The C-fibre receptors, as their name suggests, send their information in small-diameter non-myelinated (C) fibres.

The two types of receptor that have been most investigated are slowly adapting (PSR) and rapidly adapting (RAR).

Rate of **adaptation** describes the way a receptor (in the lungs, or anywhere else in the body) responds to a stimulus.

If a constant stimulus is applied to a receptor it 'gets used to it' and the frequency of the receptor discharge (in action potentials per second) decreases even though the stimulus does not change (Fig. 10.8).

The rate at which this happens defines receptors as *slowly adapting* – i.e. the frequency of discharge returns only slowly to the rest frequency, and *rapidly adapting* – i.e. the frequency rapidly returns to normal.

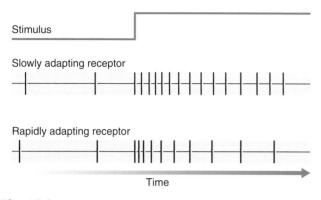

Fig. 10.8
Adaptation. The way slowly adapting (pulmonary stretch receptors in the lung) or rapidly adapting (irritant or deflation receptors in the lung) adapt to a sustained change in stimulation.

Slowly adapting pulmonary receptors (pulmonary stretch receptors)

These receptors are situated in the smooth muscle which makes up a large part of the walls of the trachea and bronchi, and so are affected by factors that influence bronchial tone (tension). Their specific stimulus is tension. The tension in the airways walls is influenced by **lung volume**: the more the lung is inflated the greater will be the stretch of the structures within it, including the airways. Thus pulmonary stretch receptors signal the volume of the lungs at any instant. This signal is in the form of action potentials: the greater the volume the higher the frequency of action potentials. During inspiration the lungs increase in volume and the frequency of discharge increases. It is thought that when the frequency reaches a certain 'threshold' it operates some kind of neural 'off switch' which switches off inspiration. This 'threshold' falls during each inspiration (the off switch becomes more sensitive (Fig. 10.9)) and is reset back to its original sensitivity during expiration while the inspiratory neurons are not active.

The effect of stretch receptors on pattern of breathing is most dramatically seen in the **Hering–Breuer Inflation Reflex**. When the lungs of an anaesthetized animal are kept inflated it ceases to make inspiratory efforts for some time (Fig. 10.10). Students are sometimes confused by the demonstration of this reflex into thinking breathing is being physically obstructed by the inflating pressure, rather like preventing someone breathing by putting your arms round their chest and squeezing. Not so: inflating the lungs is producing a reflex. The subject is not even trying to breathe, as demonstrated by the absence of phrenic activity

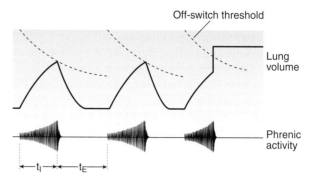

Fig 10.9
The off-switch threshold. Lung inflation is signalled to the brain by pulmonary stretch receptors. When this signal reaches a certain threshold it switches off inspiration and expiration begins. The brain becomes more sensitive to this signal (the off-switch threshold falls) through a single respiratory cycle. Once the off-switch has operated its sensitivity is reset to begin a new cycle. If the lungs are artificially inflated to above the threshold at any time inspiration is immediately switched off in what is known as the Hering–Breuer Inflation Reflex.

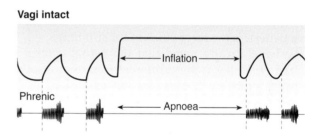

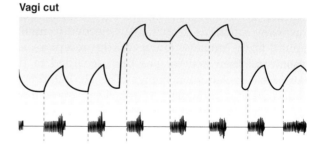

Fig 10.10
The Hering–Breuer Inflation Reflex. When the lungs are artificially inflated increased pulmonary stretch receptor activity (which signals lung volume) operates the inspiratory off-switch which terminates inspiration. This is the Hering–Breuer Inflation Reflex. That its afferent arm is in the vagus nerves is demonstrated by cutting the nerves. The reflex is abolished. This reflex is very weak in man.

during the lung inflation. Eventually, however, CO_2 builds up in the blood and forces breathing to restart.

Pulmonary stretch receptors are still active while the lungs are deflating during the start of expiration, and some are active throughout the respiratory cycle. It is important to look at what stretch receptors do to both phases of breathing. They are generally described as terminating inspiration and limiting tidal volume. Equally importantly, they extend expiratory time. This is what you see in the Hering–Breuer inflation reflex. This aspect of their action is important because the expiratory phase of breathing is usually the longest at rest, and so is the most important phase in determining rate of breathing.

The activity of stretch receptors is not essential for rhythmic breathing: breathing continues even if the vagi are cut. Nevertheless, in animals at least, stretch receptors modify the pattern of breathing. This modification makes breathing more efficient in terms of energy required to produce a given ventilation. The stretch receptors 'take note' of the mechanical properties of the lung and inform the central control mechanisms, which alter the pattern of breathing accordingly. For example, if the compliance of the lungs is reduced stretch receptors will discharge more vigorously (reduced compliance means stiffer lungs, which pull more strongly on the stretch receptors). The more vigorous discharge will switch off inspiration earlier and breathing will become shallow and rapid. This pattern is the most efficient for stiff lungs.

We have already noted that the neural control of human breathing is very different from that of other animals, probably because of the evolution of the power of speech. This difference is particularly true for the part played by stretch receptors. These receptors play a paramount role in the control of breathing in animals, yet their importance in the control of quiet breathing in humans is in dispute. For example, much larger lung inflations (over 1 L) are needed to inhibit inspiration in humans. However, the receptors are present and their activity has been recorded in the vagus nerves of human beings. The Hering–Breuer reflex is present in humans during sleep, and is more powerful in babies than in adults.

During exercise lung inflation is more rapid, which augments stretch receptor activity and may cause them to operate the off switch earlier than normal, which may be one of their roles in humans. That stretch receptors reflexly dilate the airways and accelerate the heart may also be an advantage in reducing airways resistance and increasing cardiac output in exercise. Stretch receptors are primarily mechanoreceptors, as their name implies; they are, however, inhibited by an increase in P_{CO_2} (and blocked completely by the even more acid gas SO_2). This response to CO_2 may play a part in the shortening of expiration (perhaps owing to removal of their lengthening effect), seen when inhaled CO_2 accelerates breathing.

Rapidly adapting (irritant) receptors

These mechanoreceptors respond to a sustained physical stimulus with a discharge whose frequency rapidly returns to the rest level (see Fig. 10.8). For this reason, in breathing where the stimulus is constantly changing, their discharge is highly erratic and difficult to quantify. These receptors can be powerfully stimulated by the inhalation of irritating gases and vapours such as ammonia or cigarette smoke, and this gives rise to the name **irritant receptors**, one of their many alternative names. They are also stimulated by procedures that distort the lung, such as pneumothorax (air in the pleural space, which causes lung collapse), and have occasionally been called 'deflation receptors'. These are obviously not the physiological stimuli the receptors would encounter under normal conditions, and therefore **rapidly adapting receptors** is a more suitable name. The physiological stimulus of these receptors is not lung volume, as in the case of stretch receptors, but probably the **rate of change of lung volume**, which of course is related to rate of airflow into or out of the lungs.

Rapidly adapting receptors in the lungs are free nerve endings lying close to the surface of the airways epithelium and concentrated at points where the airways divide. Their superficial position and their rapidly adapting pattern of discharge is similar to that of receptors in the larynx and trachea, which reflexly cause cough. Unlike the laryngeal cough-producing receptors, rapidly adapting receptors in the lungs reflexly produce two very different (and confusing) patterns of breathing:

1. Rapid shallow breathing, resulting mainly from a shortening of expiration.
2. Long deep **augmented breaths**, in which inspiration is about twice as long as normal (Fig. 10.11).

These augmented breaths are periodically taken by mammals (every 5–20 minutes in resting humans) to reverse the slow collapse of the lungs that takes place during quiet breathing.

Until recently it seemed paradoxical that stimulating these receptors could produce both rapid shallow breathing and the diametrically opposite pattern of the deep slow augmented breath. The explanation for this seems to be that each augmented breath is followed by a '**refractory period**' of at least 2 minutes, during which another augmented breath cannot occur and during which time rapid shallow breathing, resulting

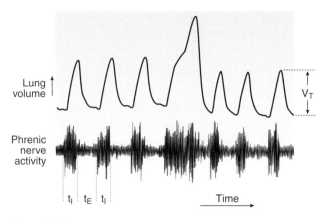

Fig. 10.11
An augmented breath. These 'sighs' occur every few minutes in man and help to reinflate collapsed areas of the lung. They are provoked by increased activity in rapidly adapting pulmonary receptors which pass to the brain via the vagus nerves.

from shortened expirations, intervenes. Your chances of provoking an augmented breath therefore depend on how recently the last one occurred.

Rapidly adapting receptors have a role in initiating the first deep gasps of newborn infants and contribute to the initiation of inspiration in adult breathing, and are possibly involved in a form of positive feedback during the accelerated breathing of exercise. As well as the irritant gases and particles that cause lung disease, rapidly adapting receptors are stimulated by the changes in lung structure that take place as a result of lung disease. They may therefore be responsible for the changed patterns of breathing seen in lung disease, and the sensation of **dyspnoea** (an overwhelming breathlessness), reflex bronchial constriction and increased airway mucus secretion that accompanies many of these pathologies.

C-fibre receptors

Thin non-myelinated afferent nerve fibres are classified as *C fibres*, and a population of those in the pulmonary vagus nerves have their endings close to the pulmonary capillaries. Hence their alternative name **J** (juxtapulmonary capillary) **receptors**. A separate group of C fibres terminate in the bronchial walls. C-fibre receptors are stimulated by increases in interstitial fluid (oedema) and by histamine, bradykinin and prostaglandins released during lung damage. The reflex response to vigorous stimulation of these receptors is apnoea, followed by rapid shallow breathing, hypotension, bradycardia, laryngospasm, and a relaxation of skeletal muscles by inhibition of spinal motor neurons. These responses would

be appropriate in an animal which has suffered severe lung damage. Although they are very numerous in the afferent vagus a clear role for pulmonary C fibres in normal human breathing has not yet been found.

Dyspnoea

Often the only or major symptom patients with lung disease complain of is dyspnoea. This condition is difficult to define, but is usually described as 'difficult breathing' or 'air hunger'. The sensation of dyspnoea arises when there is a disproportion between the demand for ventilation and its supply. The sense of respiratory effort, detected as respiratory muscle tension, is not matched by changes in respiratory muscle length and therefore ventilation.

This history of dyspnoea is important in diagnosis. Dyspnoea of sudden onset is associated with an acute cardiopulmonary event – pulmonary embolism or left ventricular failure, for example. Chronic dyspnoea of slow onset is usually associated with respiratory disease – COPD, asthma, pulmonary fibrosis – but can be the result of cardiac diseases, particularly those that cause pulmonary venous congestion.

Other reflexes

Reflex changes in pattern of breathing produced by non-pulmonary sources are important in humans and other animals. Those that transmit emotion, amicable or otherwise, to our peers are important in non-verbal communication, for example. The changes in breathing that occur when one stubs one's bare toe, and the hilarity of such an event, changes the pattern of breathing in callous observers. Thus emotion and pain can change pattern of breathing via nervous pathways from higher regions in the central nervous system.

The nose and pharynx

Most of the reflexes arising from this region protect the lower airways against the ingress of foreign objects and damaging gases and vapours. Many and varied reflexes arise from the upper airways, and many of these have secondary effects on other systems. The cardiovascular system and the skeletal muscles of posture, for example, are affected by a sneeze.

Sneezing is usually provoked by the stimulation of bare nerve endings in the nasal mucosa which send their information to the brain in the trigeminal nerves. A sneeze is a rather stereotypical response, consisting of a deep inspiration followed by closure of the glottis, against which pressure builds up until rapid opening of the glottis and expiratory effort produces airflow whose velocity can approach the speed of sound and ejects the offending stimulation. The sneeze has many features in common with the cough, but it is interesting to note that, unlike a cough, a sneeze is difficult to mimic and almost impossible to suppress. Sneezing can be provoked by stimuli applied to regions of the body other than the nose. In some people it is provoked by bright light, and in an unfortunate few by sexual orgasm!

The nasopharynx lies behind the soft palate and cranial to the oropharynx, which connects it to the larynx. This region of the upper airways reflexly produces sniffs and the similar but more powerful **aspiration reflex**. This consists of powerful inspiratory efforts with the glottis held open. These efforts tend to pull any material blocking the nasopharynx on to the oropharynx, to be swallowed or spat out.

Swallowing

Although usually associated with food, the swallowing reflex can be initiated by other stimuli applied to the dorsum of the tongue, soft palate and epiglottis. During swallowing respiration is inhibited in whatever phase of breathing the swallowing is initiated. This aspect of the reflex prevents the inhalation of food. It is interesting that in newborns water, sugar solutions and milk can provoke swallowing, but saline and amniotic fluid will not. The advantage of this to an individual who has spent the last 9 months surrounded by amniotic fluid are obvious. The anatomy of a baby's upper airways predisposes it to nose breathing, which is an advantage when suckling. (It was once thought that babies were obligate nose breathers, but this is not the case.) When one considers that babies may swallow four times per second while suckling, at the same time as breathing, the very precise integration of these reflexes becomes clear.

The chest wall

Unlike the diaphragm the skeletal muscles of the chest wall have **muscle spindles** as part of a spinal feedback mechanism. Like other muscle spindle reflexes, this mechanism seems to provide a rapid load-detecting system. Any increase in load caused by decreased compliance or increased resistance applied to the respiratory system is rapidly compensated for by an

increased drive to the intercostal muscles, which maintains ventilation.

Cough

The upper airways, particularly the larynx and upper trachea, contain superficially situated **rapidly adapting nerve endings** which provoke cough. Unlike the rapidly adapting receptors deeper in the lungs, whose action is to produce rapid shallow breathing, cough receptors produce a reflex rather similar to a sneeze, with a slow deep inspiration followed by an explosive expiration. Cough receptors provide a clear demonstration of the undemocratic nature of neural control of breathing. Stimulation of a single cough receptor will overpower the activity of all the other receptors in the lungs to produce a cough.

Somatic and visceral reflexes

Visceral or somatic pain generally produce opposite effects on pattern of breathing. Stretching the intestine or distending the gallbladder or bile ducts inhibits breathing, whereas somatic pain generally causes rapid shallow breathing.

A shower of cold water on the bare skin produces a gasp and an increase in minute ventilation by a mechanism that is independent of the unpleasant nature of the experience. Immersing the face in water, particularly cold water, causes an apnoea and cardiovascular changes which are called 'the diving reflex', and which are seen in more exaggerating form in diving mammals such as seals.

There is still much debate about what exactly causes the increase in ventilation that occurs during exercise. Reflexes from active or passive movements of the limbs (in anaesthetized subjects) may be responsible, in part, for this increase.

Further reading

Acker H. Po_2 chemoreception in arterial chemoreceptors. Annual Reviews in Physiology 1989;62:389
Bruce EN, Cherniack NS. Central chemoreceptors. Journal of Applied Physiology 1987;62:389
Eyzaguirre C, Zapata P. Perspectives in carotid body research. Journal of Applied Physiology 1984;57:931
McQueen DS, Pallot DJ. Peripheral arterial chemoreceptors. In: Pallor DJ, ed. Control of respiration. London: Croom Helm, 1983

Self-assessment case study

Opioid drugs such as morphine and diamorphine are frequently used to control pain. Although they are very effective analgesics, they have a number of side-effects including drowsiness, nausea, vomiting, constipation and respiratory depression.

Opioids act on opioid receptors that are found throughout the central nervous system, including the spinal cord and the brainstem as well as higher centres. There are three subtypes of opioid receptor, μ, δ and κ. The μ receptors are probably the most important in mediating analgesia, but unfortunately they are also the most important receptors in mediating respiratory depression. The respiratory depressant effect of opioids drugs is compounded by their sedative effect: patients who have received a relative overdose of opioids are often very sleepy and their airway may obstruct.

From your knowledge of the nervous control of ventilation, you should be able to attempt the following questions about opioid induced respiratory depression.

① Where in the central nervous system do you think opioids act to cause respiratory depression?

② What precaution could you take in a patient who is receiving intravenous opioids such as morphine after surgery to limit the effects of any respiratory depression that may occur?

③ How would you recognize respiratory depression in a patient receiving opioids?

④ How would you treat a suspected case of respiratory depression in such a patient?

Answers see page 179

Self-assessment questions

① Why is respiratory centre not a very precise term?

② Where are the majority of neurons associated with breathing located in the CNS?

③ List the three main types of receptor found in the lungs, and the type of fibre in which each sends its information to the brain.

④ What would blocking conduction in the vagus nerves do to pattern of breathing, and why?

⑤ What types of receptor provokes cough, and which part of the airways is most densely populated with them?

⑥ What is dyspnoea?

Answers see page 180

LUNG FUNCTION TESTS – MEASURING DISABILITY

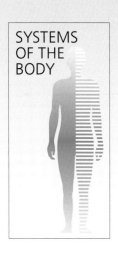

SYSTEMS OF THE BODY

Chapter objectives

After studying this chapter you should be able to:

① Appreciate that lung function tests quantify disability of function; diagnosis is usually on the basis of clinical history.

② Explain spirometry and outline the changes in static and dynamic measurements caused by restrictive and obstructive disease.

③ Describe how flow/volume loops are obtained and what changes you would expect to COPD.

④ Outline the principles and advantages of plethysmography.

⑤ Explain blood gas analysis.

⑥ Describe washout techniques for measuring $\dot{V}/\dot{Q}$ inequalities.

⑦ Explain the need for exercise testing.

Introduction

The respiratory system presents a uniquely vulnerable aspect of our bodies to the outside world. It is, for example, the only place where capillaries continuously come into direct contact with the outside air. Admittedly, that air is well conditioned before being presented to the respiratory surface, but attacks on the respiratory system and its function are extremely common. It is to be hoped that our readers will never suffer from coronary heart disease or renal failure, but which of us will go through life without a disease of the respiratory system, if only the common cold?

Most malfunctions of the respiratory system are reliably diagnosed by clinicians after taking a history of the patient's complaint and making a clinical examination. Radiological examination at appropriate levels of sophistication, microbiological and cytological investigations, blood tests, lavage, bronchoscopy, and a pantheon of other ingenious tests are available to confirm or refute the original diagnosis.

Such a diagnosis is, however, usually qualitative. It does not quantitatively measure the effect the disease is having on the functioning of the respiratory system, and hence on the quality of life. This is the province of the lung function test.

These tests range from the relatively simple to those that are the province of the specialized lung function laboratory. We have placed the tests roughly in increasing order of exoticism.

Spirometry

A simple spirometer (Fig. 5.2, p. 67) will provide much useful information about a patient's lungs. Large people have larger lungs than small people and age exerts its malign effect. Extensive study of these relationships has provided us with tables which, for example, relate vital capacity to height (see Appendix).

Measurements made on a spirometer may be classified as:

- *static*, where the only consideration is the volume exhaled, or
- *dynamic*, where the **time** taken to exhale a certain volume is what is being measured.

Although such measurements as inspiratory reserve volume (IRV) and expiratory reserve volume (ERV) can be informative, the most usual and useful static spirometric test is the *forced vital capacity* (FVC). This is 'forced' because the subject is enthusiastically urged to breathe in as far as he can and out as far as he can (Fig. 11.1). This test, which can be classed as static

because it does not involve an element of time, is often combined with a dynamic test, the FEV:

- *Forced expired volume in one second* (FEV_1) The subject is urged to breathe in as far as he can and breathe out as fast and far as he can. The volume he breathes out in 1 second is the FEV_1.

FEV_1 is commonly expressed as a percentage of FVC. This takes into account the problem that a very small person (with very small, perfectly healthy lungs) would never be able to breathe out the same amount in 1 second as a very large person, whose lungs may not be so healthy. You can expect a healthy person to force out at least 70% of his vital capacity in 1 second. Using this percentage alone can create problems in restrictive lung diseases, which restrict the expansion of the lungs: both VC and FEV_1 are reduced, therefore in those cases that percentage may be normal. For this reason both absolute values and percentage are measured. Many years ago a ratio of 70% VC was considered acceptable, but that was when smoking was considered normal.

Characteristic traces in normals and patients with chronic obstructive (emphyzematous/bronchitic) or restrictive (fibrotic) lung disease are shown in Figure 11.1.

Although emphysema is the 'classic' obstructive lung disease it can only be diagnosed with certainty at post mortem (pathologists are the only people who invariably make the perfect diagnosis, but by then it's too late). We therefore describe obstructive patterns of lung disease as asthma (reversible) or chronic obstructive pulmonary disease (COPD, irreversible).

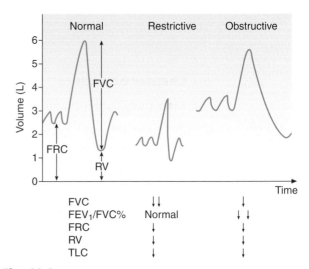

Fig. 11.1

Spirometry. Changes in lung volumes measured by spirometry that occur due to restrictive or obstructive disease.

• *Functional residual capacity* (FRC) and *residual volume* (RV) Because a subject cannot breathe out all the air in his lungs plethysmographic (see below) and dilution methods have to be used to measure these two lung volumes. RV and FRC are frequently increased in diseases such as asthma, bronchitis and emphysema, when airways resistance is increased, and RV is particularly increased in air-trapping emphysema.

In **helium dilution method** the principle is simple. The patient breathes out to FRC or RV, whichever is being measured, and is connected to a spirometer of known volume containing helium (He) at known concentration. The patient breathes normally for an appropriate length of time and the dilution of the He by the RV or FRC in his lungs is measured. The level of the trace of his breathing is carefully watched and oxygen added at the same rate as it is used up to keep the overall volume in lungs + spirometer constant (Fig. 11.2).

An interesting disparity is often seen between RV measured by plethysmography and by dilution. This arises because air trapped in the lungs, which is not in contact with the mouth, is measured by the plethysmographic method but does not take part in the dilution of He.

Restrictive lung diseases decrease TLC, FRC, RV and VC. Frequently RV is first to be affected. Care should be taken in interpreting results from obese patients, where the outward recoil of the chest wall is reduced, resulting in lower FRC.

Obstructive lung diseases show an increasing RV as gas is trapped behind the collapsed airways (see above). Increased FRC and TLC in these patients is the result of reduced lung recoil and breathing at increased lung volumes in an instinctive attempt to keep the airways open.

Flow measurements

Peak expiratory flow is the maximum expiratory flow $(L.s^{-1})^{1}$ that a subject can produce. Of course this is dependent on the subject's motivation even with healthy lungs. The advantage of this measurement is that it can be made with simple apparatus – where the subject blows against a paddle or propeller which records flow. Although not precise this has been found to be an useful domecillary measurement in asthma with the patient keeping a diary of his progress.

Flow-volume loops. With the subject breathing through a pneumotachograph (Fig. 4.6, p. 49) which measures flow, and by integrating that flow to provide volume, loops of inspiratory and expiratory flow-volume relationships can be recorded. (Fig. 11.3). These loops are constructed by having the patient breathe from total lung capacity down to residual volume several times. They are particularly useful in assessing chronic obstructive airways disease (COPD) where the inspiratory part of the loop has a normal shape, although being of reduced volume, while the expiratory part of the loop has a characteristic 'scooped out' shape as flow is restricted by airway collapse.

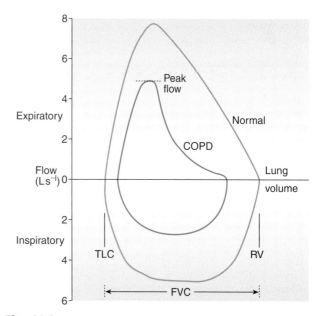

Fig. 11.3
Flow/volume loops. Plotting flow against volume while a patient takes a maximum inspiration and maximum expiration through a pneumotachograph produces a loop whose shape is very useful in diagnosis.

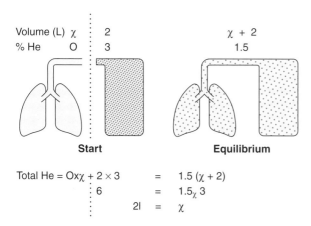

Fig. 11.2
Helium dilution. Helium dilution is used to measure lung volumes that cannot be measured by direct spirometry (FRC and RV).

Plethysmography

This instrument is described in Chapter 4 and consists of an airtight box in which the subject sits. To understand the principles on which this instrument works, consider the subject's chest as a syringe with the diaphragm represented by the plunger.

The subject first pants against a closed shutter – the neck of the syringe is blocked.

In terms of gas law the situation is as in Figure 11.4a, where a large enclosed volume of gas (the contents of the box) surrounds a small enclosed volume of gas (the air in the lungs) which increases and decreases in volume as it is compressed or decompressed. This change in volume of the syringe compresses and decompresses the air in the box, and so the pressure in the box changes proportionately and in the opposite sense to the pressure in the lungs.

Measuring the pressure changes in the box while the subject pants against a closed shutter enables us to measure lung volume, and is usually used to measure **functional residual capacity** (FRC) and **residual volume** (RV).

Plethysmography is also used to measure lung volumes (TLC) in patients with severe airflow obstruction in preference to the usual helium (He) dilution technique. This is because in these patients air trapping is so bad that the He cannot get to closed off volumes in the lungs, which are therefore not registered. In plethysmography, however, these closed off volumes are still subject to the gas laws (see the Appendix) on which this technique is based.

The principle of the relationship between box pressure and lung airway pressure does not depend on the 'syringe', which represents the lungs, being closed. In Figure 11.4B the narrow tube represents the resistance of the airways, and although air is being forced in to or out of the syringe the relationship between this driving pressure and box pressure still holds. In this case, measuring the driving alveolar pressure (by measuring box pressure) and flow (using a pneumotachograph), we can measure **airways resistance**.

Plethysmography offers an almost ideal way of measuring a number of pulmonary variables. One of its major limitations is that many subjects object to being locked inside an airtight box. This may reflect the incidence of claustrophobia in the population, or the mistrust in which respiratory physiologists are held.

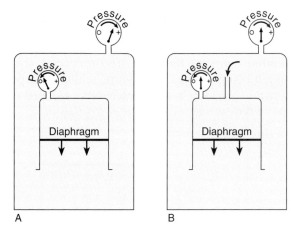

Fig. 11.4

The principle of the plethysmograph. The plethysmograph is an airtight box in which the subject sits. It can be used to measure air pressure within the subject's lungs. To understand the principle on which it works, consider the subject's chest as a 'syringe' in which the diaphragm represents the plunger and the 'neck' of the syringe represents the conducting airways of the lungs. In (A) the neck of the syringe is closed off (mouth closed). Lowering the plunger reduces the pressure in the lungs and compresses the air in the box, raising its pressure. Raising the plunger has the opposite effect. By measuring airway pressure and box pressure simultaneously while the subject pants against a closed shutter, the relationship between box and pressure within the lungs can be established. This relationship holds even when air is flowing in to or out of the lungs (B) and enables us to measure air pressure within the lungs simply by measuring box pressure.

Lung mechanics

Compliance

The variables required to calculate compliance of the lungs are volume, and the pressure that is producing that volume (intrapleural pressure). Pressure in the oesophagus is a good estimate of intrapleural pressure, and changes in oesophageal pressure are a very good estimate of changes in intrapleural pressure. Pressure in the oesophagus is usually measured using a small balloon on the end of a catheter, which is swallowed into the stomach and then withdrawn about halfway up the oesophagus. The subject breathes in to total lung capacity in a series of steps, holding his breath for a moment between steps. The volume breathed in at each step is measured using a spirometer and the oesophageal pressure at each step measured. The subject then breathes out in a series of steps, with the same measurements being made.

Because compliance depends on lung size, because the curves are not linear (Fig. 11.5) and because there is hysteresis between the inflation and deflation curves, it

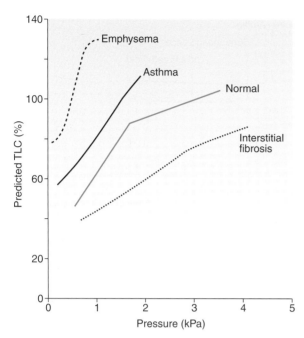

Fig. 11.5
Lung compliance. Compliance is the relationship between pressure and volume of the lungs. By measuring intrapleural pressure (as intraoesophageal pressure) and lung volume (as % predicted TLC) these characteristic curves are obtained.

is conventional to measure volume as a percentage of predicted TLC and to report compliance on the deflation limb of the curve 1 L above predicted FRC.

Resistance

The most usual way of measuring airways resistance these days is using a whole-body plethysmograph, as described above. Alternatively, the variables needed to measure resistance (airflow and the pressure producing that flow) can be obtained with a pneumotachograph (flow) and an oesophageal balloon (pressure), as used to measure compliance. Flow, oesophageal pressure and lung volume are usually measured, so that the contribution made by the elastic recoil of the lungs can be included. This type of measurement is usually called pulmonary resistance, and includes the effect of tissue resistance.

Transfer factor (diffusing capacity)

The theory behind the method of measuring transfer factor was outlined in Chapter 6 (p. 89). Methods of indirectly measuring transfer factor for O_2 which are

based on a number of questionable assumptions have been developed, but are really only of theoretical interest.

Transfer factor is now measured using carbon monoxide under steady-state or single-breath methods, both of which require us to know the partial pressure driving CO from the inhaled air into the blood, and the rate of uptake of CO.

Steady-state method

As with the single-breath method the time for which the lung is exposed to CO is fairly easily calculated. The difficulty is determining the driving partial pressure from alveolar air into blood. In this method the subject breathes a gas mixture containing approximately 0.2% CO until a steady state of removal is reached. The partial pressure of CO in the alveoli fluctuates throughout the respiratory cycle, and so cannot be measured directly. It is calculated by partitioning the concentration in the expired gas into alveolar and dead-space (which does not take part in transfer) compartments. The size of the dead-space compartment is calculated from the amount of CO_2 in the expired air using the relationship:

$$V_D/V_T = (P_{A,CO_2} - P_{E,O_2}) / (P_{A,CO_2} - P_{I,CO_2})$$

where V_D and V_T are the physiological dead space and tidal volume, and P_I, P_A and P_E are the partial pressures of CO_2 in inspired alveolar and expired gas, respectively. This method depends on estimating CO_2 in alveolar gas and, partly because of the inaccuracies this introduces, has been superseded by the single-breath method.

Single-breath method

In this method the subject exhales to residual volume then inhales a vital capacity breath containing 0.2% of CO and a known percentage (about 10%) helium (He). The subject holds his breath for 10 s and then breathes out through a gas analyser (Fig. 11.6). The first 750 mL of the expirate is abandoned to clear the dead space and the sample analysed for CO and He. The dilution of the CO by gas already in the lung is obtained from the fall in He concentration.

As the results obtained by this method are influenced by the volume of lung taking part and the amount of haemoglobin in the blood (to mop up the CO), lung function laboratories correct for both by expressing transfer factor for CO as TCO per litre of lung volume (kCO) corrected to a standard blood haemoglobin concentration.

LUNG FUNCTION TESTS – MESURING DISABILITY

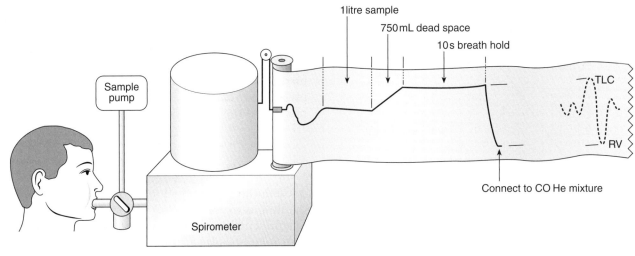

Fig. 11.6

Transfer factor. Volume manoeuvres to measure transfer factor by the single breath method. The subject breathes out to residual volume and then takes a maximum breath of the CO He mixture. He holds his breath for 10 seconds and then breathes out past a sample pump. The first 750 mL is rejected to avoid dead space and the next 1 litre sampled.

The steady-state and single-breath methods of measurement each have features to commend them that are beyond the scope of this book.

Interpretation of a low transfer factor is difficult because a number of factors, such as uneven ventilation, uneven perfusion, uneven emptying and diffusion properties, may be involved. This emphasizes the fact that lung function tests are more important for quantifying disability than for making an accurate diagnosis. In general, however, we find that transfer factor is reduced in emphysema, where respiratory surface has been lost, but less affected in bronchitis, where there has been little destruction of tissue.

Blood gases

It is the business of the respiratory system to 'condition' arterial blood for the benefit of the tissues it perfuses. Measuring the properties of arterial blood with the subject at rest and, if necessary, during the increased demands of exercise, tells us whether the respiratory system is up to the job.

Where arterial blood samples are available P_{O_2}, P_{CO_2} and pH are measured by bringing the blood into contact with electrodes whose resistance to current or whose accumulation of H^+ is determined by the P_{O_2}, P_{CO_2} and pH of the blood being tested. By bringing the blood into contact with standard gas mixtures and carrying out a variety of calculations, modern blood gas analysers calculate other variables, such as **standard** **bicarbonate** and **base excess/deficit**. These instruments have displaced all other methods of measuring blood gases and pH, but they still depend on the operator presenting a sample which has been correctly collected. The causes of error in collection are mainly due to contamination of the sample by air; delayed analysis, which results in oxygen being consumed within the stored blood; and secondarily, the effect of temperature, a drop in which can result in the measured P_{O_2} being less than the P_{O_2} of the blood when it was in the subject (most modern instruments get round this problem by automatically ensuring that the blood is kept at body temperature during analysis).

Obtaining a sample of arterial blood is not a trivial or unskilled procedure, and capillary blood from a pinprick can be used with techniques that do not need more than 0.1 mL to measure CO_2 tension, haemoglobin saturation and lactic acid. A number of non-invasive alternatives have also been developed.

Oxygen saturation used to be measured photometrically by monitoring light of the appropriate wavelength for oxygenated or deoxygenated haemoglobin transmitted through the finger or earlobe. The problem with this technique was that the blood being monitored was mainly venous or capillary, rather than arterial. This technique has now been almost completely replaced by **pulse oximetry**. In this technique, light of appropriate wavelengths is monitored as it passes through the earlobe or finger and related to the pulse pressure wave in the vessels under the sensor. The difference between the extra light signal at the peak of the pulse and that between pulses is due to the inflow of blood and reflects arterial saturation.

Another approach is to apply miniature O_2 and CO_2 electrodes to heated skin. The plan being to measure the gas tensions in the blood in the dilated vessels below the electrodes. These transcutaneous (Tc) measurements are more successful in neonates, who have thin well-vascularized skin (as soft as a baby's bottom), than in adults where $TcPO_2$ is approximately 80% PaO_2 and $TcPO_2$ is greater than $PaCO_2$.

Gas washouts

The uniformity of distribution of inspired air throughout the lungs is important to their efficient function (assuming that blood is also uniformly distributed). The uniformity of ventilation can be investigated by measuring the appearance of an inhaled inert gas at the lips in a single- or multiple-breath test.

Single-breath washout curves

In this test a single breath of O_2 is inspired and the N_2 concentration is continuously measured at the lips during the following expiration. Better-ventilated regions of the lung will have their residual volume (which contains air from the breath before the single breath of O_2) more diluted by O_2 than poorly ventilated regions. In healthy subjects residual N_2 in the expiration starts at zero (dead-space gas, phase 1; Fig. 11.7).

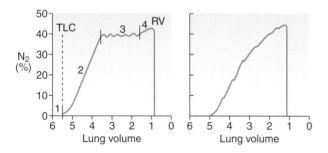

Fig. 11.7
Single-breath washout curves. After taking a breath of pure oxygen the subject breathes out past a rapidly responding nitrogen metre. In healthy subjects the concentration of nitrogen left in the expired air rises rapidly to a plateau. In patients with uneven distribution of ventilation the trace is as shown with no distinct plateau.

Nitrogen concentration then increases rapidly after the dead space is cleared (phase 2), and continues to rise very slightly (phase 3) in a plateau whose slight slope is due mainly to differences in the ventilation of different regions of the lung. Disease can cause gross abnormalities of regional ventilation which flatten phase 2 and cause a conspicuous slope of the plateau phase 3.

In normal subjects there is a slight upturn at the end of the plateau as lung volume approaches RV. This is due to airway closure in the lower lobes causing a disproportionate amount of gas to come from the upper regions which contain a higher percentage of N_2. The lung volume at which this starts is the critical closing volume (p. 40), which increases in obstructive airways diseases.

Multiple-breath washout curves

In this test the subject, after breathing room air, is connected to a system of one-way valves which cause him to inhale from a bag of pure O_2 and exhale through an N_2 meter. With each breath the concentration of N_2 is seen to fall as the residual N_2 is washed out of the lungs. This is the same process as repeatedly rinsing a piece of cloth which has been dyed: the colour of the water in each successive rinse becomes lighter and lighter. The concentration of N_2 (or dye) falls in an exponential curve. If we plot the log of concentration against the number of breaths of O_2 taken, the graph is nearly a straight line for healthy subjects, with complete washout of N_2 in 5–7 minutes (Fig. 11.8).

In less uniform distribution, as found in disease, the line becomes less steep and more non-linear, and the time for complete washout increases.

Inert gas washout

Uneven distribution of blood flow in the lungs is the commonest cause of defective oxygenation of the blood. Unfortunately, uneven perfusion is more difficult to measure than uneven ventilation.

Various methods involving the injection of radioactive gases into the blood and measuring their accumulation in the lungs have been developed to measure regional perfusion, but many of these are the province of the research laboratory.

An important concept in uneven distribution of blood flow is that of the **virtual shunt**. This concept deals with the different degrees of uneven distribution as if they were a single 'shunt' of blood from one side of the lungs to the other without coming into contact

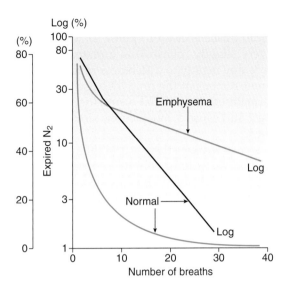

Fig. 11.8
Multiple-breath washout curves. The subject repeatedly inhales from a bag of pure oxygen and exhales past a rapidly responding nitrogen meter. As the residual nitrogen is washed out of his lungs the % in each sequential expiration falls as shown (if his lungs are healthy). If you convert this type of curve to log % you get a straight line (which is easier to quantify). The log % nitrogen plotted against breath number for an emphysematous patient is shown.

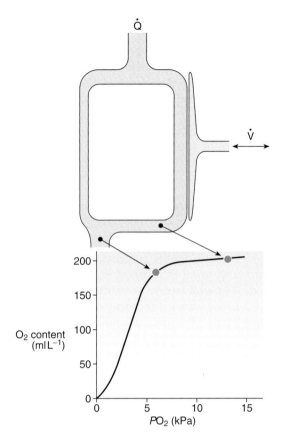

Fig. 11.9
Virtual shunt. If blood 'shunts' past or through the lungs without coming into contact with an effective respiratory zone it constitutes venous admixture to the arterial blood. Adding oxygen to the inspired air does not help this situation because this only brings oxygen into contact with blood which is already fully loaded with oxygen and so can carry no more. In practice reduced oxygen content of arterial blood is more likely to be the result of poor $\dot{V}/\dot{Q}$ ratios than this extreme condition, nevertheless virtual shunt is a concept used to construct isoshunt diagrams which help clinicians to estimate how much oxygen to add to a patient's inspired air.

with alveolar air (Fig. 11.9). The important point is that a subject with such a shunt will not improve the oxygenation of his arterial blood even if he is given pure O_2 to breathe. Blood in the shunt cannot be reached by the O_2 and continues to make a 'venous admixture' to the arterial blood.

Blood in the alveolar capillaries, on the other hand, is fully loaded and cannot take much more O_2. Therefore, because of the flat upper part of the O_2 dissociation curve the P_{AO_2} is considerably depressed, irrespective of whether the subject is breathing air or pure O_2. Normograms are used clinically to estimate the 'virtual shunt' a patient is suffering from (Fig. 11.10). This is the calculated shunt based on the assumption that the arterial/mixed venous O_2 content difference is 50 mL/L.

These 'isoshunt' diagrams are used clinically for adjusting the inspired O_2 concentration administered to patients to obtain a required arterial P_{O_2}.

Multiple inert gas washout

Estimates of shunt do not describe the *distribution* of $\dot{V}/\dot{Q}$ ratios (in terms of how much of the lungs has a particular ratio) throughout the lungs. This would

provide valuable information as to the nature of a defect resulting from disease.

A method of measuring how much blood flow and how much ventilation goes to 'compartments' with different $\dot{V}/\dot{Q}$ ratios has been developed using inert gases. In this method the lung is considered as consisting of a number of compartments (usually 50). Each compartment is considered independent of all others. A mixture of several (usually six) inert gases of different solubilities is continuously infused into the blood, and their concentration are measured or calculated in expired air and arterial and venous blood. The gases will partition

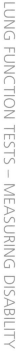

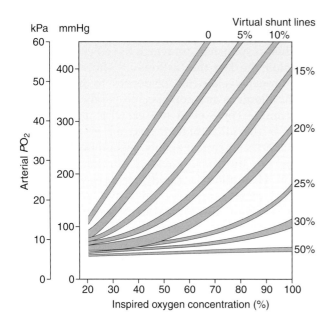

Fig. 11.10

Isoshunt diagram. Using the concept of a virtual shunt based on an assumed arterial/mixed venous blood oxygen content difference of 50 mL/litre it is possible to construct isoshunt diagrams which, assuming the shunt remains the same, relate Pao_2 to inspired oxygen concentration. This enables clinicians to achieve a required Pao_2 without administering excessively high levels of oxygen. For example if administration of 90% O_2 produces Pao_2 of 41 kPa the patient has 15% virtual shunt and to achieve a Pao_2 of 12 kPa requires an inspired oxygen concentration of 40%.

themselves between the alveolar air and the blood of each compartment. The retention (ratio arterial to venous concentration) and excretion (ratio expired to venous concentration) for each gas is plotted against the solubility of the gas in question. The retention/solubility plot yields the distribution of blood flow with respect to $\dot{V}/\dot{Q}$, and independently the excretion/solubility plot yields the distribution of ventilation with respect to $\dot{V}/\dot{Q}$. A plot for a normal subject is shown in Figure 11.11A. Note that the $\dot{V}/\dot{Q}$ ratios for the lung compartments are on a log scale, which spreads out the low $\dot{V}/\dot{Q}$ ratios. The distribution of ratios for the patient (Fig. 11.11B) shows many compartments with low $\dot{V}/\dot{Q}$ ratios, and 5% of the total blood flow (calculated separately) going to unventilated compartments (shunt).

Exercise testing

Exercise tests are generally safe because they do not, as might be assumed, involve striving to maximum effort

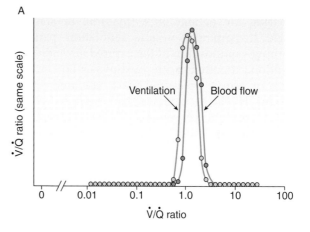

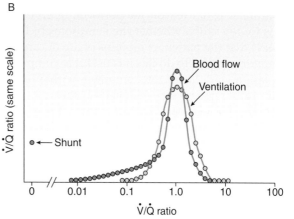

Fig. 11.11

Multiple inert gas washout. In this type of analysis the lung is divided into 50 compartments. A mixture of 6 inert gases dissolved in saline is continuously infused into a vein. At equilibrium the retention or excretion of each gas, when plotted against their solubility, yields the quantitative distribution of perfusion or ventilation against the $\dot{V}/\dot{Q}$ ratio of that particular compartment. A plot for a normal subject is shown (A) with one for a patient (B) in which 5% of total blood flow is shunted ($\dot{V}/\dot{Q}$ ratio 0) and many compartments have low $\dot{V}/\dot{Q}$ ratios.

but are aimed to provide information at loads which the patient can perform reasonably comfortably. Nevertheless, this form of testing should have a physician in attendance as cardiac dysrhythmias are not infrequent. An electrocardiogram should be continuously taken from patients suspected of cardiac disease and all subjects over 40. Walking with the patient or asking him to climb stairs are traditional and useful guides to incapacity and assessment of fitness for surgery.

Because the respiratory system has such enormous reserves many of the tests outlined above are carried out when the increased demands of exercise are being placed on it. More sophisticated exercise tests involve exercising the patient on a treadmill or stationary bicycle. In particular, minute ventilation, pattern of breathing, composition of the expired air and O_2 consumption, together with cardiovascular measurements of blood pressure, heart rate and ECG at different levels of exercise, can help to assess a patient's disability. Assessment of exercise capacity is measured as maximum O_2 uptake per minute ($\dot{V}O_{2\,max}$). This is obtained directly by increasing the exercise level until the patient can no longer continue. Because the relationship between heart rate, cardiac output and oxygen consumption is linear this information can be projected from submaximal responses in vulnerable patients.

The most usual reason for performing an exercise test is to determine whether the symptoms of breathlessness that the patient complains of are of cardiac or respiratory origin. To do this it is useful to compare the ventilation and heart rate obtained with predicted values from age and size matched normals.

Patients with impaired heart valves, for example, reach normal maximum heart rates at lower than normal workloads.

Patients with airflow obstruction have higher than expected minute ventilation for the level of exercise, which reflects wasted ventilation. Patients with restrictive diseases respond in the same way, except that their increased minute ventilation is made up of a pattern of high frequency and low V_T.

Challenge tests

For good diagnosis we wish to see the patient's complaint under the best (or, from his point of view, worst) condition. This is very clearly seen in asthmatic patients who are remarkably normal when not in status asthmaticus. Frequently the exercise tests described above will provoke an asthmatic attack in these patients but there are a variety of other challenges to which they can be put. These include tests of bronchial responsiveness which have been developed to exploit the fact that asthmatics show abnormally large bronchoconstrictor responses to inhalation of specific allergens and non-specific chemical and physical stimuli. Thus, even the exercise test described above or the inhalation of cold air may trigger an attack. Of the chemical agents, histamine and methacholine are the most popular, administered as an aerosol. Histamine is rapidly metabolized and so repeated doses are not cumulative. Methacholine seems to be more discriminatory between normal subjects and asthmatics. An aerosol of saline is first administered as saline is the vehicle in which the histamine or methacholine is administered and we wish to see if the saline itself produces an effect. The histamine or methacholine in saline is then administered in increasing doses (usually starting with about 0.003 mg mL^{-1} histamine acid phosphate and doubling with each administration). After 2 minutes of breathing the aerosol and 3 minutes for the drug to take effect the subject's FEV_1 or specific airways conductance is measured. The procedure is repeated at 10 minute intervals doubling the concentration each time until FEV_1 falls by more than 20%. The concentration which produces a 20% fall is then interpolated and this provocation concentration is reported as PC 20.

Further reading

Cherniack NS, Widdicombe JG Control of breathing. In: Farhi LE, Tenney SM, eds. Handbook of physiology. The respiratory system, Vol 2, Section 3. Bethesda, MD: American Physiological Society, 1986

Porter R (ed) Breathing: Hering–Breuer Centenary Symposium. Ciba Foundation Symposium. London: Churchill Livingstone, 1970

Whipp BJ (ed) The control of breathing in man. Manchester: Manchester University Press, 1987

Self-assessment questions

① What is the primary purpose of lung function tests?

② Which lung volumes cannot be measured by direct spirometry, and why?

③ State two methods of measuring RV.

④ What instrument is used to measure flow and construct flow/volume loops?

⑤ Which gas is used to measure transfer factor?

⑥ What test could you use to measure uneven ventilation of the lungs?

Answers see page 180

APPENDIX
SOME BASIC SCIENCE

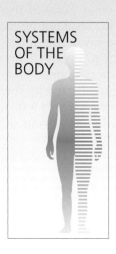

SYSTEMS
OF THE
BODY

APPENDIX

States of matter
The matter in the world around us can be considered to be made up of particles (*molecules*) which exist in three *states*: solids, liquids and gases. The respiratory system involves all three.

In solids
The molecules are strongly attached to each other and are very tightly packed. Their movement within the solid is highly constrained. Very few molecules escape from the surface of a solid.

In liquids
The molecules are freer to move within the bulk of the liquid, and the most rapidly moving may escape into the space above the liquid to form a gas which exerts a *vapour pressure*. Molecules in a liquid are, however, quite powerfully attracted to each other and those on the surface of a liquid are attracted into the bulk of the liquid by those underneath. This effect forms a skin which has *surface tension* (Fig. Appendix 1). This is why drops of rain form spheres and drops of liquid on a surface that is not wetted by the liquid do not spread out to form a thin film. Of particular interest to us is the situation when a liquid forms a bubble or lines the tiny bubbles (alveoli) of the lungs (see Surface tension and bubbles below).

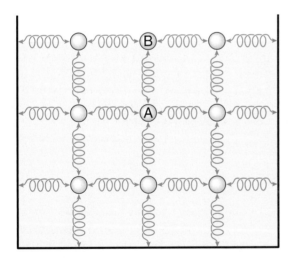

Fig. Appendix 1
The origin of surface tension. Molecules attract each other. In a liquid they have freedom to move in any direction within the bulk of the liquid. Molecule A is equally attracted in all directions so any slight imbalance will cause it to move. Molecule B, on the surface, is attracted only below and to the sides which retains it on the surface of the liquid. The forces in the horizontal plane give the surface tension like a sheet being pulled at all corners.

In gases
Molecules are free to move throughout the vessel containing them (they do this at considerable speed, molecules of room air are moving at about 500 ms⁻¹, the speed of a respectable revolver bullet; we do not feel their impact because they are so light). Because they are so far apart, the attraction between gas molecules is relatively weak. The impact of these molecules on the walls of the vessel containing the gas exerts a pressure which depends on the temperature (which determines the velocity of the molecules) and the number of molecules present.

An interesting fact is that in a mixture of gases each of the constituents of the mixture behaves entirely independently of the other gases, it exerts its pressure as if the others were not there. This *partial pressure* that a particular gas in a mixture exerts is part of the total pressure exerted by the mixture and is numerically proportional to the amount of the gas present. For example it is intuitively obvious that in a cylinder containing only O_2 (100% O_2) 100% of the pressure is due to O_2. It is not so obvious that in a cylinder containing, say, 25% O_2, 25% of the total pressure, whatever that may be, is due to O_2 (see Dalton's Law p. 169)

The molecules of a liquid that escape into the space above the liquid exert a partial pressure. This pressure is proportional to temperature because the higher the temperature the more molecule have enough energy to escape; but unlike the partial pressure of gases, this *vapour pressure* is independent of the total pressure over the liquid. This effect is particularly important in terms of the effects of water and volatile anaesthetics. Water at body temperature exerts a partial pressure of 6 kPa. That means within the lungs, where the air is saturated with water, if the atmospheric pressure is 100 kPa (about normal at sea level) there is only

$$100 - 6 = 94 \text{ kPa}$$

remaining to be made up by the other gases of the atmosphere. This is no problem at sea level but when you go to altitude the temperature inside the lungs stays the same so water in the lungs still exerts 6 kPa but the total pressure falls so that the component due to water has a bigger effect (being unaffected by the total pressure). This is particularly important in terms of O_2 supplies to the body. Similarly, the vapour of substances used as anaesthetics (e.g. chloroform) can exert partial pressures which dangerously reduce the pressure remaining to be occupied by O_2.

Elasticity – and scarred lungs
One of the properties of solids which it is important, in understanding how the respiratory system works, is

that of *elasticity*. The definition of an elastic material or object is one which returns to its original shape when a distorting force is removed. Perfectly elastic bodies obey Hook's Law, that the force (F) applied to a body is directly proportional to its extension (x) (or compression).

F = Kx (where K is the stiffness constant)

An important concept is that energy is stored in a distorted elastic body and is released to return it to its original shape.

When we distort a body:

Stress is the force (F) per unit area (a) applied to the body (and has the units Nm^{-2}).

Strain is the increase in length per unit length produced by a stress (as both increase in length (e) and unit length (l) have the same dimensions strain is dimensionless).

Hook's Law can be expressed in a different way for a body made of a particular material:

$$\frac{Stress}{Strain} = \frac{F/a}{e/l} = \text{A Constant (Young's Modulus of Elasticity for that material)}$$

Be careful not to confuse the terms elastic and elasticity. A material is said to be perfectly elastic if it gives up all the energy put into it by distorting forces to return to its original shape, without sequestering any as heat. A high modulus of *elasticity* on the other hand is frequently a property of materials that in everyday speech we do not usually refer to as elastic.

Thus Young's Modulus (in Nm^{-2}) for:

Steel = 2×10^{11}
Rubber = 2×10^{6}
Elastin (a component of connective tissue) = 6×10^{5}.

The highly elastic nature of steel is clearly seen if a steel ball is dropped on a steel plate. The ball returns to nearly the height from which it was dropped, showing it has given up almost all the kinetic energy which was used to distort it on impact with the plate in returning to its original shape. That is one of the reasons why the balls in the 'Newton's Cradle' executive desk-top toy are made of steel not putty.

It is the elasticity of the respiratory system that brings about normal quiet expiration by restoring the lungs and chest wall to the end-expiratory position. This elasticity is reduced in fibrosing lung diseases where the lungs are scarred and stiff: this makes breathing more difficult. In emphysema elasticity changes to make the lungs more 'floppy', which causes them to collapse, trapping air in the lungs.

The gas laws

Just as the elastic properties of solids can be mathematically defined, the pressure volume and temperature of a fixed mass of gas are related with mathematical precision by what are known as the gas laws. It is these laws by which we measure loss of lung function in disease:

Charles' Law   The volume (V) of a mass of gas at constant pressure varies directly with its absolute temperature:

$$V \propto T$$

Boyle's Law   The pressure (P) of a mass of gas at constant temperature is inversely proportional to its volume (V):

$$P \propto 1/V$$

These two laws can be combined to describe the relationship between pressure, temperature and volume of a mass of gas under different conditions. This is called *The General Gas Equation*:

$$P_1V_1/T_1 = P_2V_2/T_2$$

where 1 and 2 are the two different conditions being considered.

The General Gas Equation is invaluable when we wish to take into account of what happens to the volume of inhaled cold air when it is warmed in the lungs. This correction is essential when measuring the amount of gas breathed in lung function tests (see Chapter 11) because the temperature and pressure at which the exhaled gas was measured will vary depending on the temperature of the room and the barometric pressure on that day. The temperature of the gas within the lungs, on the other hand, will be a fairly constant body temperature of 32°C. The general gas equation is also used when we wish to calculate what is happening in a plethysmograph (pp. 50, 160), which is an instrument used to record pattern of breathing.

Dalton's Law of Partial Pressure   Each gas in a mixture of gases exerts the same pressure as it would if it alone occupied the same volume as the mixture. This is another way of saying that gases in a mixture have no effect on one another; they 'ignore' each other. Another way of expressing the partial pressure (P) of a gas which makes up a % of a mixture which exerts a total pressure (T) is:

$$P = \% \times T$$

Thus if the atmosphere exerts 100 kPa and contains 21% O_2 the partial pressure of O_2 is:

$$100 \text{ kPa} \times 21/100 = 21 \text{ kPa}$$

This law is absolutely fundamental to understanding the monitoring of patients in intensive care, patients being anaesthetised or in diagnosing many lung diseases. Composition of gases administered to patients and the composition of gases sampled from patients' lungs is frequently reported in terms of partial pressures.

Graham's Law of Diffusion   Describing the fact that lighter molecules travel faster than heavier ones, Graham's Law states: the rates of diffusion (D) of two gases at the same temperature and pressure are inversely proportional to the square roots of their molecular weights (MW).

$$D_1/D_2 = \sqrt{MW}_2/\sqrt{MW}_1$$

Where 1 and 2 refer to the two gases.

Because the molecular weights of the three main gases in the air (O_2, N_2, and CO_2) are about 32, 28 and 44 daltons respectively, their rates of diffusion in the gases in the alveoli of the lungs are not very different. This does not mean that the ease with which the respiratory gases are taken up and released by the blood is about the same because other factors are involved (see below).

Fick's Law of Diffusion   The rate of diffusion of a substance through a membrane is proportional to the area of the membrane (A), the solubility (S) of the substance in the membrane, the concentration gradient ΔC, and inversely proportional to the thickness of the membrane (t) and the square root of the substance's molecular weight:

$$\text{Rate of diffusion} = AS\,(\Delta C)/t \cdot \sqrt{MW}$$

Evolution has resulted in the lung exploiting Fick's law by evolving a thin wall of large area between air and gas and a system of ventilation and perfusion that ensures a steep concentration gradient. Carbon dioxide is 23 times more soluble in tissue fluid than O_2 and even though it has a greater molecular weight, it will diffuse 20 times more rapidly down the same concentration gradient. This is why, when the respiratory membrane across which diffusion takes place in the lungs is reduced or damaged by disease, uptake of O_2 is usually impeded before loss of CO_2.

Henry's Law   This describes diffusion across a gas–liquid interface. It states that at equilibrium the amount of a gas dissolved in a given volume of the liquid at a given temperature is proportional to the partial pressure of that gas in the gas phase above the liquid.

The situation under physiological situations is slightly more complicated because, although the amount of a single gas dissolved is always proportional to its partial pressure, obeying Henry's Law, different gases have different solubility coefficients and therefore different absolute amounts dissolve at the same partial pressure (more CO_2 than O_2 for example).

Also complicating the situation is the fact that a gas taken up in chemical combination with other substances in the solution is 'locked away' and not involved in the equilibrium, only that in free solution is considered. For example O_2 must dissolve in blood plasma before it can reach its most important carrier in the blood haemoglobin. The solubility coefficient for O_2 in blood without haemoglobin is very much lower than with haemoglobin. This storage phenomenon alters the amount carried. It does not alter the partial pressures involved and at equilibrium the partial pressure of a gas dissolved in a solution is the same as the partial pressure of the gas above the solution.

The flow of gases (which may be impeded in disease)

Flow of fluids (liquids and gases) takes place from a region of high pressure to a region of low pressure. During this flow pressure falls because energy is being used up in producing the flow. This using up of energy is the result of *viscosity*, which Sir Isaac Newton described as a 'lack of slipperiness' between concentric layers of the fluid. Flow can be generally considered as one of two types *lamina* or *turbulent*. In laminar flow the fluid moves parallel with the walls of the conducting tube in organized layers called laminae. The action is something like closing of an old fashioned telescope where the tubes slide one within the other. It is the sort of flow you see in a gently flowing river. The 'lack of slipperiness' means there is a resistance to flow which depends on the rate of flow ($\dot{V}$), the viscosity of the fluid (η) the length of the tube containing the fluid (l) and the radius of the tube (r).

Poiseulle's Law states that in such a situation where the tube is relatively long and smooth a pressure difference (ΔP) between its ends will produce a flow-

$$\dot{V} = (\Delta P)\,\pi r^4/8\eta l$$

This law strictly applies to straight circular rigid tubes of considerable length with smooth walls in which flow is constant. This does not apply to many tubes in the body. However, it makes a good approximation of what is happening under many circumstances, such as flow in the airways of the lungs and blood vessels and does not have the disadvantage of the intimidating mathematics associated with turbulent flow. This law is of outstanding importance to understanding what is happening to asthmatic patients where, during an attack, smooth muscle constricts their airways, reduces their radius and so has a profound effect on the air-flow through them.

Lamina flow becomes turbulent in the long straight smooth tube mentioned above when the flow exceeds

a certain rate. In this perfect tube it is possible to calculate when this will happen by calculating *Reynold's number (N)*:

$$N = \rho \, vD/\eta$$

where ρ is the density of the fluid, v is the velocity of flow and D is the diameter of the tube. When N exceeds 2000, flow becomes turbulent.

Long straight round smooth tubes do not exist in the body and turbulent flow does occur. In turbulent flow a significant percentage of the movement of the fluid is not along the axis of the conducting tube, eddies take place with flow moving at all angles, even backward, against the general direction of flow. Turbulent flow is what you see in a rushing mountain stream. It is more difficult to propel a turbulent stream of fluid than a laminar one. If all other things are kept the same, to double a lamina flow you need to double the driving pressure; to double a turbulent flow you need to square the pressure. Turbulence is very important in causing particles to be deposited in the nose, and so protecting the lungs from pollution.

Surface tension and bubbles: why lungs tend to collapse in premature babies

The respiratory surfaces our lungs are moist – they are lined with a film of liquid which exhibits the properties of surface tension. The tubes and surfaces are curved (the major respiratory surface, the alveoli, are roughly spherical). This causes them to behave like bubbles. A bubble remains as a sphere because the air pressure inside it is greater than the pressure outside. This excess pressure resists the tendency of the bubble to collapse due to surface tension. In the case of a bubble, unlike the flat liquid surface considered in Figure Appendix 2, the attraction between the molecules is resolved in toward the centre of curvature.

Laplace's Law states that the pressure (P) inside a sphere of liquid of surface tension T is inversely proportional to the radius (R) of the sphere:

$$P = 2T/R$$

The excess pressure (P) inside a bubble is:

$$P = 4T/R$$

because there are two air/liquid surfaces to a bubble.

For a cylinder, like the airways of the lungs, where the surface only curves in one dimension and has only one air liquid surface:

$$P = T/R$$

The relationship between pressure and surface tension has important consequences for compliance of the lung (see Chapter 3) and is of particular importance in the treatment of premature babies whose

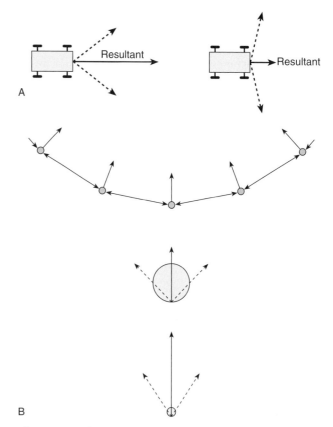

Fig. Appendix 2
Pressure in a bubble. If two people are pulling a cart with ropes (A), part of the tension in the ropes is exerted in the direction in which they want the cart to move. This is called the resultant of the two tensions or forces. The nearer they are to the required direction, the greater the effect (no-one would attempt to move something by pulling at right angles to the direction you want it to go). The same effect exists in a bubble (B) where the pull between molecules at its surface would cause the molecules to move in, collapsing the bubble if it was not for an excess pressure inside the bubble resisting the movement. You can see there is a bigger resultant (pressure) in a smaller bubble.

lungs tend to collapse because they are not yet making sufficient of a surfactant which reduces surface tension.

Measuring gas volumes: to measure the extent of disease

The air around us is relatively cool and dry compared with the air in our lungs. From the laws we have listed we can expect the temperature and/or pressure of a volume of gas we inhale to change when it passes into the conditions inside our lungs. This creates difficulties when we are accurately measuring the size of a breath (it has a different volume before and after you have breathed it in than when it is inside you).

As with most measurements it doesn't matter much which measuring system you use so long as you make it quite clear which you are using. The two most usual systems of expressing volume in respiratory physiology are: BTPS (**B**ody **T**emperature and **P**ressure, **S**aturated with water vapour) which is the condition of air within the lungs or immediately leaving them; and STPD (**S**tandard **T**emperature and **P**ressure **D**ry),

which refers to the condition when the gas has all water vapour removed and is measured at 0°C (273° Kelvin) and 100 kPa (1 atmosphere, 1 bar, 760 mmHg). Although expressing the properties of a fixed amount of gas using these two systems would result in very different figures, this difference does not affect the systems described in this book. Therefore we do not mention it further except to repeat the warning that if you are carrying out quantitative measurements it is essential to specify what conditions the measurements were made under.

Males of European descent

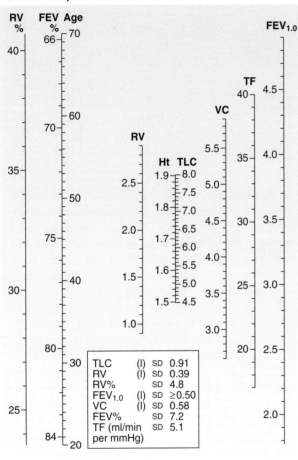

A

Females of European descent

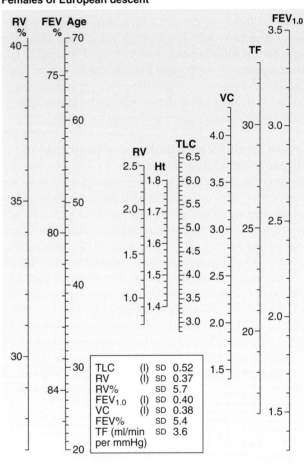

B

Fig. Appendix 3

Normograms. These have been constructed from considerable amounts of collected data and enable an estimate of a normal value of a lung variable by drawing a line from the age and height of the subject to the scale of the variable required. (A) Normal adult males of Western European descent. The RV% and the FEV% are related only to age and the TLC only to height. (B) Normal adult females. The RV% and the FEV% are related only to age. (Source: Adapted from Cotes JE, Leathart GL. Lung function: assessment and application in medicine. Edinburgh: Blackwell Science, 1993)

ANSWERS

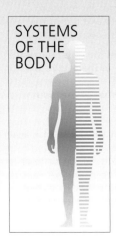

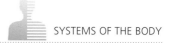

Chapter 1
Self-assessment questions

① Define homeostatis.
The maintenance of a constant internal environment.

② Approximately how many times does your heart beat, and how much blood flows through your lungs during each breath when you are at rest?
At rest you take approximately 12 breaths per minute and your heart beats approximately 60 times, forcing 5 L blood through the lungs. There are therefore 5 beats per breath and 416 mL of blood flow through the lungs.

③ What is the vapour pressure of water at body temperature?
6 kPa

④ Write the general gas-equation.
$P_1V_1/T1 = P_2V_2/T_2$

⑤ What is the partial pressure of O_2 in air (21% O_2) at an altitude where the air pressure is 50 kPa?
21% of 50 = 11.5 kPa

⑥ What is the formula for the excess pressure inside a bubble?
The Laplace relationship states P = 4T/R, where P = the excess pressure, T is the surface tension and R is the radius of the bubble. 4 is in the relationship because a bubble has two surfaces.

⑦ What is the symbol for partial pressure of carbon dioxide in arterial blood?
$PaCo_2$

Chapter 2
Self-assessment case study

① Why is food usually swallowed instead of being inhaled?
Food is usually swallowed as a result of the swallowing reflex. As swallowing is initiated the larynx is lifted up, making the angle between the oropharynx and the airway very acute, which tends to prevent food entering the larynx. The soft palate is raised up and blocks the entrance to the nasopharynx, which prevents food from going up into the nose.

② Why does choking sometimes occur?
Choking occurs if this reflex is not coordinated. Often a subject may happen to inhale with food in their mouth, which tends to draw the food into the airway.

③ During choking, where in the respiratory tract would you expect the foreign body to lodge?
The foreign body tends to lodge in the larynx above or between the vocal folds. The gap between the vocal folds (the glottis) is usually the narrowest part of the upper airway. Smaller foreign bodies (for example peanuts) may pass through the larynx and usually lodge in the main bronchi, which are the next narrowest part of the respiratory tract after the larynx. If a foreign body lodges in one of the main bronchi, it usually does so in the right main bronchus. This is because the angle between the trachea and the right main bronchus is much less acute than that between the trachea and the left main bronchus.

④ Why did the man in this case become cyanosed?
Total blockage of the airway means that oxygen is unable to reach the alveoli and therefore the blood becomes deoxygenated.

⑤ How did striking the man's back cause the foreign body to be dislodged?
Striking the thorax causes gas within the lungs to be compressed. The pressure builds up behind the obstruction and may thereby dislodge it. Another technique to dislodge foreign bodies is the 'Heimlich manoeuvre', named after a Cincinnati physician. A sudden thrust to the xiphisternum causes a reflex increase in intrathoracic pressure which may dislodge a foreign body.

⑥ Do you know another name for the syndrome of choking, based on the location where it often occurs and the appearance that the victim frequently has?
An episode of choking is also sometimes known as a 'café coronary', because it frequently occurs in cafés (or anywhere else where eating takes place) and the appearance often resembles that of a myocardial infarction, popularly called a 'coronary'!

Self-assessment questions

① What are the three mechanisms by which particles are deposited in the lung, and to what size particles do they apply?
Once a particle touches the wall of the airways it sticks there by surface tension and is not released. The deposition of particles can be described in terms of the diameter of a drop of water which has equivalent aerodynamic properties. These properties determine whether deposition takes place due to:

- *Impaction (> 5 μm equivalent diameter) when the rapid change in direction (turbulence) causes these large particles to be thrown out of the airstream*
- *Sedimentation (1–5 μm) when the particle falls out of the airstream because of gravity*
- *Diffusion (< 5 μm) when the particle is battered about by Brownian motion of the air particles until it touches the airway wall, where it sticks.*

The equivalent aerodynamic diameter for minimal deposition (most particles going into and out of the lungs without touching the sides) is about 0.5 μm

② What resistance to breathing resides in the nose, compared to the mouth and the total resistance of the respiratory system?
The resistance of the nose is twice that of the mouth and half the total resistance.

③ How does the diameter and number of airways at each level of the bronchial tree change as you move into the lung? What effect does this have on the velocity of the airflow?
The diameter of individual airways decreases with each generation, but their number increases at a rate that overpowers this effect and causes an enormous increase in total cross-sectional area. This causes a slowing of inspired air and acceleration of expired air.

④ Define the Reid Index and give its normal value.
The Reid Index is the fraction of bronchial wall thickness taken up by gland tissue. In healthy lungs it should be < 40%.

⑤ What are the two circulations of the lungs, and what are their functions?
The pulmonary circulation arterializes blood passing from the right to left sides of the heart.
The bronchial circulation is the nutrient circulation of the lungs and is part of the systemic circulation.

Chapter 3
Self-assessment case study

① What do you understand by the term 'low compliance'?
Low compliance means 'stiff lungs'. In other words, a high inflation pressure is needed to inflate the lungs with a given volume of gas.

② Why is the pressure needed to inflate the patient's lungs higher than normal?
In ARDS, the low compliance of the lungs means that ventilation requires high airway pressures.

③ Why do you think there is a maximum pressure set on the ventilator?
There is a maximum pressure set on the ventilator because high airway pressures cause further lung damage, and may even result in a pneumothorax.

④ What effect do you think a low compliance will have on the tidal volume that a ventilator can deliver?
To administer a given tidal volume the ventilator will need to produce a higher airway pressure in the face of decreased lung compliance. However, if this pressure is greater than the maximum pressure that is set on the ventilator, it will not be possible to deliver that volume. There is therefore an effective upper limit on tidal volume.

⑤ What effect will this have on gas exchange?
Because the airway pressure and tidal volume are both limited in patients with ARDS it is often necessary to alter normal ventilator patterns in order to maximize the lung ventilation. Sometimes it is necessary to accept a relative underventilation of the lungs (and therefore a high $PaCO_2$) in order to prevent further damage to lungs with a very low compliance.

Self-assessment questions

① Describe the origins and nature of intrapleural pressure.
Intrapleural pressure is the pressure in the small amount of fluid between the visceral and parietal pleurae. This pressure is normally negative relative to atmospheric and alveolar because it is generated by elastic recoil of the lungs and chest wall in opposite directions. In the upright (standing or seated) subject, it is less negative the lower in the chest it is measured because of the pressure of overlying tissue, which acts as a fluid with a density one quarter that of water. Intrapleural pressure can become negative during cough or forced expiration due to compression of the chest contents by the expiratory muscles.

② Define lung compliance.
The lungs are elastic, i.e. they return to their original form when distorting forces are removed. They show elasticity.
Stress is a measure of the cause of a distortion: if the distortion produces a change in the volume of the object involved,

$$Stress = \frac{Change\ in\ pressure}{Change\ in\ volume}.$$

Strain is a measure of the extent of a distortion: if the distortion produces a change in volume

$$Strain = \frac{Change\ in\ volume}{Original\ volume}.$$

Elasticity =

$$Stress/strain \quad \frac{\dfrac{Change\ in\ pressure}{Change\ in\ volume}}{\dfrac{Change\ in\ volume}{Original\ volume}} = \frac{Change\ in\ Pressure}{Change\ in\ volume}$$

Compliance is the reciprocal of elasticity, therefore:

Compliance =

$$\frac{Change\ in\ volume}{Change\ in\ pressure\ to\ produce\ the\ change\ in\ volume}$$

In other words, compliance is a measure of how easily the lungs can be stretched.
The tendency of the lungs to return to their original shape is due to elastic recoil.

③ What is the origin and function of pulmonary surfactant?
The phospholipid surfactant of the lung is produced by type II pneumocytes in the alveolar walls. Its functions are to:
- *Reduce surface tension and so make breathing easier*
- *Reduce the fraction of alveolar pressure required to resist surface tension, and so allow more of that pressure to be used to prevent oedema*
- *Equalize pressure in large and small alveoli*
- *Produce hysteresis, which stabilizes the lungs by 'propping open' the alveoli.*

④ To what and in what proportion is the elastic recoil of the lungs due?
About half of this is due to the elastic nature of the tissues and about half is due to the surface tension of the liquid that lines the air spaces of the lungs.

⑤ A patient has one of his lungs removed. Assuming both lungs were the same volume and of the same mechanical properties, what would happen to his measured compliance? How does the concept of specific compliance address this problem?
Although the mechanical properties of his remaining lung may not change, its compliance would appear to be half his original compliance. This is because

$$compliance = \frac{\Delta\ Volume}{\Delta\ Pressure}$$

and the amount of lung tissue available to increase in volume was halved. Specific compliance addresses this problem by dividing measured compliance by maximal lung volume, and so takes into account the amount of lung tissue present.

ANSWERS

Chapter 4
Self-assessment case study

① As a bronchogenic carcinoma increases in size, what effect will it have on gas flow through the adjacent airway?
As the tumour increases in size the airway becomes increasingly narrowed. Eventually, the airway may become completely obstructed by the tumour.

② What effect will this have on the ventilation of the regions of lung supplied by the affected bronchus? What symptoms may this produce?
Ventilation to the regions of lung supplied by the affected bronchus will be increasingly reduced and eventually will cease altogether. If a region of lung is no longer ventilated, the gas in that region is absorbed into the blood and the alveoli collapse. In the chest X-ray, you can see where this has happened. This collapse of the lung may lead to the symptom of dyspnoea.

③ What effect may a bronchogenic carcinoma have on gas exchange and why?
The collapse of a region of the lungs that still has blood flowing to it leads to hypoxia as a result of ventilation/perfusion mismatching (see Chapter 7).

Self-assessment questions

① What will be the effect of doubling the radius and the length of a tube in which laminar flow is taking place?
Laminar flow in a tube is described by Poiseuille's Law, which states that:

$$\dot{V} = \frac{(\Delta P)\ \pi\ r^4}{8\ \eta l}$$

Where $\dot{V}$ represents flow, (ΔP) pressure gradient, (η) viscosity, (l) length of the tube and (r) its radius.
Taking both the radius and length as 1 and keeping all other independent variables constant, the starting conditions are:

$$\dot{V} = everything\ else\ constant\ (K) \times \frac{(1)^4}{1} = 1K$$

Doubling the radius and the length:

$$V = (K) \times \frac{(2)^4}{2} = 8K$$

Flow will increase eight times, which demonstrates the profound effect of radius of a tube on its resistance to flow.

② What is the most likely reason and consequences of flow being limited during a cough?
In cough the glottis is first closed and the pressure throughout the chest made positive compared to atmosphere by contracting the abdominal and internal intercostal muscles. The glottis is suddenly opened and pressure inside the trachea falls rapidly, causing a high-velocity flow of air out of the lungs. Pressure around the airways remains positive during the cough, causing collapse, particularly of the bronchi not sufficiently supported by cartilage. This collapse reduces airflow and hence the efficiency of cough in clearing material from the airways. This is particularly unfortunate for people with lung disease, which make the airways more flaccid

and produce large amounts of mucus that need to be coughed up.

③ What is the significance of the total cross-sectional area of the airways of the lung?
The lung airways are an irregular dichotomously branching series of tubes. They can be represented as about 23 'generations', each member of each generation dividing into two of the next. With each generation the diameter of individual members is smaller than those of the previous generation, but the number of members is greater.
The total cross-sectional area of each generation is the sum of the cross-sectional areas of all its members. Because the number of members of each generation increases much more rapidly than the diameter of individual members, the total cross-sectional area of successive generations increases rapidly as we penetrate the bronchial tree. The functional consequences of this are that the large-diameter airways of the early generations offer the maximum resistance to flow, and airflow slows down as it penetrates the bronchial tree, being almost stationary by the time it reaches the alveoli. The final movement to the alveolar wall is by diffusion.

④ When is intrapleural pressure positive with respect to atmospheric pressure?
Only during forced expiration or cough.

⑤ Which branch of the nervous system is most important in producing bronchoconstriction?
The parasympathetic branch of the autonomic system.

⑥ What is the 'equal pressure point' in the airways, and what is its significance?
The equal pressure point is the place in the airways where the pressure outside is the same as the pressure inside. Normally pressure inside intrathoracic airways is greater than pressure outside and holds them open. At an equal pressure point only structural support holds the airway open, and if this is reduced by disease they tend to collapse.

Chapter 5
Self-assessment case study

① Why was a segment of Mr Jones' chest moving in the opposite direction to the rest of his chest?
A flail segment is an area of the ribcage which has become partially or completely detached from the rest as a result of trauma. During inspiration the intercostal muscles cause the ribcage to expand, but in contrast the flail segment is 'sucked' into the thorax by the increase in negative intrapleural pressure generated during inspiration.

② Why might Mr Jones have had a pneumothorax?
The sharp ends of the rib fractures that Mr Jones sustained may have punctured the underlying lungs, causing a traumatic pneumothorax.

③ Why was Mr Jones finding breathing difficult?
Breathing is difficult with a flail segment because it causes severe pain as the fractured ends of the ribs move against each other. In addition, if the flail segment is large it may impair ventilation of the lungs.

④ Why, when he was on a ventilator, did the flail segment of Mr Jones' chest now move in the same direction as the rest of his chest during breathing?

During mechanical ventilation, the lungs are inflated by a positive pressure applied to the airways. This positive pressure inflates the lungs and expands all parts of the ribcage, including the flail segment if there is one.

Self-assessment questions

① Which of the following lung volumes cannot be measured with a spirometer alone, and why? (a) residual volume, (b) tidal volume, (c) functional residual capacity, (d) vital capacity, (e) total lung capacity?

(a) (c) and (e), because they all contain residual volume (a), which by definition is the residual air that cannot be breathed out – into the spirometer.

② What is the relationship between anatomical dead space, physiological dead space and alveolar dead space? To what might the physiological dead space of a healthy subject be approximately numerically related?

Physiological dead space = Anatomical dead space + Alveolar dead space

Alveolar dead space is zero in a healthy subject and so

Physiological dead space = Anatomical dead space

which is approximately equal (in mL) to the subject's weight in pounds (1 lb = 0.45 kg).

③ What is the major type of inhomogeneity of ventilation in the healthy subject, and by what is it caused?

The major type of inhomogeneity of ventilation in a healthy subject is regional, in which the base of the lungs is better ventilated than the apex. This is caused by the gravity-dependent gradient of pleural pressure 'squeezing' the base of the lungs more forcefully than it squeezes the apex, and so more completely emptying it at the end of expiration.

④ What is the value of alveolar dead space in healthy subjects?

Zero.

⑤ What is FEV_1?

Forced expired volume in 1 second. Used to measure airways obstruction.

⑥ Define respiratory exchange ratio.

Rate of CO_2 output/Rate of O_2 uptake.

Chapter 6
Self-assessment case study

① Why do you think that the pressure in this patient's alveolar capillaries is high?

Failure of the right ventricle means that it has a higher filling pressure for a given cardiac output. This increase in filling pressure is reflected in an increase in pulmonary vein pressure and hence an increase in alveolar capillary pressure.

② What effect do you think the build-up of fluid in the alveolar walls will have on gas exchange, and why?

The rate of diffusion of oxygen and carbon dioxide is reduced by fluid in the alveolar wall. However, a failure of diffusion is only important in the early stages of pulmonary oedema. As the fluid in the lungs increases, the alveoli themselves become flooded and so no gas flows into them. This results in a failure of ventilation of the alveoli.

③ What do you think is the rationale for the treatment that this patient was given?

Oxygen helps to limit the hypoxia by increasing the diffusion gradient across alveolar walls containing a lot of fluid. It can also, to a limited extent, help to ameliorate the hypoxia caused by fluid-filled alveoli that are no longer being ventilated. Diuretics probably act by decreasing the venous pressure filling the right heart, thereby reducing the cause of the oedema.

Self-assessment questions

① Write the equation for diffusion of a gas across a membrane and define the terms used.

Fick's Law defines this situation as follows:

$$\text{Rate of diffusion} = \frac{A \times S\,(\Delta C)}{t\,\sqrt{MW}}.$$

where A is the area of the membrane available for diffusion. (S) is the solubility of the gas in the membrane, (Δ C) is the concentration gradient – brought about by the differences in concentration (or partial pressure) on either side of the membrane – (t) is the thickness of the membrane and (MW) is the molecular weight of the gas.

② Would it be reasonable to measure transfer factor in a patient with lung disease using CO in 100% O_2 to help his difficulties with breathing?

It would not be reasonable because the O_2 would compete with the CO for the storage sites on haemoglobin. All the standards for normal transfer have been obtained with atmospheric level of O_2.

③ What factors determine Pa_{CO_2}?

Pa_{CO_2} is the result of the balance between CO_2 added to the blood and CO_2 removed. CO_2 diffuses so readily that the alveolar membrane must be very impaired before it limits transfer from blood to air. The major factor determining removal of CO_2 from the body is therefore alveolar ventilation. In extreme cases no ventilation – breath-holding – means no loss of CO_2. Metabolism is the source of CO_2 added to the blood, so Pa_{CO_2} is a balance between metabolism and alveolar ventilation.

④ What is the single physical phenomenon that moves gas from alveolar air into the blood, and vice versa?

Diffusion.

Chapter 7
Self-assessment case study

① What effect do you think that chronic hypoxia will have on the blood vessels within his lungs?

Chronic hypoxia in this man's lungs will lead to a widespread vasoconstriction of the vessels in his lungs as a result of hypoxic pulmonary vasoconstriction.

② What effect will this have on the resistance of the blood vessels within his lungs?

Vasoconstriction results in an increase in resistance to blood flow within the vessels concerned. Usually, hypoxic pulmonary vasoconstriction is limited to hypoxic regions of the lungs and therefore results in blood being redirected to better ventilated regions of lung with higher partial pressures of oxygen. If the pulmonary vasoconstriction occurs throughout the lungs because of widespread hypoxia then there will be an increase in resistance to blood flow through the pulmonary circulation as a whole.

③ How might his right ventricle be affected?

Because the resistance of the pulmonary circulation is increased, the right ventricle will need to generate an increased blood pressure to achieve the same blood flow. High pressure in the pulmonary circulation is termed pulmonary hypertension. As we have seen in this chapter, the right ventricle is not adapted to generating a high pressure, as the pulmonary circulation is usually a low resistance, low pressure system. In the face of pulmonary hypertension, the right ventricular muscle may hypertrophy to some extent, but in severe cases of pulmonary hypertension, the right ventricle may start to fail.

④ How might all this be related to the swelling of his ankles?

As the right ventricle starts to fail, the ventricular pressure at the end of systole starts to rise, leading to an increase in systemic venous pressure.

Self-assessment questions

① What is the normal arterial blood pressure in the systemic and pulmonary circulations?

In young, healthy individuals, the normal systemic arterial blood pressure is about 120/75 mmHg. The normal pulmonary arterial blood pressure is about 25/12 mmHg.

② What is the normal blood flow through the systemic and pulmonary circulations?

The pulmonary and systemic circulations are in series, so the blood flow through them both, on a minute-to-minute basis, must be the same. In healthy resting individuals this flow is about 5 litres per minute.

③ What are the main anatomical differences between the systemic and pulmonary circulations?

The systemic circulation is a high pressure system, reflecting its role in organ perfusion, whereas the pulmonary circulation is a low pressure system. The right ventricle has a much thinner wall than the left ventricle and the pulmonary artery has a much thicker wall than that of the aorta. In the systemic circulation, flow to different organs is regulated by arterioles which represent the site of highest resistance to blood flow, whereas there are no similar vessels in the pulmonary circulation. In the pulmonary circulation, blood flow is significantly influenced by gravity whereas this is not the case with the systemic circulation. Although there are differences in the blood pressure between the systemic and pulmonary circulations, the blood flow is the same.

④ What factors influence the distribution of blood within the lungs?

Because the blood pressure in the pulmonary circulation is low, gravity has a significant effect on the distribution of blood flow in the lungs, tending to direct blood towards the lung bases. However, even at a given height above the lung bases there is quite a wide variation in blood flow different lung regions. Some authors think that this variation may be due to the that fact that when large blood vessels divide, they often give rise to smaller vessels of unequal size. What is important is that in any given lung region, ventilation is matched to blood flow.

⑤ What are the consequences of a mismatch in ventilation and perfusion?

Throughout the lungs, ventilation and perfusion are relatively well matched. A relative over-ventilation (high $\dot{V}/\dot{Q}$ ratio) results in an increase in physiological dead space and a relatively high partial pressure of oxygen and low partial pressure of carbon dioxide. A relative under-ventilation (low $\dot{V}/\dot{Q}$ ratio) results in an increase in shunting an relatively low partial pressure of oxygen and a high partial pressure of carbon dioxide. Overall, a mismatch in ventilation and perfusion causes a reduction in arterial oxygen concentration. This is because the blood leaving the under-ventilation regions of lung has a low oxygen content. Although the blood leaving the over-ventilated lung regions is coming from a region of relatively high oxygen partial pressure, the oxygen content of the blood is not elevated. This is because the haemoglobin leaving lung regions with a normal $\dot{V}/\dot{Q}$ ratio is 97% saturated. The haemoglobin in blood leaving lung regions where the partial pressure of oxygen is higher can therefore carry very little additional oxygen.

⑥ What are the important sources of shunt?

Anatomical sources of shunt are blood vessels which add deoxygenated blood to the oxygenated blood in the systemic circulation. This includes the deep bronchial veins that drain venous blood from the bronchial into vessels of the pulmonary circulation. In addition, the thebesian veins drain blood from the myocardium into the chambers of the heart. The thebesian veins that drain into the left ventricle and atrium form a shunt. Shunted blood also comes from relatively underventilated lung regions.

Chapter 8
Self-assessment case study

① What effect will anaemia have on the carriage of oxygen by the blood?

Anaemia will result in a reduction in the ability of the blood to carry oxygen. Over 97% of the oxygen carried in the blood is bound to haemoglobin. A reduction in the haemoglobin concentration of 1 gramme per litre results in the blood being able to carry roughly 3mL less of gaseous oxygen. However, the body has quite a substantial 'reserve' of haemoglobin and a quite large reduction in haemoglobin concentration can take place before overt tissue ischaemia occurs.

② How might the cardiovascular system respond to anaemia?

The haemodynamic response to anaemia is to increase the cardiac output. Although there is less oxygen being carried per litre of blood, if the cardiac output increases, the oxygen delivery to the tissues will be maintained as more blood is flowing through the tissues per minute.

③ What adaptive changes to anaemia might be seen in the red cell?

Chronic anaemia results in an increase in the red cell concentration of 2,3 DPG which causes the oxygen-haemoglobin dissociation curve to be shifted to the right. This shift means that oxygen is more readily given up by haemoglobin in the tissues.

Self-assessment questions

① List four factors that would displace the oxyhaemoglobin dissociation curve to the right.

1. Increased CO_2
2. Increased $[H^+]$
3. Increased temperature
4. Increase 2,3,diphosphoglycerate

② In carbon monoxide poisoning what values would you expect for

a) arterial Po_2, b) arterial O_2 content, c) arterial O_2 saturation?

(a) Normal *(b) Low* *(c) Low*

③ In which direction does chloride ions (Cl^-) move across the red cell membrane, a) at the tissues, b) at the lungs?

(a) In *(b) Out*

④ Write the Henderson–Hasselbalch equation and define the terms used.

$$pH = pK' + log \frac{[HCO_3^-]}{\alpha \; Pco_2}$$

where pH is $-log [H^+]$ (acidity)
$[HCO_3^-]$ is the concentration of bicarbonate ions
α is the solubility of CO_2 in plasma, and
Pco_2 is the partial pressure of CO_2.

⑤ Which enzyme catalyses the reaction $CO_2 + H_2O \Leftrightarrow H_2CO_3$, and where is it found in the blood?

Carbonic anhydrase found in the red blood corpuscles.

⑥ At the same Po_2, which is more saturated, fetal or adult haemoglobin?

Fetal, which means it has a greater affinity for O_2 and will take it from adult haemoglobin.

Chapter 9
Self-assessment case study

① Why is there an initial hyperventilation on ascent to altitude?

There is an initial hyperventilation on ascent to altitude because hypoxia stimulates the peripheral chemoreceptors.

② Why is this hyperventilation less than would be expected, given the severity of the hypoxia that occurs?

Hyperventilation increases the Pao_2 but decreases the $Paco_2$. The reduction in $PaCo_2$ causes a respiratory alkalosis. This alkalosis limits the hyperventilation by reducing the stimulation of the central chemoreceptors which essentially respond to the pH of the CSF. The

respiratory alkalosis is reduced over time by the kidneys which increase the excretion of bicarbonate.

③ Why are drugs such as acetazolamide effective in treating acute mountain sickness?

Acetazolamide increases the acidity of the blood and therefore tends to limit the respiratory alkalosis. This means that the degree of hyperventilation in response to the hypoxia is greater.

④ Do you know what other symptoms may develop in acute mountain sickness?

Other problems associated with acute mountain sickness include pulmonary oedema and cerebral oedema.

Self-assessment questions

① What are the roles and time scales of operation of chemical and neural control of breathing?

The two types of control of breathing are called chemical and neural. This division is rather artificial but those elements involved in chemical control of breathing exert homeostatic control on the chemical composition of the blood (arterial PO_2; CO_2 and pH) over a relatively long time scale (minutes). Neural control of breathing is related to the form of individual breaths and so must exert its influence in a fraction of a second. Its role appears to be ensuring that breathing is energy efficient.

② What are the names and anatomical sites of the sensors involved in the chemical control of breathing?

They are called central and peripheral chemoreceptors. Central chemoreceptors are found on the ventrolateral surface of the medulla of the brain where their environment is cerebrospinal fluid. Peripheral chemoreceptors are found on the aortic arch (aortic receptors) and at the bifurcation of the common carotid arteries (carotid bodies). The peripheral chemoreceptors monitor the composition of arterial blood.

③ Define three types of stimulus to breath that can be produced by changing the composition of inspired air.

a) Hypoxia – when the partial pressure of O_2 in the air is reduced.
b) Hypercapnia – when the partial pressure of CO_2 in the air is increased.
c) Asphyxia – when O_2 partial pressure is decreased and partial pressure of CO_2 is increased.

④ What is meant by 'the hypocapnic brake'?

When pure hypoxia stimulates breathing the increase in ventilation washes out CO_2 from the blood. This reduces the drive to breath from CO_2. Ventilation therefore becomes inappropriately low. This effect is seen in acute mountain sickness when a subject travels rapidly to altitude where the total atmospheric pressure, and therefore partial pressure of O_2 is reduced.

⑤ How do the respiratory responses to hypoxia and hypercapnia differ when applied singly and combined?

Even a small increase in the inspired partial pressure of CO_2 provokes an increase in ventilation. There is almost a linear relationship between the two until quite high levels of CO_2 are reached. On the other hand decreases in partial pressure of O_2 have to be quite profound (to

ANSWERS

about 10 kPa) before breathing is stimulated. Below this level however hypoxia is a powerful stimulus until it begins to exert a depressing effect on breathing. The combination of hypoxia and hypercapnia (asphyxia) exerts a more powerful influence than the sum of the effects of the two components.

Chapter 10
Self-assessment case study

① Where in the central nervous system do you think opioids act to cause respiratory depression?
Opioids cause respiratory depression by their action on receptors in the brainstem. It is thought that they act on the central chemoreceptors as well as the respiratory centres.

② What precaution could you take in a patient who is receiving intravenous opioids such as morphine after surgery to limit the effects of any respiratory depression that may occur?
It is common practice to administer oxygen to patients who are receiving opioids such as morphine postoperatively, particularly if these drugs are being administered intravenously. This will tend to reduce the likelihood of hypoxia occurring should there be any respiratory depression. It is also common practice to monitor the haemoglobin saturation using a pulse oximeter.

③ How would you recognize respiratory depression in a patient receiving opioids?
Respiratory depression is usually evident by a slow respiratory rate. The patient is usually quite drowsy because of the sedative effects of the opioids. If the patient is not receiving oxygen, he may be centrally cyanosed.

④ How would you treat a suspected case of respiratory depression in such a patient?
The treatment of opioid-induced respiratory depression depends largely on its severity. If necessary the patient's airway should be opened and oxygen administered to the patient. If the respiratory depression is very severe it may be necessary to ventilate the patient's lungs. In less severe cases it may be sufficient to administer oxygen by a facemask and discontinue the opioid infusion.
Naloxone is an opioid antagonist which will reverse the opioid-induced respiratory depression. Unfortunately, it also antagonizes the analgesic effects of opioids.

Self-assessment questions

① Why is respiratory centre not a very precise term?
Because there are no clearly defined anatomical 'centres' or structures in the brain that can be associated

with breathing. There are, however, populations of neurons, concentrated in certain regions, which are all active together at the same time in each respiratory cycle. These groups are what is generally referred to as respiratory 'centres'.

② Where are the majority of neurons associated with breathing located in the CNS?
The pons and the medulla.

③ List the three main types of receptor found in the lungs, and the type of fibre in which each sends its information to the brain.
- *Slowly adapting pulmonary stretch receptor – PSR (myelinated)*
- *Rapidly adapting (irritant) receptor – RAR (myelinated)*
- *Juxtapulmonary capillary – J receptor (unmyelinated).*

④ What would blocking conduction in the vagus nerves do to pattern of breathing, and why?
It would produce slow deep breathing because information from stretch receptors which triggers the inspiratory off switch would have been cut off.

⑤ What types of receptor provokes cough, and which part of the airways is most densely populated with them?
Cough receptors are a type of rapidly adapting receptor that most densely populate the larynx and upper trachea.

⑥ What is dyspnoea?
A sensation of breathlessness – 'air hunger'.

Chapter 11
Self-assessment questions

① What is the primary purpose of lung function tests?
To measure degree of disability of some aspect of the respiratory system. Diagnosis of disease is usually made mainly from the clinical history.

② Which lung volumes cannot be measured by direct spirometry, and why?
Functional residual capacity (FRC) and residual volume (RV) because RV cannot be breathed out into a spirometer.

③ State two methods of measuring RV.
Helium dilution spirometry or plethysmography

④ What instrument is used to measure flow and construct flow/volume loops?
A pneumotachograph.

⑤ Which gas is used to measure transfer factor?
Carbon monoxide (CO).

⑥ What test could you use to measure uneven ventilation of the lungs?
Single- or multiple-breath inert gas washout.

GLOSSARY

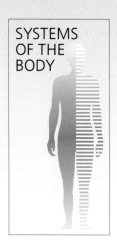

GLOSSARY

α₁-antitrypsin – any of a group of glycoproteins migrating in the α_1 region on serum protein electrophoresis and capable of inhibiting trypsin and such other proteolytic enzymes.

acetylcholine – an important neurotransmitter. It is produced by the vagus and other parasympathetic nerves.

acidaemia – an abnormally low pH of whole blood.

acidosis – a disturbance of the acid-base state of the body towards the acid.

adenosine triphosphate – a phosphate donor in biochemical systems. It functions as an energy store and is used up in muscular work, ion pumping, and many other energy-requiring reactions.

adrenalin – a proprietary name for epinephrine.

aerosol – a suspension in the air or other gaseous medium of minute solid and/or liquid particles having a negligible falling velocity.

airways resistance – the resistance to flow of gas presented by the airways of the lungs. Analogous to the electrical resistance of a wire to flow of current.

alkalosis – a disturbance of the acid-base state of the body in which arterial pH is higher than 7.45.

alveolar dead space – that alveolar region of the lung that is ventilated but not perfused. This is not an absolute state. Alveoli may be relatively under-perfused for their ventilation. This type of dead space should be minimal in healthy subjects.

alveolar gas equation – defines the relationship between the alveolar concentration of a gas, its inspired concentration, its output or uptake and alveolar ventilation.

alveolar sac – the last generation of air passages in the lungs. They are similar in structure to alveolar ducts except that they are blind-ended. Both ducts and sacs bear about half of the total alveoli each.

alveoli – the blind-ended terminal sacs of the airways where the majority of gas exchange takes place and the majority of lung volume resides.

anoxia – lack of oxygen in the circulating blood or in the tissues.

aortic body – peripheral chemoreceptors situated near the aortic arch.

apneustic – prolonged breath-holding at full inspiration.

aspiration – the act of drawing foreign material into the lungs.

augmented breath – a sigh, a deep breath having an inspiratory duration about one and a half times normal.

baroreceptor – a sense organ responsive to the stretch of large blood vessel walls, signalling blood pressure.

base – a substance that can combine with protons and so neutralize acids.

blood–brain barrier – the functional isolation of cerebrospinal fluid from blood plasma.

Bohr shift – shift of the oxyhaemoglobin dissociation curve caused by a chance in pH (due mainly to CO_2) which facilitates O_2 loading at the lung and unloading at the tissues.

bronchi – airways between the trachea and the alveoli.

bronchial tree – a phrase which draws attention to the similarity of the branching of the conducting airways of the lung to that of a deciduous tree in winter.

bronchiolus – one of the numerous subdivisions of the intrapulmonary secondary bronchi in which the diameter diminishes to 1 mm or less.

bronchoconstriction – narrowing of a bronchus caused by contraction of bronchial smooth muscle.

bronchopneumonia – inflammation of the lung producing patchy and often widespread consolidation.

buffer – a system that keeps relatively constant the concentration of some constituent, (usually hydrogen ions).

canaliculus – a small groove or channel (pl. canaliculi). A very narrow, fine canal or channel.

carbaminohaemoglobin – the normal complex of haemoglobin with carbon dioxide that transports carbon dioxide in the blood.

carbonic anhydrase – an enzyme found in red blood cells which accelerates equilibrium of the reaction $CO_2 + H_2O = H_2CO_3$.

carina – the ridge between the proximal ends of the two principal bronchi.

carotid body – peripheral chemoreceptors situated near bifurcation of the common carotid artery.

cartilage – a relatively nonvascular, specialized connective tissue comprising cartilage cells, young chondrocytes, occupying lacunae in a matrix of amorphous ground substance surrounding a network of collagen fibres.

central chemoreceptors – chemosensitive regions of the medulla whose activity promotes breathing. (See peripheral chemoreceptors)

central pattern generator – neural networks in the pons and medulla, as yet poorly defined anatomically, which generate the basic pattern of breathing.

chloride shift – the movement of chloride ions into or out of red blood cells to compensate for the movement of bicarbonate ions and to maintain electrical neutrality.

closing volume – as lung volume is reduced towards residual volume there is a point at which airways begin to close; this is called closing capacity. Closing volume is closing capacity minus residual volume.

compliance – the ease of stretching of the lungs or chest wall. Reciprocal of elastance. Units = $L:kPa^{-1}$ or $L:cmH_2O^{-1}$.

conductance – the ease with which gas or liquid can be made to flow down a tube. Reciprocal of resistance.

conducting airway – those airways involved in the conduction of air to the respiratory regions of the lung. They largely make up the anatomical dead space.

COPD – chronic obstructive pulmonary disease.

countercurrent – two streams flowing in an opposite directions in such a way as to maximize the exchange of chemicals or heat.

cyanosis – blue/grey/purple colour of the skin caused by the presence of abnormal amounts of deoxygenated haemoglobin.

degranulation – the process of shedding granules from cell cytoplasm to the exterior.

detoxification – the inactivation of the toxic properties of substances in the body by enzymic action.

diaphragm – the dome-shaped musculofibrous partition between the thoracic and abdominal cavities.

diffusing capacity – the ability (capacity) of the lungs to allow gas to diffuse from air to blood and vice versa.

diffusion – the process whereby a substance is transported along a concentration gradient by the random movement of molecules.

double Bohr shift – a Bohr shift (see above) occurring in both foetal and maternal blood caused by the same carbon dioxide produced by the fetus and enhancing its supply of oxygen.

drive to breathe – Physiological changes (e.g. increased CO_2 or decreased O_2) which increase ventilation.

dynamic airway collapse – collapse of the airways provoked by the phenomena which bring about flow. Thus increasing flow as in a cough provokes more collapse.

dynamic compliance – compliance measured while breathing is taking place.

dyspnoea – the sensation of breathlessness or 'air hunger'.

elastance – the reciprocal of compliance.

elastic recoil – the tendency of the lungs, being elastic, to resist stretching.

elasticity – the tendency to return to normal shape when a distorting force is removed.

elastin – an elastic protein.

emphysema – a condition where there is dilatation of the pulmonary alveoli distal to the terminal bronchioles with destruction of their walls.

endoderm – the inner layer of the embryo, giving rise to the primitive intestine and the yolk sac.

epiglottis – an unpaired, leaflike plate of elastic fibrocartilage situated behind the root of the tongue and the hyoid bone and in front of and overhanging the inlet of the larynx.

equal pressure point – during forced expiration, that point in the airways at which intraluminal pressure equals external lung pressure and when collapse is likely to occur.

erythrocyte – an anucleate cell, normally the most common formed element in circulating blood, filled with haemoglobin and shaped as a biconcave disk. Also red cell, red blood cell, red corpuscle, red blood corpuscle.

expiratory flow limitation – expiration is brought about by forces that tend to collapse the airways. With age and some diseases the airways collapse more easily than normal tending to limit expiratory flow.

expiratory muscle – expiration is passive in quiet breathing. Forceful expiration, as in exercise, enlists muscles which directly or indirectly compress the chest. These include the restus abdominus, external intercostals, external and internal obliques and transversalis.

expiratory reserve volume – that part of the functional residual capacity that can be voluntarily exhaled.

forced expiratory volume in 1 second (FEV$_1$) – the volume of air that a subject can blow out in 1 second making a maximum effort from a maximum inspiration. This lung function test is used to assess airways resistance.

forced vital capacity (FVC) – the largest breath a subject can take making maximal effort.

free radical – a highly reactive radical frequently of oxygen.

functional residual capacity – that volume of air remaining in the respiratory system at the end of quiet expiration.

generation – order of airways within the bronchial tree. The most usual convention is to call the trachea generation 0, the main bronchi are generation 1, the lobar bronchi are generation 2 and 3, the segmental bronchi generation 4 and so on to the alveolar sacs, which are generation 23.

haemoglobin – a complex molecule by which most of the oxygen in the blood is carried.

haldane effect – displacement of the CO_2 dissociation curve upwards in deoxygenated blood, enabling blood to carry more CO_2 from the tissues.

heat of vaporization – the amount of heat required to change 1 g of the substance in question from the liquid to the gaseous state. The latent heat of vaporization is high in the case of water which makes evaporation of water a good way to keep cool.

helium dilution method – a method of measuring residual volume (RV) and functional residual capacity (FRC, which is RV+ERV, expiratory reserve volume). The subject breathes out to RV and then breathes from a bag containing a known volume and concentration of helium. The dilution of the helium by the RV enables RV to be calculated.

Henderson–Hasselbalch equation – equation relating blood pH to blood CO_2 and bicarbonate.

hilum – a small gap or hollow in an organ where vessels, nerves, and ducts enter or leave it.

homeostasis – the relative stability of the internal environment of a normal organism which is preserved through feedback mechanisms despite the presence of influences capable of causing profound changes.

hypercapnia – an elevated level of carbon dioxide in the blood.

hypocapnia – an abnormally low concentration of carbon dioxide in the blood.

hypotension – abnormally low tension or pressure, especially blood pressure.

hypoventilation – insufficient ventilation of the alveoli of the lungs to maintain normal levels of oxygen and/or carbon dioxide in arterial blood.

hypoxaemia – reduced oxygen concentration in arterial blood.

hypoxia – inadequate oxygen supply in body or tissues.

hysteresis – characteristic 'loop'-shaped graph describing the relationship between two variables, where the value of one variable at a given value of the second depends on whether the latter is increasing or decreasing.

immunoglobulin – a family of proteins having antibody activity. There are five classes of immunoglobulins (IgA, IgD, IgE, IgG, IgM).

impaction – the collision of a moving particle with another or a stationary object.

in series – elements (tubes or components) are in series when they are connected 'one after the other'. Flow is therefore the same in all series elements.

intercostal – between the ribs.

interstitial fluid – the fluid in the interstices or interspaces of a tissue or organ.

intrapleural – within the pleura or pleural cavity.

irritant receptor – free endings of small myelinated afferent nerves found in the airway walls. They provoke cough, rapid shallow breathing and augmented breaths depending on their site and the stimulus they receive (also called-rapidly adapting receptor; deflation receptor).

laminar flow – the condition when fluid moves parallel to the walls of the conducting tube in an organized pattern, as if in layers.

Laplace relationship – relates excess pressure (P) within a bubble to it radius (R) and the surface tension (T) of the liquid of which it is made. $P = 2T/R$.

laryngospasm – reflex spasm of the laryngeal sphincter, particularly the glottic sphincter, initiated typically by the threat of inhalation of foreign material.

larynx – a tubular organ which extends vertically from the root of the tongue opposite the hyoid bone to the trachea and is composed of a framework of cartilages held together by ligaments and membranes.

leukotrienes – a group of icosanoid compounds derived from 5-hydroperoxy-6,8,11,14-icosatetraenoic acid, and thus ultimately from arachidonic acid, that are mediators of the inflammatory reaction.

loading region – the flat upper portion of the oxyhaemoglobin dissociation curve. This region of the curve represents conditions in the lung where oxygen is loaded into blood.

lung volumes – internationally agreed names for the volumes that make up breathing and other respiratory manoeuvres. Lung capacities are the sum of two or more lung volumes.

macrophage – a cell found in many tissues in the body which is derived from the blood monocyte and which has an important role in host defence mechanisms. It phagocytizes and kills many bacteria.

mechannoreceptor – receptors which are sensitive to mechanical stimulation. In the respiratory system these include receptors in the chest wall and diaphragm, as well as slowly adapting and rapidly adapting receptors in the airways which are sensitive to stretch as well as mechanical stimulation of the respiratory mucosa.

mediastinum – a median septum or partition between two parts of a cavity or an organ.

medulla oblongata – the caudal portion of the brainstem that extends between the pons and the most rostral part of the cervical spinal cord.

GLOSSARY

mesoderm – one of the three primary germ layers of the embryo. From this layer are derived the majority of the skeletal system, the circulatory system, the musculature, the excretory system and most of the reproductive system.

methaemoglobin reductase – an erythrocyte enzyme that converts methemoglobin to haemoglobin while oxidizing NADPH.

minimal air – the small amount of air left in the lungs taken out from the body and allowed to collapse.

motor cortex – posterior part of the frontal lobe of the brain anterior to the central sulcus from which impulses for voluntary movement arise.

mucopolysaccharide – a polysaccharide that contains amino sugars or monosaccharides They occur either alone or in combination with proteins.

multi-unit smooth muscle – smooth muscle made up of individual fibres not connected by gap junctions.

muscle spindle – a proprioceptor which detects striated muscle length and rate of shortening.

n parallel – elements (tubes or components) of a circuit are in parallel when they are connected to each other and the rest of the circuit at both ends. Flow divides itself inversely as the resistance of the elements.

peripheral mechanoreceptor – receptors which are sensitive to mechanical stimulation. In the respiratory system these include receptors in the chest wall and diaphragm, as well as slowly adapting and rapidly adapting receptors in the airways which are sensitive to stretch as well as mechanical stimulation of the respiratory mucosa.

pharynx – the space behind the nose and the mouth leading to the larynx and the oesophagus.

phosphoric acid – an important intracellular buffer. Also, an acid which is excreted by the kidneys as part of maintaining acid/base balance.

phrenic nerve – the nerve which originates from the cervical spinal cord and innnervates the diaphragm.

physiological dead space – the volume of gas in the respiratory system which does not equilibrate with blood. It includes the volume conducting airways (the anatomical dead space, see above) plus an additional volume relating to alveoli which have a high $\dot{V}/\dot{Q}$ ratio.

pneumotachograph – instrument for measuring gas flow.

pneumotaxic centre – respiratory area of the pons whose discharge is thought to cut short inspiration.

pneumothorax – gas entering into intrapleural space causing the underlying lung to collapse.

pons – area of the brainstem above the medulla.

prostaglandins – regulatory substances derived from arachidonic acid which have a range of actions on nearby organs, e.g. prostaglandins released from cells in the immune system can cause bronchoconstriction or bronchodilaration in the respiratory system.

proton – positively charged subatomic particle found in the nucleus of an atom. A term often used synonymously with a hydrogen ion, H^+ (when the electron is removed from a hydrogen atom, all that remains is a proton).

pulmonary circulation – the part of the circulation involved in carrying blood to and from the alveoli.

pulse oximetry – a method of monitoring the oxygenation of peripheral blood. Light is shone through a peripheral extremity, such as the finger or ear-lobe, and the pattern of absorption of the light indicates the degree of haemoglobin saturation.

radial traction – in the respiratory system, radial traction is the outward pull of the lung parenchyma which tends to 'hold open' smaller airways and aveoli.

rapidly adapting nerve ending – a nerve ending whose response to a stimulus decreases quickly with time, even though the stimulus is still present.

rapidly adapting receptor – receptors in the airways which respond to dynamic changes in lung volume or to irritants in the respiratory tract.

recruitment – the process in the pulmonary circulation whereby additional blood vessels open up and carry blood when there is an increase in cardiac output.

refractory period – the quiescent period following activation during which tissue such as nerve and muscle cannot be fully stimulated again.

Reid Index – the proportion of the total airway thickness that is made up of mucous glands. Is normally less than 40%.

residual volume – the volume of gas that is left in the lungs at the end of maximum expiration.

respiratory airway – airways from which alveoli branch directly.

respiratory exchange ratio – ratio of CO_2 output to O_2 input (also called respiratory quotient).

shunt – deoxygenated blood which passes from the right hand (venous) side of the circulation to the left, without becoming oxygenated in the alveoli. By doing so, it reduces the oxygen content of arterial blood.

shunt equation – equation used to calculate the shunt fraction or venous admixture.

sickle cell disease – inherited abnormality of haemoglobin characterized by a change in shape of red blood cells (sickling) in response to hypoxia. So called because the shape of the deformed blood cells is thought to resemble a sickle.

smooth muscle – involuntary muscle such as that found in the bronchial walls, the digestive system etc.

spirometer – instrument for measuring and recording lung volumes.

standard bicarbonate – the theoretical concentration of bicarbonate in the plasma at a normal $PaCO_2$, calculated from the pH and the measured (actual) $PaCO_2$.

sternum – the 'breast bone' situated in the front of the ribcage in the midline to which the costal cartilages attach.

strong acid – in physiological terms, an acid which dissociates almost completely at body pH, making it a poor buffer.

surface tension – surface tension results from greater than normal attraction between molecules on the surface of a liquid. This force tends to cause droplets of liquid to assume a spherical shape and also tends to cause alveoli, which are lined by a thin film of liquid, to collapse.

surfactant – phospholipid secreted by type II alveolar cells which reduces the surface tension of the alveoli and increases lung compliance and stability; dipalmitoyl phosphotidylcholine.

sympathetic nervous system – part of the involuntary nervous system. Fibres from the sympathetic nervous system innervate organs which are not under voluntary control such as the heart, airways, digestive organs etc.

Thalassaemia – inherited group of diseases characterized by a reduced production of one or more of the molecules making up haemoglobin. This can lead to severe anaemia in badly affected individuals.

Thebesian vein – veins the myocardium which drain blood into the underlying atrium or ventricle.

tidal volume – that volume of air passing into or out of the respiratory system in each breath.

total cross-sectional area – the sum of the cross sectional areas of all the airways at a given distance into the lung.

total lung capacity – the sum of the tidal volume, inspiratory reserve volume, expiratory reserve volume and the residual volume, i.e. the volume of gas that is in the lungs at maximum inspiration.

trachea – the 'windpipe'; the tube which connects the larynx to the two main bronchi.

transfer factor – in respiratory physiology, the transfer factor for a gas is the rate movement of the gas across the alveolar membrane divided by the difference in partial pressure of the gas across that membrane.

transmural pressure – in respiratory physiology this usually refers to the difference between the alveolar gas pressure and the intrapleural pressure.

turbinates – bony, mucosa-covered projections into the nasal cavity. There are three on each side. Sometimes also called conchae.

turbulent – flow of a fluid through a vessel whereby the particles making up the fluid move in lines that are not parallel.

vagus nerve – parasympathetic nerve which arises from the brainstem and which innervates many of the internal organs, including those of the respiratory system.

vapour pressure – the gas pressure exerted by a vapour.

vasoconstriction – the reduction in diameter of a blood vessel as a result of the action of smooth muscle in its walls.

venous admixture – the theoretical volume of mixed venous blood that would need to be added to blood leaving the alveoli per unit time in order to produce an oxygen content equal to that actually seen in aortic arterial blood.

ventilation – the volume of air leaving the respiratory system in 1 minute.

ventilation/perfusion ratio – for any given part of the respiratory system, the ratio of gas leaving the region per unit time divided by the blood flow through that region.

VIP – vaso-intestinal polypeptide. A neurotransmitter found in the respiratory system.

visceral pleura – the innermost of the two layers of pleura; i.e. the one lying directly over the lung.

vital capacity – the maximum volume of air that can be passed into or out of the respiratory system in one breath.

vocal folds – also called vocal cords. Paired folds of tissue in the larynx which vibrate when air passes between them producing a sound from which the voice is generated.

volatile acid – acid that is formed by the solution of a gas in water. The most important volatile acid in respiratory physiology is carbonic acid, formed when carbon dioxide dissolves in water.

voluntary control – the ability to control an organ at will. Skeletal muscles are under voluntary control, smooth muscles of the respiratory tract are not.

work of breathing – the energy exerted by the respiratory system on its surroundings in unit time. It is not equal to the total energy used up by the respiratory system, because not all of that energy is transferred to its surroundings.

INDEX

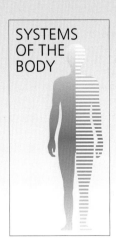

SYSTEMS
OF THE
BODY

INDEX